HUMAN SICKNESS AND HEALTH

A Biocultural View

CORINNE SHEAR WOOD

California State University, Fullerton

MAYFIELD PUBLISHING COMPANY

Library of Congress Catalog Card Number: 78-71608
International Standard Book Number: 0-87484-418-5

Manufactured in the United States of America
Mayfield Publishing Company
285 Hamilton Avenue, Palo Alto, California 94301

This book was set in IBM Baskerville by Trend Western
Technical Corporation and was printed and bound by
Haddon Craftsmen. Sponsoring editor was C. Lansing
Hays, Carole Norton supervised editing, and Lieselotte
Hofmann was manuscript editor. The book was
designed by Nancy Sears, cover by Joan Brown and
line drawings in text are by Barbara Stewart.
Michelle Hogan supervised production.

CONTENTS

iv

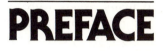

PREFACE

This book emerged out of the need to lessen the frustrations of teaching classes of medical anthropology with texts that satisfy some requirements but leave wide gaps in numerous areas. As one of the newest branches of anthropology and medicine, the subdiscipline of medical anthropology has arisen in part as a response to a major dilemma: the persistance of many illnesses and diseases in spite of effective technological means for eradication or at least alleviation. The vigorous growth of medical anthropology over the past decade owes much to the enthusiasm of students of many health-related disciplines who view this relatively new field as a commingling of the social sciences and medicine. This book attemps to bridge the chasm still existing between the two by focusing on the intimate interactions between culture and health around the world, both in the past and today.

If it does nothing more than show that the study of human societies must incorporate considerations of the health conditions of the people involved, this book will have accomplished a substantial part of its goal for the student of the social sciences. If it should convince any of the agencies of medical delivery systems that even the most subtle aspects of human culture set limitations on the health of a society as well as on a people's ability to accept many aspects of health care, then the book will indeed have justified its existence.

The "message" is my own but in it are reflected the sentiments of many others who have also spent time "in the field" where the disturbing world of fevers, bugs, and boils intrudes into every day's work. My hope is that there may be some help beyond sympathy for those altruistic souls who labor within unfamiliar cultures, trying to bring remedies that they know can solve so many problems but meeting on every hand resistance that frustrates their aims.

Although any errors, inaccuracies, over- and understatements are accepted—and regretted—as my own full responsibility, much of the positive spirit of the book derives from many persons, mostly friends and colleagues, whose help, patience, and wisdom I gratefully acknowledge. Many Native Americans of Southern California and people of Western Samoa were kind enough to accept me into their worlds for a time; their problems and hospitality did much to provoke the thinking that led to the writing of this book. My students through the past five years have been an invaluable source of the ideas offered and approaches attempted here. I salute them all.

The editor, Lieselotte Hofmann, was particularly helpful in ferreting out innumerable sins of omission as well as commission. Her ability to transform clumsy, ill-stated thought to cogency and clarity has been a joyful educational process for me. My own writing ability is inadequate to express my gratitude to her. Barbara Stewart, the artist whose work adds to many of the pages that follow, contributed much more than her obvious talent. She has been the epitome of the involved collaborator, imparting an informed enthusiasm that makes working with her a delight. Sala Ponnech had a big hand in preparing the glossary and the index and was consistently helpful with criticism and suggestions.

Many colleagues and friends read sections and offered welcome advice. The convolutions that some of their suggestions have been turned into are my own doing and I hope do not displease them too much. To them—Gene Anderson, Churchill Carmel, Joan Critchlow, Mary Edgecomb, Ngapare Hopa, E. T. Jacob-Pandian, Anne Jennings, Leroy Joesinck-Mandeville, Hans Leder, Logan Moore, Rose Tyson, Carole Venditti, Christine Wilson, Jack Zahniser, and others—I extend my gratitude and, where appropriate, my apologies.

The staff of the Mayfield Publishing Company was most helpful and encouraging. To them, especially to Alden Paine, I offer my sincere thanks. To my family—Bill, Gina, Carl, Roberta, David, and Anita—who had to live with or put up with me during this, my longest gestation period, I offer a promise to wait a bit before beginning another.

INTRODUCTION

Traditionally, anthropologists devote long, hard years to living in "the field" among people with whom they share little common experience, often under conditions of considerable communication difficulty. Their contacts are, by necessity, the flourishing, rarely the languishing, members of the group. As a result, we have the popular concept of the "carefree savage," the "natural man." In reality, normal life for the vast majority of people in human history has meant a short life, punctuated by intermittent encounters with an interminable list of biological jeopardies. In this book, culture, and disease are shown to be inextricably coupled, tied to each other in an intimate, feedback relationship.

The material presented supports and reinforces the premise that human cultures and human biological propensities have evolved in response to environmental forces. But it goes a step farther and demonstrates that disease is one of the most critical components of environmental stress. Indeed, an inseparable dialectical process can be discerned in which disease subtly molds fundamental elements of a society and, in turn, many aspects of human cultures determine the prevalence, and even the existence, of particular disease patterns. And the roles of cause and effect often interchange as a result of given circumstances.

The argument pursued is that studies of human lives must devote serious consideration to the health and disease expectations of the people under scrutiny. For, to an extent seldom appreciated, the presence or threat of disease has shaped, and continues to shape, all human cultures and societies. Investigations of human institutions are incomplete, even deceptive, unless they reflect the real world in which people live. Using the perspective of medical anthropology, the social scientist enhances the understanding of this real world, providing insights rarely attainable through traditional anthropological, sociological, religious, political, or ecological analysis alone.

In every society the sick person is a person out of rhythm with his or her culture. As Sigerist (1951) stresses, "Sickness isolates." This accounts for the rather distorted view obtained from classic ethnographies, where, except for the briefest incidents, one encounters only societies in which all members are functioning in their appropriate roles. Everyone feels well; each has arrived at his or her present maturity through an uneventful infancy and childhood, unscathed except for the celebrated *rites de passage*. Much of this book performs the unhappy task of shattering that dream world.

Chapter 1 is concerned with the antiquity of disease. Fossilized bones give us a fleeting glimpse at some of the forms of life that preceded humans by many millions of years. This source offers two primary lessons: first, ancient life was subject to many of the same forms of disease that continue to afflict life today; and second, powerful physiological and biochemical responses to the assault of parasites evolved very early and apparently have barely changed since.

The evidence validates Sigerist's claim (1951:65) that disease "must be as old as life itself because it is life, a manifestation of life, a reaction of a living organism to abnormal stimuli." The fossil record testifies that all life has evolved in continuous confrontation with parasitism and disease. As a result, our common phyletic heritage has benefited from the selections made long before anything like humans appeared on the landscape.

Through the powerful forces of evolutionary selection, humans have inherited impressive abilities to withstand attacks from the vast majority of the world's parasites. As Majno (1975) points out, it is not easy to prevent a wound from healing; in fact, it is frequently acknowledged, even by profit-oriented practitioners of Western medicine, that, given a modicum of care, 85 percent of all human ailments will heal spontaneously in time. John Fry (in Dingle 1973) points out that major diseases, the potential killers, account for only some 5 percent of all illnesses.

There is no society known that has not had to accommodate to the presence or threat of illness at some time in its history. By and large, the basic immunological responses are panhuman, with only minor variations related to specific environmental pressures. But, with the emergence of true humans, a vital ally sprang into the battle against disease—human culture. From that point on, disease patterns were forced into new adjustments, some flourishing where human cultures provided favorable conditions for maintenance of the parasites, others waning, occasionally even disappearing, where human societies were able to muster effective social and technological weapons. More often, it was when social conditions inadvertently acted against their continued transmission that diseases decreased to the point of near eradication—only to attack with renewed energy when social conditions unwittingly acted again in their favor.

Shaped by the ever-present forces of disease, human cultures often produced supernatural as well as more mundane interhuman behavioral rationales to explain the onslaughts of these invisible enemies. Less obvious cultural responses are evident in the basic human ability to cooperate and exhibit "humane behavior" in times of medical emergency. Indeed, the recognition of human interdependency and the display of concern in times of medical stress can be said to distinguish the species *Homo sapiens* from all other forms of life.

Throughout this book it is proposed that the ability of humans to give health care is itself a product of our evolutionary history. Even though an individual's survival depends ultimately on his or her immunological defenses against invasive substances, the afflicted person must be able to rest and receive nourishment. If the society is to survive, other members of the group must be able to take over the sick person's functions; still others must provide comfort and care.

As reflected in Chapter 2, observers of the behavior of our nonhuman primate relatives (cf. Lawick-Goodall 1971) frequently are dismayed by the inability of even the quite highly structured anthropoid groups to extend the most rudimentary care to the stricken companion. The sick or injured baboon or chimpanzee, unable to keep up with the daily activities of the group, is soon dead, either picked off by omnipresent predators or starved to death because healthy comrades are incapable of sharing their food.

Round-the-clock rest, a primary requisite for the mending of a sick body, was not usually feasible until a uniquely human institution, the home base, was adopted. A base implies not only the opportunity to rest but also the chance to benefit from another exclusively human attribute, the sharing of food. Adoption of these two truly revolutionary innovations was a prerequisite for *Homo sapiens* to thrive almost everywhere on earth. Thus, although Chapter 2 shows that human and nonhuman primates share almost all of the same diseases and the same physiological responses, the medical prognosis for the human primate is distinctly different, thanks to human cultural innovations.

The brief glimpse at segments of the medical histories of some of our nonhuman primate kin gives significant hints of the evolutionary bonds shared. In these histories we see disease confronted with only the weapons derived through biological evolution. This biologically impressive but psychologically meager arsenal has telling effects on the ability of these anthropoids to cope with sickness. Lacking the reinforcements of developed cultures, they are at a distinct disadvantage. Each, in a sense, is on his own when illness strikes—alone in a way that no member of human society can ever be.

It has been argued that human cultural attributes became feasible only after protohumans acquired a taste for meat. Recent studies (cf. Lawick-Goodall 1971) reveal that occasionally chimps, and more rarely baboons, obtain meat through deliberate capture or chance encounters with small mammals. They then share the kill. The concentrated protein in meat makes feeding more efficient, permitting satiation and fulfilling nutritional requirements with comparatively small amounts of food. The holding power of meat also permits longer periods of comfort without food than is possible with a purely vegetarian diet. Carnivores regularly fast for several days with no apparent ill effects, whereas an herbivorous animal must shovel in prodigious amounts of leaves, roots, fruits, and grasses through most of its waking hours, leaving little time for cultural development even if the propensity were present.

Once meat eating or, more accurately for humans, an omnivorous way of life became established, populations could, for the first time in the history of animal life, succor their wounded, deliver and care for their newborn, and have food brought to the injured or ill at fixed locations. Freedom from the need for continuous stuffing gave the emerging hunters, with their rapidly expanding brains, the leisure to use their intellectual potential to develop cultural means of caring for the sick and, eventually, to search for explanations of illness and death. Concomitantly, the demands of a hunting way of life provoked the evolutionary selection of a brain quite different from that required for simple foraging, a brain that permitted further elaborations in the cultural responses to disease.

In addition, the evolutionary trend toward an omnivorous diet prompted the migrations so characteristic of emerging *Homo sapiens.* These migrations, carrying protohumans more than a million years ago to southern Europe, Asia, the Near East, and much of Africa, were not deliberate attempts to arrive at a particular destination (actual rates of travel have been estimated at approximately one mile per year). Rather, they probably evolved from a way of life tied to the movements of the hunters' quarry and less bound to a given territory than is the life of the essentially herbivorous nonhuman primate. In the migratory process, new foods, new diseases, and new cultural adaptations were added to the human repertoire.

Chapter 3 develops these ideas and extends them to review many puzzling aspects of human behavior in regard to food. The relationship between food beliefs and nutritional requirements, as well as the biological impact of various deficiencies, is considered in some depth. In examining the conflict between biological nutrition needs and social practices, it is noted that food prohibitions of some sort exist panculturally; but particularly deleterious taboos seem to be directed disproportionately against the most vulnerable segments of populations.

There is apparently no population that completely utilizes all the potential nutrients in its environment. As shown in Chapter 3, intensive study over the past decades has produced reliable scientific data on human nutrition requirements. By and large, the problems that exist stem most glaringly from our inability to translate this knowledge into usable form for the mass of poorly nourished populations in the world today. Chapter 3 argues that in the field of nutrition, more than any other aspect of human health, intensive input from the social sciences is in order.

The seemingly maladaptive cultural practices and beliefs concerning nutrition apply especially to women and their offspring. As a sequel to the bewildering findings discussed in Chapter 3, Chapter 4 offers a more detailed medical-anthropological examination of women and their reproductive role. Because of their critical dependence on adequate health conditions and cultural support for the proper functioning of their reproductive role, women are particularly appropriate subjects for a study that is bioculturally oriented.

Female functions such as childbirth and lactation have been fundamental to the development of human cultures and, as might be anticipated, are inextricably tied to cultural attitudes. Indeed, it is reasonable to postulate that it was the critical health needs and dependency of new or potential mothers that provided the major thrust for the emergence of human cultures.

As Dubos (1968:70) notes, "Many of the diseases known today have long existed and probably have been coeval with human life." The biological uniformity of *Homo sapiens* assures that all humans are subject, at least theoretically, to the same diseases. Likewise, the panhuman processes of growth, reproduction, aging, and death are physiological constants. But a medical-anthropological perspective of the medical histories of females in their reproductive role reveals that the biological as well as the medical manifestations of the events of reproduction are quite different from society to society. It is hypothesized that the attitudes of a woman's culture toward her reproductive functions vitally determines how she experiences these events. On the other hand, the histories of many societies—certainly their ability to perpetuate themselves through time—are directly proportional to the ability of their women to reproduce in healthy circumstances. Chapter 4 proposes, then, that a biocultural examination of the females of a given society provides invaluable information about the state of that society. Likewise, the status of women in the society is shown to depend on the attitudes and material conditions presented to them by their culture.

A striking example of the interdependence of material or technological developments and social accommodation can be seen in the changing roles of women in several industrialized societies today. Women's liberation movements have behind them a long history of struggle for equality and dignity, but until only recently, as is shown throughout Chapter 4, biological factors, which in turn shaped deleterious cultural attitudes, stood in the way.

Immunization against the traditional childhood diseases and the subsequent virtual eradication of these diseases have now given women in advantaged societies reasonable expectations that the children they produce will survive into adulthood. In addition, powerful antibiotics have altered the historical role of mother and wife as the main source of care during what were once inevitable and long family illnesses.

The increased assurances of the survival of all or most children and a coinciding technological improvement in birth control devices have at last made it possible to plan families—quality can eliminate the need for quantity. Lacking these advances, a woman's fate was, and in many places still is (cf. Ramalingaswami 1975), continuous childbearing and repeated lactation periods, with frequent miscarriages, stillbirths, and high rates of infant mortality—or, as some have put it, a twenty- to thirty-year sentence of ongoing, frequently fruitless reproduction. Chapter 4 demonstrates how the cultural and biological aspects of women's reproductive lives constitute two sides of the same coin. It attempts to show that only where efforts are made to unite medical science with cultural change in attitudes is there any possibility of enabling women to join with men in aspiring to a full life experience.

Clearly, the medical destinies of individuals have been directly tied to the position assigned to them by their society on the basis of their biological roles. But the medical destinies of societies have largely been determined by their geographic location. Since early in their evolutionary history, humans have populated vastly different areas of the earth. Every ecological niche presents its own particular hazards to human survival. Those humans who have met the demands of their environment satisfactorily have necessarily had to structure their societies to cope with the specific syndromes menacing them. The fossil record of extinct human populations, touched on in the first chapter, provides us with many examples of those who failed to meet the demands. It is proposed that among the overwhelming pressures were diseases for which biological responses had not been primed.

It is difficult for the modern, technologically sophisticated person to identify with the health status of these ancient forebears. Indeed, it is hard to identify with those who preceded us as recently as fifty years ago, or even with the vast numbers of people today who still do not have access to the fruits of modern medical advances. For all such people, the hold on life was, and is, quite tenuous—in constant jeopardy from mysterious attacks from unseen agents. This point is tragically underscored in Chapter 5, which examines the record of the indigenous populations of the New World through the perspective of their unique medical history.

The special circumstance of a people migrating to a vast continent devoid of any other human life, and then remaining isolated for millennia, provides a unique opportunity to examine geographic factors as determinants of human medical events. The lack of contact with other humans, and particularly other human viruses, is seen to underlie the catastrophic inability to cope when the conquering parasites borne by peoples from other continents eventually descended on the New World. Immunological virginity was also mirrored in the lack of cultural experience with the unfamiliar diseases. The result was social disruption, shattered cultural supports, and loss of human life on a scale that approached annihilation.

Chapter 5 also attempts to dispel some of the myths frequently associated with pre-contact peoples. Particularly, the ancient Maya are examined from an ecological and medical perspective, with strong reliance on the "biographies written in the bones." They emerge as a people beleaguered by problems that led inevitably to serious deterioration of health and living conditions. Some of the unassimilated peoples living in hunting-gathering or incipient agricultural economies in the New World today are also presented from a perspective that reveals a portrait quite different from the usual ones.

In order to provide concrete examples of the dynamic interactions of human cultures and pathological parasites, Chapters 6 and 7 offer in-depth examinations of two widespread diseases, syphilis and malaria, within the context of evolutionary processes. In Chapter 6, syphilis, like malaria, is shown to be a disease with a fascinating, albeit controversial, association with human life. Here both the fossil record and historical accounts become sources of valuable information about the various forms through which the responsible parasite has evolved. Like malaria protozoa, the spirochetes of syphilis were profoundly altered in their evolutionary course by many conditions of human existence. For our purposes, one of the basic differences between syphilis and many other diseases is that reliable evidence of its presence or absence has been recorded in human bones. Through this powerful source of information, it is possible to derive solid data pertinent to the continuing controversy over the origin as well as the probable evolutionary course of a particular constellation of diseases.

As a disease with strong cultural as well as biological ramifications, syphilis demands study by students of human behavior. Eradication of both syphilis and malaria is technically feasible but not yet in sight—primarily because of unresolved cultural problems.

Malaria emerges, in Chapter 7, as one of the most critical diseases interacting with human evolution. This is a disease whose transmission depends on an incredibly complex cycle of events. Indeed, the recitation of all the requirements for its maintenance gives cause to wonder that it should even exist. Nevertheless, the many activities and vagaries of human societies, particularly since the introduction of agriculture, have, with tragic frequency, provided exactly the configurations of the improbable that have assured the success of malaria parasites.

As in the examples of other diseases that are considered, an overview of malaria and human cultures elucidates how cause and effect intermittently switch roles when tangible material factors interact with the more elusive cultural forces. For students of human life, malaria is the best-documented disease for which biological variations in the host have been evoked through evolutionary selection. For students of the microscopic world, malaria provides an excellent illustration of how the human host can shape the evolutionary history of a parasite. For all students, the portrayal of the many societies whose histories have chronicled malaria's impact manifests that this is a disease with many lessons to offer.

The search for explanations of illness and death, as well as for some rational course of action to follow, has helped mold cultures wherever sickness has threatened or appeared. The final chapter examines some of the traditional healers and proposes that the continuous presence of oppressive diseases has contributed heavily to the propensity of all human cultures to fill their worlds with gods, souls, magical powers, and associated supernatural forces. The beliefs, and the leaders that arose to interpret and enforce them, represented a cultural response that augmented the invisible immunological abilities slowly acquired during our evolutionary past. Individuals emerged who were deemed able to interpret and thwart the frightening threats to life and bodily integrity. These became the healers, mentors, and leaders who were forged by the crises of their peoples' health.

It is shown that these healers—the shamans, herbalists, diviners, and others—have often constituted the main source of judicial and creative power in their societies. Even in "advanced" societies, patients are seldom satisfied with the explanation that their illness is the result of a chance encounter with an opportunistic microscopic organism. For them the world consists of pain, fever, chills, and, often, dread. The inevitable reaction is, "Why me?" In every case, sickness touches the inmost core of human existence. Scientifically oriented victims seek answers in possible violations of their culture's health rules: they have not been eating properly, have not gotten enough sleep, have permitted themselves to become chilled, or have committed some culturally defined excess of behavior. Earlier people, lacking a germ theory of disease, similarly sought explanations in their own behavior. In the recitations of people offended, rules broken, and traditions violated, the healers reinforced the norms of their societies.

The hunter-gatherer and the agricultural villager explained their illnesses primarily through extrapolations of the world with which they were familiar, the world of interpersonal relations. Logical progression led to the belief that illness stemmed from transgressions against kin, neighbors, or cultural rules. Ghosts, sorcery, or other supernatural visitations from angered or deceased tribal members accounted for attacks that would reduce a sound body to pain and helplessness.

As the final chapter illustrates, the development of early intellectual leadership and, eventually, of power in the hands of individuals was intimately shaped by unnerving assaults on health. In keeping with the dialectics of the process, it is suggested that these healers-leaders significantly influenced the development of the situations that created them, mediating the cultural impact of disease and indirectly maintaining the very social conditions that permitted the diseases to flourish.

To the extent that the aim of this book—to offer an account of the sensitive interrelationship between human culture and disease—has succeeded, it may be argued by some that it has been at the cost of a disturbing degree of overstatement. But the medical histories of human societies in the past, and to an appalling extent still today, argue strongly for the need for heavy input from the social sciences, which up to now have been seriously remiss in studying this critical aspect of human life.

HUMAN SICKNESS AND HEALTH: A Biocultural View

THE MEDICAL
HISTORY IN
THE FOSSIL
RECORD

DISEASE BEFORE MAN

For evidence of the presence of disease in prehistoric animals and humans we are dependent almost entirely on the record provided by bone fragments and teeth. Except for the exceedingly rare preservation of soft parts of the body through entrapment in peat bogs or natural mummification in singularly dry, bacteria-free environments (Fig. 1–1), and even more rare capture in conditions of near-instant freezing, bones and teeth are the only parts of animal bodies that are amenable to preservation in forms that can be "read" by future generations.

A fossilized bone is actually a replica of the living organ. In order for fossilization to occur, the animal must die somewhere removed from all the predators, scavengers, and microorganisms provided by a tidy Nature. Suitable minerals must be present at the site of death, and there must be a carrying agent such as water to propel the minerals through the bone maze, eventually replacing all the organic material of the once living bone with inorganic minerals. In spite of the limitations presented by the unlikely occurrence of the fossilizing process, through the science of paleopathology a surprising fund of information has accumulated concerning the diseases that afflicted animal life throughout evolution.

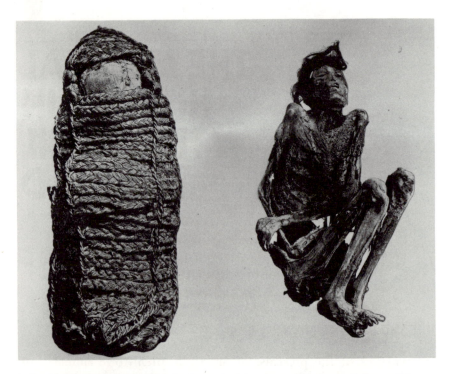

1-1 Ritual preparation of the dead practiced by the ancient Incas. *Left*: an elaborate mummy bundle. *Right*: unwrapped desiccated body. An arid environment provided excellent preservation conditions for this comparatively rare archeological find. (Courtesy of Field Museum of Natural History, Chicago.)

From these sources we have gained knowledge regarding the possibility of changing characteristics of disease through time. The fossil record suggests that in ancient times, as today, some diseases were species-specific, whereas others appeared to be common afflictions of all animals. Finally, we are able partially to assess to what extent physiological responses to disease have developed throughout evolution.

ANTIQUITY OF PARASITISM
More than three billion years ago, long before there were any bones to become fossils, bacteria lived and died, some conveniently leaving traces of their existence in rocks scattered throughout the world. Studies of coal formations, coprolites of fishes and reptiles, and,

Table 1-1
Geological and evolutionary timetable

ERA	EPOCH	MILLION YEARS B.P.*	DURATION (million years)	FAUNAL EMERGENCE
CENOZOIC	PLEISTOCENE	10,000 – 2 million	2	Hominids, large mammals, modern marine invertebrates
	PLIOCENE	2-6 million	4	Hominids, camels, giraffes, bovines, dogs, hyenas
	MIOCENE	6-23 million	17	Hominoids, grazing mammals, mastodons
	OLIGOCENE	23-36 million	13	Modern families of mammals (cats, primitive anthropoidea)
	EOCENE	36-54 million	18	Modern orders of mammals (tarsiers, lemurs, horses, whales)
	PALEOCENE	54-65 million	11	Archaic mammals (lemurs), modern birds, marine invertebrates
MESOZOIC		65-145 million	80	Toothed birds, pouched and placental mammals, modern insects, "Age of Reptiles"
Paleozoic				Amphibians
Proterozoic				Water life, insects, trilobites
Archeozoic				One-celled animals, bacteria, algae
Azoic				No evidence of life

*B.P. = Before Present. Accept these dates as rough approximations — guides, not gospel. As you dig into the relevant literature you will find other proposals and much controversy.
Source: Based on Ernst Mayr, 1978. Evolution. *Scientific American,* 239, no. 3:46-55.

more recently, teeth and jaws of mammalian fossils verify the presence of many types of bacteria among the earliest forms of life. As more complex forms of life developed, the record shows that some opportunistic microorganisms evolved mechanisms that permitted them to live at the expense of other forms of life. The classic works of Ruffer (1921), Moodie (1923), Pales (1930), and others offer concrete evidence that as animals and plants emerged (see Table 1–1), diseases resulting from infestations by microorganisms were awaiting them. Parasitism had arrived on the earth's scene.

Fossilized bones indicate that many animals must have suffered periostitis (infections of the outer bony layer) and osteomyelitis (infections of the inner marrow cavity) (Fig. 1–2). These bone infections, now relatively uncommon where penicillin and related antibiotics are available, result from pus-producing microorganisms, most often *Staphylococcus*. It is possible that these same ubiquitous bacteria were responsible for many of the deformed bones found in the fossil record.

The physiological responses found throughout nature appear to be a fundamental sequence of events that have evolved through con-

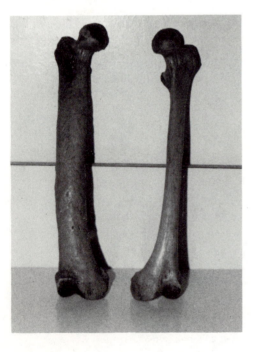

1–2 *Left*: femur of an ancient American showing effects of a severe case of osteomyelitis, with cylindrical enlargement of the bone. *Right*: unaffected femur. (Courtesy of San Diego Museum of Man. Photo by Joyce Taylor.)

tinuous interaction with foreign organisms that activate immunological mechanisms in the host. Bones invaded by bacteria introduced through an infected wound, fracture, or systemic assault will invariably respond by swelling from the mustered armies of white blood cells that constitute the bulk of pus-filled channels—a universal immunological reaction by the animal body as it attempts to destroy the invading parasites.

THE WOES OF ANCIENT REPTILES

There is clear evidence from 200-million-year-old reptiles and from many other long extinct animals that infections occurred during their lifetimes. The Edaphosauri (Fig. 1–3) are a fertile source of information. Moodie (1923:116) pictures them as "one of the most bizarre of all the ancient reptiles and they abounded in grotesque forms [with a] brain case no larger than the ball of one's fingers in a skull

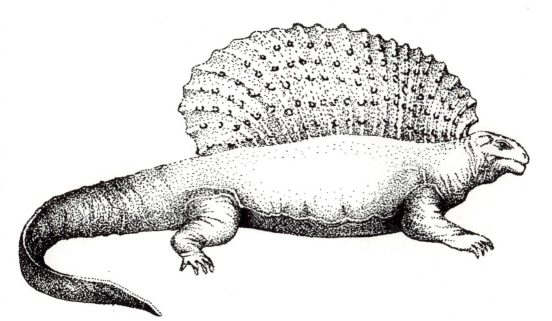

1–3 Edaphosaurus, a swamp-dwelling, herbivorous animal whose appearance fit well into its ancient environment of ferns and primitive tree-like plants of more than 150 million years ago. Its eleven-foot length was augmented by comb-like spines along the back, which were actually an extension of their vertebrae. Remains of these creatures in Europe and North America show evidence of injury, infection, and healing, particularly in the vulnerable spines. (Adapted from Augusta 1960.)

twelve to fourteen inches long." One of these creatures suffered several fractured spines, one spine showing two breaks. In addition, the left radius had a complete but simple fracture that had healed in its time with little or no shortening. Still another of these creatures experienced a broken rib that had healed completely within its lifetime. Another dinosaur, a nine-foot Dimetrodon found in Texas, broke one of its dorsal spines. Microscopic examination across the fossilized spine revealed the structure to be expected in an infected bone riddled with pus-filled sinuses. The fossilized remains indicate that the healing processes were well established; the reptiles' fancy, fanlike back tells the story of infection and subsequent recovery. Perhaps the most vital information derived from these medical relics is the proof that nature had established, more than two or three hundred million years ago, a method for repair of fractures and subsequent infections that remains essentially the same today.

Among the most gigantic dinosaurs, the Apatosauri, one suffered a fracture on the right member of the fifth pair of ribs, a break that did not heal well. The adjoining rib had a similar fracture that did not heal at all. One wonders, along with Moodie, what tremendous impact could have broken these massive structures and must conclude that only another creature of at least equal size could have been responsible.

From the same era, we have been left a fossilized horned dinosaur that died at a site in present-day Edmonton, Canada, after enduring an oblique fracture of the humerus. Moodie (1923:123) calls this "the sickest looking fossil bone known." Extensive infection prevented satisfactory healing, producing instead an enormous abscess capable of holding several liters of pus. Thus, some 150 million years after the event, we are able to bear witness to a battle even more catastrophic than the one suggested above. And in this case, a huge dinosaur was defeated by bacteria too small to be seen by the naked eye!

In the same Cretaceous time there lived an unfortunate phytosaur. It was related to many fellow aquatic reptiles distributed through North America, Europe, and East India. They all had very long heads with nostrils set far back on a snout that was just in front of the eyes. The end of the snout was fitted with long teeth, perhaps foreshadowing present-day sharks. As projected by Moodie, one of these phytosaurs, either in an unfriendly encounter or perhaps in an attempt to burrow under a large stone, managed to break its snout. The formation of abundant callus and extensive necrotic sinuses that had worked their way through the surrounding bone tells an ancient story of an infected fracture that slowly, and perhaps painfully, eventually healed.

Living along with the dinosaurs and even earlier were the mosasaurs, aquatic reptiles that achieved lengths of fifty feet and left skeletal remains throughout much of the world (Fig. 1–4). Their fossil remains add to the picture of ancient trauma. Moodie reports several cases of osteoperiotitis as well as evidence of a tumor on the

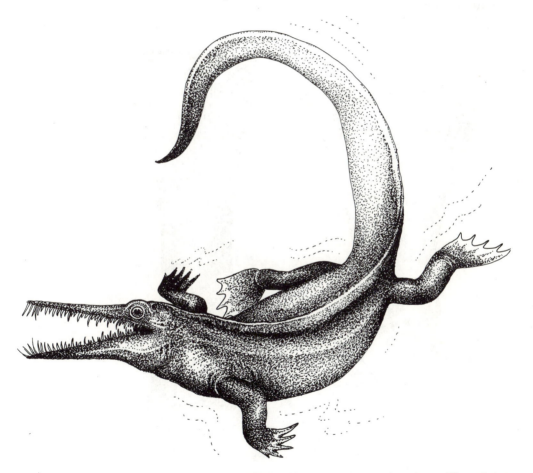

1–4   A mosasaur, an aquatic reptile that lived and became extinct many millions of years ago. Skeletal remains of mosasaurs are found in numerous places around the world and often reveal evidence of infected fractures, osteoperiositis, tumors, and arthritis. (Adapted from Moodie 1923.)

8

lower end of a vertebra and an extensive overgrowth of the vertebral junction that he believed to be indicative of further bony tumors. Additional mosasaur finds suggest some of the earliest evidence of multiple arthritis (Fig. 1–5). In one specimen each successive joint of the toe is "deformed, enlarged, necrotic, with the articular ends of the phalanges lipped similar to the lipping observed in human skeletons" (Moodie 1923:172). Further arthritic lesions are reported from another mosasaur, this one with characteristic deformities involving the limb bones.

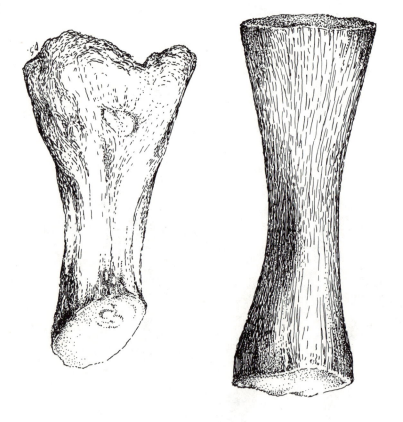

1–5   *Left*: diseased metatarsal of a mosasaur found in Kansas. The bone is notably shortened, and broadened from deforming arthritic lesions, carious roughening, and a large terminal necrotic sinus. *Right*: normal, unaffected metatarsal of the same animal. (Original in Kansas University Museum of Natural History.)

Although we find no evidence of dinosaurs by the end of the Mesozoic era, the mammals that took over, rapidly filling in the niches left empty, were subject to the same kinds of attacks by microorganisms as well as trauma and inflammation following injuries inflicted by larger enemies. In South Dakota are fossilized remains of a large horned mammal, brontops, that recovered from injuries and subsequent infections by means of the same immunological responses manifested by the bones of dinosaurs that preceded it (see Fig. 1–6).

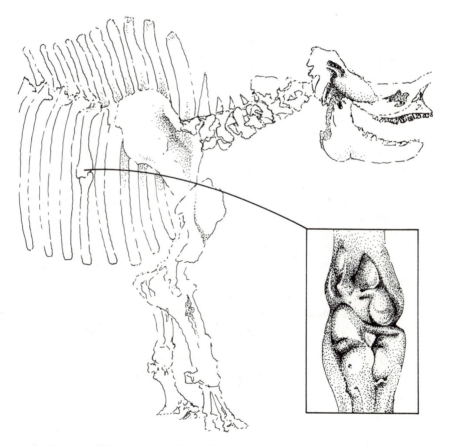

1–6   Brontops (*Titanotherium robustum*), a large horned mammal that lived over twenty-five million years ago; found in South Dakota. Somehow the fifth rib was broken and became seriously infected. It eventually healed with the consequent distortion shown here. (Adapted from Moodie 1923. Original in American Museum of Natural History.)

SPECIAL PROBLEMS OF THE CAVE BEARS

Another permanent record of injury and subsequent healing was reported as early as 1774 by a German minister and naturalist, E. J. C. Esper (Sigerist 1951), who described the femur of a cave bear with a considerable tumor, later identified as a callus resulting from the healing of an infected fracture. In 1825, Philip von Walther described eleven diseased bones from cave bears and lions dating from the Pleistocene epoch, about one to three million years ago; in 1854 F. J. Carl Mayer added descriptions of twenty-four bones from these same animals, to all of which he attributed pathological lesions; and in 1895 Rudolf Virchow contributed studies of various carnivores that revealed the characteristic cavities typical of osteomyelitis (ibid.).

These early diagnoses depended on gross examination; later techniques of microscopy and X-ray, as applied by Moodie (1926), permitted differentiation of the lesions. These modern applications of science made it possible to distinguish with a great degree of certainty those lesions, actually artifacts, that resulted from the actions of erosion, fungi, or rodents on bones long dead as distinct from lesions that in fact were caused by inflammatory and reparative processes that took place while the animal was alive. Many of the bones belonging to the cave bears, as well as one upper limb bone from a mosasaur from an earlier time in Kansas, show convincing evidence of chronic infection which stimulated the periosteum to produce new growth that adhered to the surface of the old bone, presenting a fossil with rough, ragged areas where normally smooth surfaces would be expected.

No evidence has been reported indicating the presence of rickets in the bones of prehistoric animals. But the adult counterpart of rickets, osteomalacia, apparently did take a toll among various ancient animals. Typical deformities, resulting from deficiencies of calcium and phosphorus, are reported by various investigators. Abel (1924) observed osteomalacia in a cave bear, von Walther in 1825 diagnosed it in an earlier carnivore (Sigerist 1951), and Moodie (1923) found it in bones of a carnivore that had lived nearly three million years ago.

HINTS OF TETANUS

In addition to the staphylococcus and streptococcus types of infections for which we have convincing evidence in fossilized bone changes, Majno (1975:16) suggests:

As for the problem of infection, bacteria should have been old hands at causing trouble by the time that man came around. Clostridia in particular should have been rampant, for they are able to survive in inanimate nature and also happen to cause two of the deadliest wound infections, tetanus and gas gangrene.

It is noteworthy that, much earlier, Moodie (1923:324), suggested the possibility of tetanic distress in a large number of early fossil material:

> Every student of the fossil vertebrates who is fortunate enough to collect a number of complete or approximately complete skeletons of ancient animals is almost sure to be impressed with the frequency of the peculiar curve to a backwardly bent neck and the rigid appearance of the limbs.

This clinical condition is not uncommon today; it is seen most frequently in humans in association with lockjaw (caused by *Clostridium tetani*), abscesses or trauma on the brain, severe middle-ear infections, meningitis, or strychnine poisoning. The frequent appearance of this tetanic, arched position (Fig. 1–7) is found associated with the death of prehistoric camels (*Stenomylus*) from Nebraska, several carnivorous dinosaurs, some small dinosaurs (*Struthiominus*), primitive reptiles from early Texas, many winged small reptiles (*Pterodactylus longirostris*), and a toothed bird (*Archaeopteryx*).

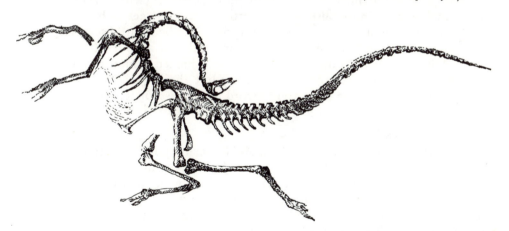

1–7 Tetanic arched position found associated with the death of many prehistoric animals. In apparent death spasm here is *Struthiomimus altus* from the Belly River Series of Alberta, Canada. (Adapted from Moodie 1923. Original in American Museum of Natural History.)

Moodie urges caution in applying a diagnosis of tetanus as the only possible cause of the death of animals found in this position. He speculates that some may have been plant feeders and their spastic distress and deaths may have been a result of having fed on poisonous plants ancestral to those that can cause tetanic spasms today. On the other hand, the distinctive spastic position cannot be dismissed as possible evidence for a very ancient history for tetanus, a disease that, until the development of effective immunization techniques, was a dreaded killer of countless humans and other animals.

CIRCUMSTANTIAL EVIDENCE OF OTHER DISEASES

An additional example of the use of circumstantial evidence to suggest the presence of a disease that does not affect the skeletal structure is the demonstration by Cockerell (1918) that several species of tsetse flies (*Glossina*) lived a million or more years ago in areas around today's Colorado. These flies, found abundantly in Africa today, are vectors of sleeping sickness, a frequently fatal disease of the blood, spleen, liver, and central nervous system. The appearance of these disease vectors coincides with the mysterious mass extinctions of many large mammals, such as horses and camels, from the North American continent. One may speculate that this sequence of events provides indirect evidence of the possibility of mass epidemics of the ungulate form of sleeping sickness.

We are still denied much information about ancient disease syndromes because most diseases that produce pathologies in bones are limited to the abscess or deficiency types described. But diseases such as tuberculosis, syphilis, leprosy, and arthritis also result in characteristic bone deformities. No available evidence demonstrates the presence of the first three syndromes; but the sequelae of arthritic inflammation have left a vivid record in the fossil material.

ARTHRITIS EVERYWHERE

Arthritis is a catch-all name given to many bone and joint conditions. As defined by Sigerist (1951:50) it encompasses "a group of chronic diseases of the joints of different origin, in the course of which the joints become enlarged, produce new bone, thus creating deformities" (Fig. 1–8). The end product of many cases is complete rigidity of the joint. The cause of most arthritis today is still not completely known. But it is commonly suspected, particularly by U.S. medical scientists, that a "silent infection," usually bacterial, or a

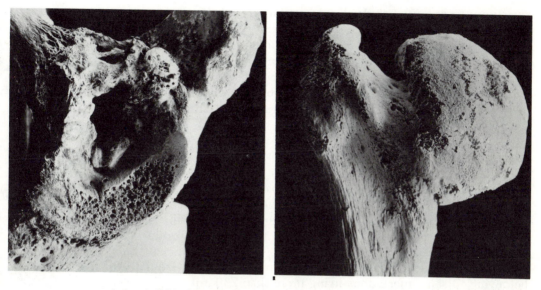

1–8 Arthritis deformans in the skeletal remains of a mummy from prehistoric Peru. *Left*: deformed pelvic bones. *Right*: characteristic changes of this crippling disease on the head of the same individual's femur. (Courtesy of Field Museum of Natural History, Chicago.)

chronic recurring one may contribute significantly to some types of arthritis.

In its many forms arthritis remains widespread throughout the animal kingdom. Apparently it was a source of crippling pain and body deformities even in the days of the dinosaurs. Moodie (1923) reported evidence of arthritic damage in bones from dinosaurs and other reptiles that lived hundreds of millions of years ago and, so far as external appearances were concerned, there had been no changes. He found frequent arthritis in some bones from mosasaurs, as well as from a sabre-toothed tiger and some mammals that lived in America during the Eocene epoch. Joining this varied company are characteristic changes in bones from a crocodile that lived in Egypt between twenty-five and twelve million years ago, in a camel from five to two million years ago, and in many mammals of more recent vintage. In fact, the disease was so prevalent in the remains of Pleistocene cave bears that a special name, "cave gout," was coined for it by Virchow in 1896.

It may be significant that except for the cave bears, all the animals mentioned lived in warm environments, a fact that raises questions regarding the usual association of arthritic lesions with cold, damp regions. However, Janssens (1970) believes that, for the cave bears, arthritis became severe and common enough to have figured importantly in the subsequent extinction of the species. The Neanderthal humans, who probably competed with bears for use of the caves as shelters, were also plagued by the crippling misery of arthritis. They, and the subsequent interaction of this one disease with all human life, are examined below.

THE ANTIQUITY OF DENTAL PROBLEMS

Although skeptics have argued that the deformities exhibited in the fossilized long bones could have been caused by agents such as fungi or protozoa acting upon the structures after death, there is no question regarding the distinctive cavities found in many fossilized teeth. No known process other than bacterial invasion can produce the carious teeth recovered from a surprising number of ancient creatures. The first documented occurrence of caries dates from teeth belonging to some mastadons living more than 230 million years ago (Janssens 1970). From the Oligocene epoch, more than twenty-five million years ago, there are fossilized remains of a primitive rhinoceros that lived, and very likely ached, in South Dakota with a tooth abscess that had penetrated to the mandibular canal. Nor were elephants exempt from the problem of carious teeth; Janssens reports the presence of caries among elephants, now extinct, that were rather widespread during the Pleistocene epoch.

Not only teeth but also gums have a long history of infections. Sigerist (1951:59) notes: "Beginning with *pyorrhea alveolaris,* we can state without hesitation that this condition occurred at all times in men, and it was found even in a few fossil animals. . . . On the subject of pyorrhea, all investigators agree." He also raises the possibility of a causative relationship between the high rates of pyorrhea and subsequent arthritis among the ancient Egyptians. A more ancient case is reported by Moodie (1923), who cites evidence for pyorrhea as well as osteitis in a fossil belonging to a forerunner of the modern horse, *Meryhippus campestris,* which lived more than one and a half million years ago.

It should not be unexpected, then, that when human forms began to evolve, dental problems awaited them. Carious teeth have been found in australopithecines who lived, probably quite uncomfortably, some two or three million years ago in Africa. Likewise, teeth belonging to Neanderthal skeletons alive between 115,000 and

40,000 years ago show characteristic signs of retreating gums and related dental distress.

One of the most poignant relics of prehistoric misery belonged to the being now dubbed "Rhodesia Man." Some thirty to forty thousand years ago, this Neanderthal-like creature must have suffered sorely: of the fifteen teeth remaining in his fossilized jaw, ten exhibited severe caries; three had progressed to abscesses, with two perforations situated in front of the left ear as a result of the abscessed petrous bone still preserved in the fossilized skull. One is tempted to speculate about the owner of this skull, found at the base of a forty-foot cliff in Rhodesia: Was the site of his death accidental or did the agonies from his multiple infections help push him over?

DISEASE IN THE LIVES OF EARLY HUMANS

WHO OR WHAT IS HUMAN?

The title "human" is not lavishly bestowed. Learned groups have filled distinguished halls with the sounds of debate on the subject. Some scholars advocate assigning a distinct genus status for every new fossil find. Others, with equal fervor, argue that *Australopithecus,* the Neanderthal finds, *Homo erectus*—all the controversial fossil finds of recent times—are human and should be welcomed into our presently exclusive genus and species. Since ours is the only self-determined category, it has always tended to remain quite select. Membership is restricted, often excluding obviously close relatives on rather flimsy pretexts: they are not quite human enough. Yet when we probe into the realm of what is human, we have great difficulty once we leave the familiar arena of beings who closely resemble humans as we know them today. Every humanlike fossil find has provoked storms of controversy, obviously of no consequence to the beings each find represented, but perhaps revealing of the fragility of the egos making the entry rules.

Consequently, when we are confronted with the task of examining the fossil record for evidence of health and disease in early humans, we have to make our own decisions, perhaps arbitrarily, on what to include. To skirt the debate and to suit our purposes, let us accept all the upright, apparently omnivorous, culture-bearing beings as at least our very close kin. Surveying the fossil record for informa-

16

tion as to how they fared in matters of health and disease should contribute to our knowledge of the human heritage.

POPULATION SIZE AND DISEASE

Cockburn (1971) and others suggest that early humans were comparatively rare creatures, probably no more numerous than present-day chimpanzee populations. The everyday life of the individual was conducted in contact with members of a band, a group probably composed of less than a few hundred individuals, with occasional interactions between members of other bands. Since agriculture was unknown until only ten to fourteen thousand years ago, the bands would have had no assured source of sustenance other than what could be hunted or gathered within the immediate environment. When supplies were exhausted, the only recourse was to move on.

The diseases that afflicted such early human groups would, by necessity, have derived from pathogens that are able to survive in small, more or less nomadic populations. Most known viral diseases, such as measles, smallpox, poliomyelitis, and mumps, have been shown by numerous studies to be dependent for continuous transmission on the presence of large, settled groups of hosts. So it is highly unlikely that these diseases were of much consequence in the early evolution of *Homo sapiens.*

Similarly, diseases dependent on complex cycles involving transmission by specific insect or animal vectors, with rigid requirements of their own, would tend to make little impact upon small groups that migrated regularly. This factor probably eliminates some of the most devastating diseases of recent human life. Bilharzia, for example, today one of the most important causes of death and debilitation on a worldwide scale, can be transmitted only under very special conditions. Transmission depends on specific snails in intimate contact with humans who must spend much of their days partially immersed in water—typical conditions among populations employing irrigation techniques for growing crops. Until agriculture was developed as a way of life, it is unlikely that diseases of this nature would have been a problem for emerging humans.

On the basis of numerous studies of living hunters and collectors of food, Weiner (1971:161) extrapolates convincingly to similar societies in ancient times:

> Infectious disease remains the overriding cause of high mortality at all ages. . . . Even in the pre-agricultural era, men were as susceptible as they are now to infections by viruses

responsible for respiratory disorders, influenza, common cold and others; amongst modern hunters and collectors there is a world-wide distribution of viral antibodies from Pacific Islanders to Kalahari Bushmen.

As discussed earlier, concrete evidence of the presence of diseases that leave no record in the fossilized material is not available for direct examination. The extrapolative approach is a less desirable alternative to the direct evidence of specific conditions provided by the fossil record and perhaps even less reliable than such indirect evidence as the hints of tetanus and sleeping sickness discussed above. Nevertheless, when all other evidence is wanting, limited speculations are in order where populations are found living today under conditions similar in many respects to those of ancient peoples.

Weiner finds that in many primitive societies females are particularly at a disadvantage during their reproductive years, primarily because of insecurity of the food supply. When there are extended food shortages and concomitant deficiencies of vitamins and of minerals such as calcium and iron, the losses could be critical to the pregnant woman and her fetus or to the nursing mother and her infant. For these and other reasons, it follows that infant mortality rates would have been extremely high and populations would have persisted only at low levels. (See Chapter 4 for the distinctive medical history of women in their reproductive role.)

The fossil record does appear to concur with the assumption of low survival rates for the very young and, consequently, small human populations for all of our existence until quite recently—until agriculture replaced hunting and gathering as the primary means of sustenance. Weiner adds to this assumption with his documentation of the widespread consistency of family sizes: nomadic groups tend to have families with four children, with fewer of the newborn surviving beyond infancy than the newborn of sedentary peoples, who tend toward families of six or more children.

LIFE SPAN OF PREHISTORIC HUMANS

That small populations were the rule during almost all of human existence was undoubtedly owing in large part to the precarious infant survivals, but facile explanations of infant morbidity and fetal wastage leave questions unanswered. According to Vallois (1923), of the more than forty Neanderthal fossils he examined, only one past the age of fifty was found. The remains of early *Homo sapiens* available during his studies yielded some 141 skeletons, of which only four had lived beyond the age of fifty. Since Vallois's investigations, many more fossil finds continue to verify his ratios of early deaths for those prehistoric humans who managed to survive the perils of infancy.

It will be shown that even today the life cut short is more the rule than the exception among hunters and gatherers. What calamities have been in operation in the lives of these peoples to reduce their life span from the "three score and ten" so commonly expected in sedentary and "advanced" societies? Can the cause be accidents, food deprivations, pathogens, predators, or some combination of these? Examinations of the fossil record provide some clues, and studies of living populations offer some insights, but it is quite likely that the complete answer, at least for our prehistoric ancestors, will remain forever shrouded by the thousands, sometimes millions, of years that intervene between their existence and the finding of their remains.

AUSTRALOPITHECUS

The earliest known creatures for whom a direct evolutionary line can be reasonably extrapolated to modern humans are represented by the expanding numbers of fossil finds lumped collectively in the genus *Australopithecus*. Most of these finds have taken place in Africa, particularly in Olduvai Gorge and Lake Rudolf in Kenya and Tanzania and in various other sites in East Africa as well as in South Africa. As the digging for more representatives of incipient humans intensifies, more will unquestionably be found.

Day et al. (1975) report the presence of a possible healed fracture in an adult right femur from the australopithecine specimen called KNM-ER 1472 and dated at 2.6 million years. They also report a tibia with an undiagnosed swelling on its medial side, belonging to another equally ancient adult with a similarly uninspiring name. Clement (1956) presents a clear case of dental decay: two bacterial infections in an upper molar of an australopithecine that had formerly been named *Paranthropus crassidens,* from Swartkrans in South Africa, and also dated several million years old.

One of the former mysteries associated with an australopithecine fossil yielded to solution through the judicious application of medical techniques. A small piece of jaw, found in 1932 in Kanam, Kenya, and dating from australopithecine times, was puzzling because it possessed a chin. No other *Australopithecus* had anything like a real chin and the ownership of one is always associated with much more recent human types. The mystery of this incongruous piece of anatomy was solved when Tobias (1962) cut into the jaw and examined it microscopically. The "chin" turned out to be an infected fracture with a callus lump grown over the break. Perhaps, more than a million years ago, this unfortunate creature had injured himself in a fall; perhaps someone or something had delivered him a nasty blow. In any case, in the slow healing process, a chinlike structure developed and subsequently fossilized to confuse paleontologists for thirty years after its discovery.

Most of the australopithecines have been uncovered only within recent years. Confusing newer finds suggest the simultaneous presence of more advanced hominids, which have been put into another category, *Homo habilis* (Walker and Leakey 1978). Thorough investigations of the hominids' possible diseases are still to come. All the evidence thus far, however, points to their disappearance approximately one million years ago. What became of these creatures who had persisted for perhaps more than five million years is still a matter of speculation. Future studies that focus on their paleopathology may shed more light on this intriguing question. An important point made by Janssens (1970:16) should be borne in mind at such time as more information becomes available and attempts are made to connect disease with the extinction of this, or any, species:

> It is not likely that virulence [of pathogens] was greater in the past than it is now, otherwise survival would have been impossible. Nevertheless, one has to be careful; it is not impossible that with the extinction of a race, the cause of that extinction, in this case, disease, has disappeared too.

HOMO ERECTUS

Many anthropologists contend that it is inaccurate to speak of the extinction of *Australopithecus*; rather, they postulate a gradual evolution into the forms of human ancestry that followed next in the fossil record—the numerous finds from Java, China, Africa, and parts of Europe—all now lumped together as *Homo erectus.* Other paleontologists argue that the australopithecines left no genes whereas the *Homo habilis* evolved into the larger *Homo erectus.* In any case, these creatures were completely upright, about five and one half feet tall (more than a foot taller than the australopithecines), and possessed brain capacities that were much greater than those of their predecessors, some in fact overlapping into the range of modern humans. With their distinctive tools, use of fire, and cooperative hunting techniques, they have persuaded today's taxonomists to open the genus door, to permit entry to *Homo erectus.*

Until the australopithecine finds had emerged, the oldest example of human pathology was attributed to an osteitis lesion in a six-inch piece of femur belonging to a *Homo erectus* from the group that lived some half a million years ago and disappeared perhaps 100,000 years B.P. Guthrie (1958) reports a large bony tumor or exostosis near its upper end. This piece of bone, along with a fragment of the dome of the skull, an upper molar, and several crude stone tools, was found in 1891 by a Dutch army surgeon, Eugene Dubois, who proposed the name *Pithecanthropus erectus* for his exciting find.

The discoveries in Java as well as those in China and other parts of the world include many individuals who appear to have died as a result of cranial injuries inflicted by violence. Janssens (1970) lists thirteen skulls that show distinctive skull fractures. He cautions that although the owners of these skulls most probably were done in during unfriendly encounters with their fellows, they could have been victims of volcanic eruptions that were common at that time. As the evidence accumulates, however, the opportunity to lay the blame on acts of nature becomes almost untenable.

Janssens reports an additional eleven skulls found near the Solo River in Java; four of these showed wounds that would be lethal. The Pekin group of *Homo erectus* remains found in the caves of Choukoutien in China included forty individuals. All of these had received severe head injuries and subsequently were decapitated—hardly the action of a volcano. At least one of the skulls had suffered two separate head wounds; the first one had healed, permitting the owner to survive until a second blow irrevocably set him or her on the road to fossil immortality.

In a cave located at a higher level, indicating more recent life during the Stone Ages, remains of four adults and three children were found. These also had been slaughtered and the murder weapons, clubs and pointed implements, left behind. We shall see, as more fossilized human finds are examined, that violence accounted for an extraordinarily high proportion of the deaths among the fossilized remains of our forebears. Among the several possible explanations, the presence of severed heads, particularly with markings at the base of the skull that could have come from scooping out the contents, suggests at least one: utilization of the brains, either for ritual purposes or, in bad times, as a source of food. Here again, some investigators would like to believe that some of the *Homo erectus* victims died from natural causes—rock falls in caves, disease, or, as mentioned above, volcanic activity—and that their deaths were followed by ritual decapitation. Until more finds and better techniques of analysis accrue, we are left with a most disquieting inheritance.

THE NEANDERTHAL RECORD
Neanderthals constitute the first known human group that struggled for existence in cold climates. Except for the cave bears, all life that we have considered thus far evolved in and adapted to tropical or subtropical environments. It follows that this new form of human life—called *Homo sapiens* by some, *Homo neanderthalensis* by the more conservative, and *Homo sapiens neanderthalensis* by the bickerers—living between 115,000 and 40,000 years ago often on the edge of glacial advances, would have confronted quite different problems of adaptation, problems that included new diseases as well as transformed old diseases. If, as is generally postulated, Neanderthals evolved from the earlier forms of hominids we have already touched upon, these cold-dwellers would have confronted the new diseases equipped with immunological responses geared toward much different, often irrelevant contexts. That they survived and more or less prospered for more than seventy-five thousand years speaks strongly of their remarkable technological and cultural development and perhaps of the pliability of human physiology as well.

Lacking the ability to grow heavy coats of fur or thick subcutaneous layers of insulating fat, humans could survive in extreme cold only by elaboration of culture. Neanderthals left eloquent evidence that this, indeed, was their survival strategy. Their repertoire included the regular use of fire; a highly developed kit of tools for sawing, scraping, and boring; impressive techniques for cooperatively hunting huge mammals; elaborate rituals based on magical or supernatural ideology; and considerable care and compassion for the sick or injured members of their groups. Neanderthals are credited with furnishing the first proofs of attempts to deal with the problem of death. Beginning with these ancient ancestors, one finds distinctive, deliberate burials, frequently in family-type groups and often accompanied by possessions and decorations that suggest a rather sophisticated concept of an afterlife.

Forced to maintain life by hunting the enormous animals of their day, equipped only with tools fashioned out of wood, stone, or bone, Neanderthals must have led a life fraught with danger. It is not surprising that injuries and infected fractures fill a large part of their fossil record. Arthritis may have been one of the sequelae of many infected wounds. But some propose that it may have developed from a primary infection such as pyorrhea, which was a fairly familiar ailment; others suggest that the harsh climate was responsible. Whatever the cause, arthritis was a common affliction of the Neanderthal humans, particularly among those who survived past their teens. One of the best known is the "old man" of La Chapelle-aux-Saints in France who, in fact, was middle-aged at best when he died. During his life, however, he was beset with crippling arthritis and severe pyorrhea that combined to produce the aged appearance in his skeletal remains that confused the early investigators.

One of the most traumatized Neanderthal skeletons was found in the Shanidar caves of northern Iraq. This being began life with a stunted arm, either from a birth defect or as a result of an undetermined illness, and then lost a large part of that same arm later in life. With only one functioning arm, he probably used his mouth to compensate in some tasks such as scraping or cutting; in any case, he ended up with very badly ground-down teeth. Later, two front teeth were lost, probably in another accident. Sometime in this tragedy of antiquity, he was delivered a sharp blow to the top of his head. Recovering from that assault, he sustained another, harder blow that smashed the left side of his face and probably destroyed the sight of his left eye. Somehow he persevered to about the age of forty, long enough for him to acquire severe arthritic crippling to add to his burdens. One would like to believe that better days were in store, but around his fortieth birthday the roof over his cave hearth collapsed, ending his saga and his troubles.

"Nandy," the name affectionately given to our hero by his discoverers, evoked more than sympathy among the many scholars who have since studied his remains. Neanderthal buffs frequently cite him as the world's first surgical patient, assuming that his arm was deliberately amputated to save him after a mangling accident* (Fig. 1–9). Others argue, sometimes heatedly, that the amputation was not the result of planned medical intervention, for, as Majno (1975:9) puts it, "there were surely more lions than surgeons in the immediate neighborhood." One might propose cave bears as the more likely

---

*Feminists should undoubtedly intervene at this point to insist that the earliest surgeon was surely the first female who severed and tied an umbilical cord.

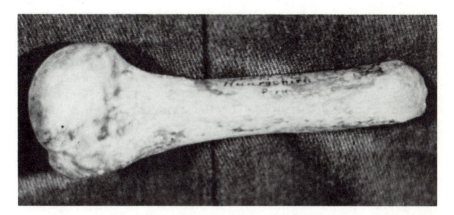

1–9 Evidence of an amputation of the upper arm of a prehistoric American—similar to the surgery associated with "Nandy." The basis for such amputations cannot be determined. The cut end of this humerus indicates that complete healing occurred. (Courtesy of San Diego Museum of Man, cat. no. 668. Photo by Mary Edgecomb.)

candidates for the times involved, but it is an excellent point nevertheless.

Arguments of this nature, while often absorbing, tend to obscure more important implications that finds such as Nandy reveal. The presence of enemies who perpetrated the skull damage is obvious, but perhaps more significant were the neighbors or kinsmen who were willing to deliver the sustained nursing that sufficed to bring him through all but the last of his traumas. Further, Nandy provides additional eloquent testimony of early man's powers to recover, repair, and persist in the face of formidable odds.

DISEASE AND THE SETTLED LIFE

Until some ten to fourteen thousand years ago, every form of life, human and otherwise, made its living by hunting and collecting such food as nature provided. If we accept the australopithecines as the first creatures verging on human, we then have almost a five-million-year history for human evolution with only the smallest, most recent fraction of that time—in geological terms, hardly yesterday—given to adaptation for a sedentary life based on deliberate food raising.

Thus, except for the present two-thousandths of our time on earth, all evolutionary selection took place in a framework of small, often migratory bands. These consisted of people who followed herds of animals and had only fleeting contact with other humans (fortunately not too fleeting to effect some gene exchange, thus maintaining *Homo sapiens* today as one species). Their life frequently required them to carry their infants as well as their few personal belongings from place to place; and their diet depended completely on the vagaries of a fickle Nature.

Somehow—the method of discovery is still hotly disputed—humans learned that plants could be cultivated and small animals could be taken from the herds to be bred deliberately in one place. Agriculture was under way, effecting so profound a change in human life that it has been called, appropriately, the Neolithic Revolution. For the first time in more than five million years of precarious existence, many generations would now live out their lives in one small area, more or less assured of a food supply, and in intimate, regular contact with large numbers of fellow humans.

INCREASED POPULATIONS, NEW DISEASES, AND NEW MODES OF RESISTANCE
In evolutionary terms our adaptations have clearly been for a way of life profoundly different from that found among almost all human populations in the world today. Although the fundamental immunological responses such as antibody production, fever, inflammation, and repair, all activated by the stimuli of parasitic invasions or injury, have persisted and continue to sustain us, the new way of life permitted the introduction of diseases for which there had been no specific immunological preparation. Among the unfamiliar problems confronting newly settled populations were the viruses and bacteria responsible for measles, smallpox, influenza, syphilis, plague, tuberculosis, and many other diseases that are dependent for steady transmission on the presence of large numbers of intimately associated people. When agricultural villages and, later, towns and cities were made possible by the shift to agriculture, these diseases became capable of epidemic ravages that in many places probably negated the many benefits derived from the new way of life.

Our continued existence testifies to a considerable flexibility in immunological responses and to the powerful human cultural potentialities that acted to counterbalance the negative pressures of the new diseases as well as the old ones that may have acquired increased virulence. The positive forces are to be found in the advantages inherent in a settled mode of living: improved supply of food with storage facilities to help carry people over the lean times; guaranteed continuous shelter with protection against the elements or more frightening invasions; leisure time and the impetus for the development of incredibly numerous technological and cultural innovations; opportunities for a broader range of gene exchange—all culminating eventually in the inauguration of the first baby boom.

Population sizes in Neolithic times did not get more than a start toward the explosive numbers harassing the world today primarily because the death rate remained extremely high. Averaging the age of death for all prehistoric human finds up to and including Neolithic remains, Moodie in 1923 found that most of the skeletal remains began their fossil careers at around fourteen years of age! Wells (1964) estimates that only one Neanderthal in twenty lived beyond the age of forty, while 80 percent perished before the age of thirty. Likewise, he shows that, of Cro-Magnon fossils dated as more recent than forty thousand years old, more than 88 percent did not survive as long as forty years.

Similarly, Krogman (1940) found, from a study of twenty-two *Homo erectus* skeletons, that fifteen had died within fourteen years of their birth; three more were dead by age thirty, and three before age fifty, leaving one stalwart soul who lived more than fifty years. Moreover, as Krogman notes, the skeletons of children do not preserve well, so the figures for early death are probably even higher. An interesting finding, whenever large numbers of human burials have been studied, is that, until the present century, women frequently died at younger ages than their male counterparts.

We continue to be handicapped by the absence of any written records throughout the early millennia of the agricultural life; we remain dependent on the fossil record and such evidence as may be deduced from archeological investigations. However, as might be anticipated, both sources are considerably richer for sedentary agriculturalists than are the scanty human remains of their preagricultural predecessors.

MORE ARTHRITIS, NEW IMPLICATIONS

In agricultural Europe and in the New World, arthritis continued to extract its crippling toll. Bones with arthritic changes have been related to populations from France, England, and Scandinavia, and to almost all early New World populations.

Possibly connected with the large numbers of arthritic deformities is the high incidence of dental problems found in the same skeletal remains. The stigmata of pyorrhea and of abscesses of the roots are reported by many investigators (Fig. 1–10). Some suggest that grit, dirt, and stone particles clinging to food combined to produce a high rate of attrition, thus opening the way for subsequent bacterial infections. However, after agriculture became established, carious teeth became more common, as indicated by larger proportions of caries in skeletal remains than ever before, particularly throughout Europe. Dietary changes, which included an increased dependency on starchy root crops, were undoubtedly an important contributing factor.

In a symposium devoted to human paleopathology (Jarcho 1966:108), Alice M. Brues observed, "Arthritis is so common in all prehistoric people that we can perhaps ignore it except where it is exceedingly severe and destructive." For our purposes, and most

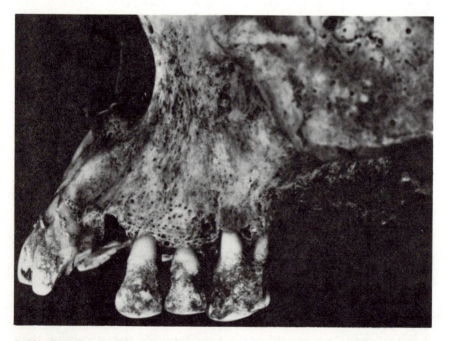

1–10   Part of a maxilla of an ancient American showing evidence of severe bacterial infection or pyorrhea as well as salivary calculus. (Courtesy of Field Museum of Natural History, Chicago.)

assuredly for the people afflicted, arthritis cannot be ignored. Sigerist (1951:51), commenting on the vast amount of material on arthritis, describes its deplorable effects:

> Under the most varied climates, under the sun in Egypt, in caves in neolithic France, in the mountains of Peru, people of all ages, but especially people of mature and old age, suffered atrocious pains in their joints and felt their spine, their hip, or knee stiffening gradually until they could hardly move. They were crippled and helpless unless their neighbors attended to them.

Pales (1930), in an examination of the sites of occurrence of arthritis, for prehistoric as well as modern humans, concluded that the affected areas of the body are those that a person moves the most. He found that prehistoric humans were afflicted mainly in the anterior lumbar spine, the most involved segment in the physically active person, whereas modern populations, living much more sedentary lives, are affected primarily in the cervical part of the spine (Fig. 1–11).

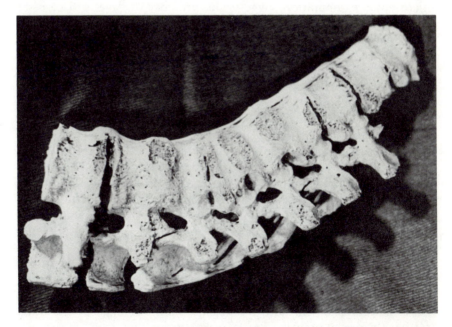

1–11 Vertebra from an ancient Peruvian who suffered from ankylosing spondylitis. This progressive, debilitating condition produces a rigid "poker spine" that crucially limits mobility, particularly restricting most bending movements. (Courtesy of San Diego Museum of Man, cat. no. 562. Photo by Mary Edgecomb.)

We have seen that since our vetebrate phylum began to populate the earth, perhaps some three hundred million years ago, virtually all of its history has been perfused with arthritis, a disease whose cause is still unknown and whose cure is yet to be realized. Arthritis continues to torment humanity and to challenge the medical scientist. For the social scientist, however, it sheds some light: the large number of deformed bones attesting to damaged humans, living rather extended years with these afflictions, implies that during the arthrítics' lifetimes there were people among them who were willing and able to nurture relatively unproductive members of their society. The presence of so many incapacitated individuals further suggests an early emergence of cultural institutions related to the care, prevention, and explanation of such painful phenomena.

In addition to the many sufferers from arthritic crippling, the fossil record has revealed skeletons of prehistoric people who survived for many years in spite of equally severe pathologies. For example, Pales (1929) reports an open sacrum, a femur from an individual with a congenital dislocation of the hip, and a femur that on microscopic examination suggests the presence of Paget's disease—all from a small population in early agricultural France. Each of these individuals would have lived with reduced capacities; nevertheless, their ages at death suggest a relatively long, albeit handicapped life. Findings such as these, along with the arthritis record, imply cultural adaptations, at early stages in human evolution, to integrate the handicapped person.

"BATTERED, SLICED OR STRANGLED"

The perpetuation of so many dependent lives, years beyond the time when they could actively contribute to the daily chores and innumerable tasks required for survival under primitive living conditions, speaks eloquently of a deeply embedded humanity as a critical factor in the survival of *Homo sapiens.* The evidence of cooperation and concern tends to counterbalance the less humane history of violence and brutality so abundant in the fossil record. Every survivor with a crippling disease, and perhaps even some of those with healed wounds or fractures as well, attests to human cooperation and peaceful interaction. This evidence is available only through extrapolation but is nonetheless real and perhaps consoling in light of the other side of our human record.

As Wells (1964:111) writes about that other side:

The long road of paleopathology is littered with the cadavers of men, women and children who have been battered, sliced or strangled to death. The muster remains unreckoned but it runs into thousands.

As one example from a potential store of many, Moodie (1923) describes a specimen of a lumbar vertebra bearing a stone arrow point deeply embedded in the ventral surface. He speculates that the individual was shot through the abdomen with great force, considering the distance the arrowhead had to travel through the abdominal wall and through the viscera to root itself in the vertebra, where it remains fixed after thousands of years.

In keeping with the propensity of humans to inflict damage on others of their species, remains of early humans abound with wounds made by blows from clubs, axes, arrow points, and spears (Fig. 1–12). The skull was apparently the main target (Fig. 1–13). Even though the skulls of earlier humans were generally somewhat thicker than those of modern humans, they proved equally vulnerable to a determined assault. The frequent scars in the skulls were often deep

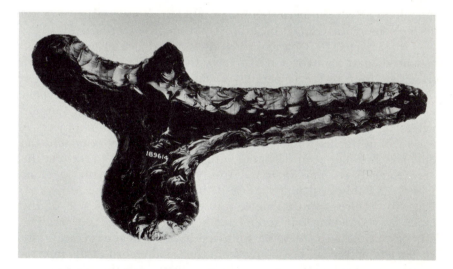

1–12   Obsidian monolithic ax from prehistoric British Honduras (Belize). Weapons and tools of this sort, which exhibit fine workmanship, may have been responsible for many of the traumatic injuries observed in prehistoric skeletal remains. (Courtesy of Field Museum of Natural History, Chicago.)

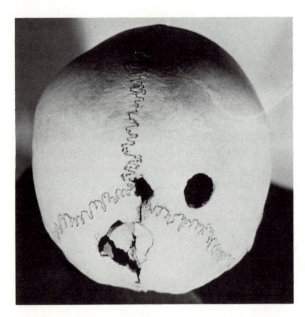

1–13 Pre-Columbian skull showing injuries that quite likely resulted in the death of the young victim. The penetrating and crushing wounds were probably made by slingshot and/or mace points. (Courtesy of San Diego Museum of Man, cat. no. 16. Photo by Mary Edgecomb.)

enough to affect the periosteum and adjacent bones, either directly through traumatic contact or indirectly through infections.

In Janssens (1970) is described the skull of an early agricultural-ist who died at about the age of forty-five or fifty and who took to his grave four severe, separately incurred head lesions. All these wounds had healed in his lifetime. The first lesion was on the right parietal bone, an impacted fracture 28 millimeters wide and 35 milli-meters long, probably caused by a blow from a blunt object. A second blow to his forehead caused a wound of approximately the same size but had been delivered with sufficient force to stave in the bone some 3 to 5 millimeters. Another blow, again from a blunt object, probably cost him the use of his left eye, but he recovered, living to receive a fourth blow, this one, on the right side of the upper jaw, knocking out several teeth and dislodging another. The last injury produced infection followed by slow healing. Once more we are left with vivid testimony from the fossil record of the impres-sive recuperative abilities of the human body and, in this case, we find evidence of a perversity within human interactions that too frequently makes this recuperative ability mandatory.

Apparently the threat of blows to the head was common enough to engender a number of special kinds of related fractures, appropriately labeled "parry fractures of the ulna." This type of break cannot be reconstructed as occurring through any natural cause. The most reasonable explanation is that it results from the action of raising an arm to avert a blow, particularly a blow aimed at the head, so that the impact of the thrust is on the presenting bone of the forearm instead.

Fortunately for our survival, the fossil record indicates that in spite of the frequent batterings and damaging altercations, healing rates were quite high, perhaps thanks to the cultural adaptation mentioned above (Fig. 1–14). Perhaps, too, as Majno (1975) suggests, earlier humans were safer than we are from the threats of infection

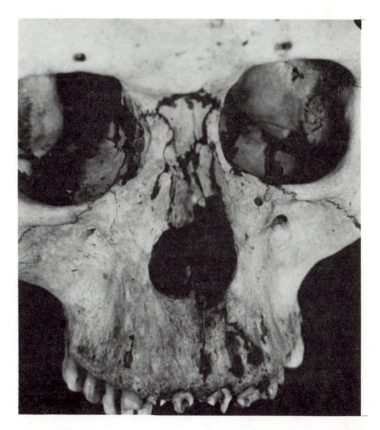

1–14 This ancient Peruvian suffered and recovered from an extensive nasal fracture. (Courtesy of San Diego Museum of Man, cat. no. 305. Photo by Mary Edgecomb.)

superimposed upon injuries, not only because of the absence of medical personnel who, in modern hospitals today, may be carriers of staphylocci but because conditions that lead to the breeding of more virulent strains of infecting bacteria may not have existed.

Moodie (1923), Janssens (1970), and others call attention to the disconcerting evidence regarding the sex of the owners of many of the damaged skulls. An overwhelming majority of the injured heads apparently belonged to females. For the New World fossil record, Janssens (1970:28) notes:

> It is extraordinary that this type of lesion—three depressed fractures of the skull are situated between lambda and the obelion, left of the sagittal suture, the other two probably delivered by one and the same blow touch each other and are situated on the occipital bone, underneath the left of lambda—appear so often on women during the Pre-Columbian period.

Were these New World women sacrificed in some unknown religious ritual? Does the choice of females as victims suggest fertility rites associated with early agriculture? Or was there a time when women were actively engaged in fighting? Or were they victims of intertribal wars? The possibilities are endless and may quite likely involve circumstances of which we are completely ignorant. Answers that may be forthcoming will have to derive from the combined efforts of paleopathologists, archeologists, cultural anthropologists, geographers, and medical historians. Or, as in so many mysteries of paleopathology, the answers may remain buried forever with the victims and their assailants.

EARLY SKULL SURGERY

Not content with bashing in one another's skulls, early humans also had holes cut deliberately into their crania. On some of the large numbers of skulls giving evidence of this it is apparent that the treatment was performed not once, but often several times in the victims' lifetimes (Fig. 1–15). This operation, known as trepanning or trephining, was first discovered in a Neolithic skull in France in 1685; another was found much later, in 1816. The holes in the skull were dismissed as wounds by the earlier discoverers. Then, in 1873, at a meeting of the French Association for the Advancement of Science, a French anthropologist, Prunières, demonstrated an oval piece of bone cut from a parietal bone that he had found on a skull

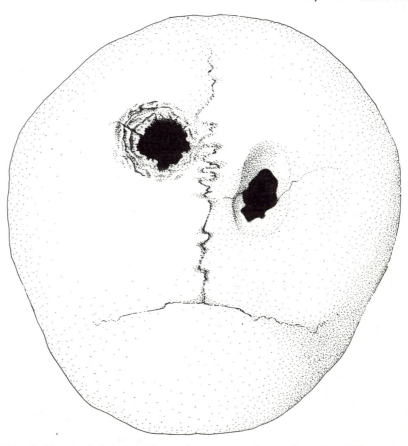

1–15 Prehistoric skull with evidence of two trepanations performed at different times. The hole on the right side shows evidence of complete, uneventful healing. The subsequent hole on the left side apparently became infected and may have been responsible for the owner's death. The skull was found at Monte Alban, in a valley on the western edge of Oaxaca, Mexico, a site occupied from 500 B.C. to A.D. 700. (Adapted from Wilkinson 1975.)

in a tomb. He suggested that this "rondelle" had been used as a charm or an amulet and had probably been worn by the owner to protect against evil or to aid in some other way.

In the years that followed, many trepanned skulls and a great many more round or oval pieces of bone cut out of skulls came to light. By 1950, more than two hundred trepanned skulls were reported from France alone; many others were found all over Europe and some in Algiers. In the New World, the numbers were equally impressive. On the other hand, no trace of this surgery in Hindu or Chinese societies has been reported, nor was it undertaken by the ancient Greeks or Romans.

As the unearthing of trepanned prehistoric skulls accelerated, reports began to appear of the same practice by lay practitioners in contemporary societies, particularly in the Balkans, among some of the Indians of Bolivia and Peru, among the Cabyls of the Atlas Mountains, and among a number of tribes of the South Pacific. Sigerist (1951) reports that the operation is done primarily as treatment for people suffering from severe chronic headaches and similar ailments.

In technologically sophisticated societies, trepanation is occasionally done to relieve pressure on the brain, notably in cases of depressed fractures or other serious injuries. The prehistoric skulls, however, rarely show any signs of previous damage; it must be assumed that the operations were performed for other reasons. Temkin (1945) suggests that ancient and medieval surgeons made openings in the skulls of persons afflicted with epilepsy and similar diseases, in order that the evil be forced out. Guthrie (1958) theorizes that trepanning was done originally in order to drive out the demon or demons that had taken possession of the individual—conditions that today might be diagnosed as, for instance, epilepsy, mental disorders, cerebral tumors, *tic doloureux*, or migraine. Basing his argument on the assumption of a belief in demons, he asks, "What treatment could be more obvious than to make an opening in the head so that the evil spirit could escape?" This reasoning involves an assumption that may or may not be valid. In any case, if the demons entered before the hole was cut, they would have access to the same route if they wanted to leave. Perhaps, more important, if the suggested maladies were the root cause, pragmatic experience would demonstrate that trepanning would not effect a lasting cure. What is obvious here is that the projection of explanations for cultural practices onto cultures other than one's own is an unsatisfactory methodology.

The record of paleopathology imposes a further contradiction in the attempts to explain trepanation as a treatment for illness. Although most of the skulls were operated upon while the victims were alive, a considerable number have been found in which the surgery was performed on the dead. In these cases, it could hardly be argued that attempts were being made to relieve symptoms of the various pathologies proposed. Thus, again, the whole story has yet to be told.

Apparently the rondelles were considered desirable and were highly coveted. Many of the small ovals are perforated, which suggests they were worn as pendants. Sigerist (1951) notes that when a successfully trepanned person eventually died, discs were cut from the skull in such a way that part of the edge of the original perforation would be included. It may be that the trauma involved in the operation and the courage to undergo it were appreciated and endowed the person, or at least his or her skull, with special powers. Or, is this again a case of culturally biased reasoning?

Experiments on modern cadavers have shown that it is relatively easy to trepan a skull with a sharp flint—the only instrument known to have been available to the prehistoric surgeons. The edges of the trepanned holes show that three primary methods were employed: the bone could be scraped or scratched; a circular incision could be gradually deepened; or a series of small holes arranged in a circle could be drilled and then the narrow bridges between them cut. Fig. 1–16 shows each of these methods and the resulting scars.

Whichever approach was used, it is certain that the process would have been excruciatingly painful. Yet, as Wells (1964:144) points out, it is "clear that the operation was undertaken with an assurance bred of familiarity." In addition, the size of some of the

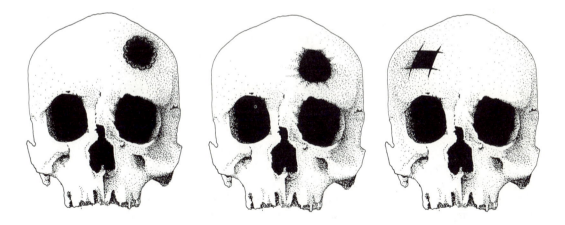

1–16   Three methods of trepanation. *Left*: Small holes were drilled close to one another in a circle and then the narrow bridge remaining between them was cut out. *Center*: The bone was scraped or scratched in a circular incision that was gradually deepened. This was the most common method used. *Right*: This geometric approach involved sharp cuts.

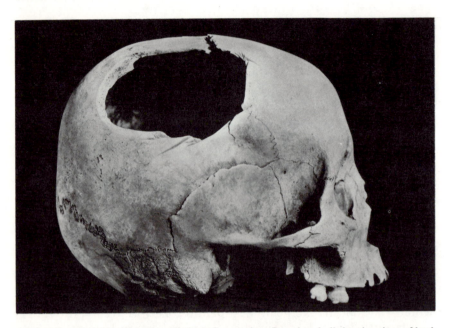

1–17 Extremely extensive trepanation of an ancient Peruvian skull showing signs of healing but suggesting that subsequently the head was permanently vulnerable to injury. (Courtesy of Field Museum of Natural History, Chicago.)

openings gives further proof of the operator's dexterity and confidence (Fig. 1–17). One of the most striking examples is seen in a skull recovered from France in which the top of the skull had been trepanned over the course of a number of operations until eighteen square inches of bone had been removed! Nevertheless, this individual had survived—with a head considerably softer than usual but presumably with a brain still fully intact.

The recovered skulls, most of them thousands of years old, represent all three surgical techniques. But the most unexpected revelation of the remains is that many, perhaps most, of the individuals on whom the mutilations were performed—in the absence, of course, of modern antiseptics or anesthesia—survived and, even more incredibly, had the operation done again. Some skulls reveal as many as a dozen trepanations, all of them healed. Most investigators concur in granting the master trepanner's award to the practitioners among the ancient Peruvians: more than three-quarters of the skulls collected in Peru indicate that the patients recovered. Collectively, however, the

ancient surgeons continue to evoke admiration from modern practi-
oners. Majno (1970:28) reflects this sentiment:

> In most cases the outer surface of the skull around the oper-
> ated site is smooth, indicating that bacteria caused no major
> complications. In only a few cases did osteomyelitis leave its
> marks.
> On the whole, therefore, skull trepanning in the brush
> has always been, and still is, a substantially safe procedure.

We know, then, that sometime after village life began, pragmatic
humans learned they could carve into one another's skulls and have a
reasonable expectation of survival despite holes in the head. The
bones reveal the methodology as well as the survival rates (Fig. 1–18).
As similarly constructed humans, we know also that to pay the price
of such trauma, the anticipated reward would have to be prodigious

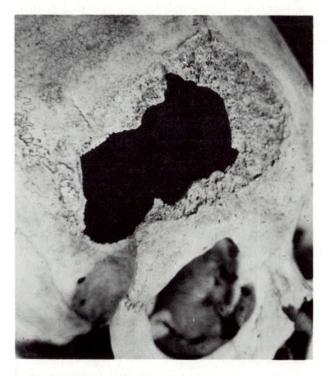

1–18 An ill-fated trepanation. The initial cutting lines are seen
in the upper area; the extensive infection that followed suggests a
poor prognosis. (Courtesy of San Diego Museum of Man, cat. no.
303. Photo by Mary Edgecomb.)

indeed. At this point, as in so much of the fossil record, we are left with a tantalizing Why.

MORE SKULL MANIPULATIONS

An additional form of skull manipulation is revealed from burials of people who had newly entered into an agricultural way of life. From dolmens, prehistoric burial monuments found frequently in Britain and France, have come some crania whose upper halves are marked by curious lesions. As described by Sigerist (1951:113), these lesions consist of a "T-shaped scar beginning on the frontal bone, running all along the sagittal suture, and branching into two parts along the posterior edge of the parietal bones." It is difficult to reconstruct a process that would achieve scars of this nature other than cauterization, cutting deeply and burning through the scalp. Most specimens came from early village settlements in northwestern France, but the practice has also been identified in central Asia, in parts of Africa, and in Peru. These mutilations, like many of the foregoing ones, have been found primarily on female skulls.

Cauterization has a long history, possibly extending as far back as 3000 B.C. Arabic curers once used it as a therapy for epilepsy and certain mental disorders. Some eye diseases were treated by cutting deeply into the forehead by Alexandrian surgeons around the third century B.C., and similar practices continued through medieval times as treatment for melancholia. As had already been discussed, and as anthropology should teach us, it is risky to accept one people's reasoning as answer for another people's practices. Therefore, even though it appears reasonable, to us, to point to the almost exclusive occurrence of these scars in women who lived in the early stages of sedentary agriculture and then deduce a relationship to magical ritual associated with fertility, this is little more than a guess. One can only hope that eventually sufficient clues will accumulate to make substantial statements possible; until such time we are again left with hints that mystify more than they enlighten.

THE RICKETS RECORD

Rickets (see Fig. 3–13) is a deficiency disease resulting from insufficient vitamin D, which leads to defective calcium metabolism. The victim of this disease frequently suffers from bowed legs, sometimes knock-knees, a pigeon breast, flattening of the pelvic bones with altered pelvic outlet, and, in extreme deficiencies, even tetany. Signs of the syndrome first become notable among the skeletal remains from early villages of Norway and Denmark. It is probable that in these areas several factors contributed to the deforming disease: heavy cloud cover for much of the year would reduce the ultraviolet rays of the sun necessary to activate the vitamin D precursors; a diet heavily committed to early agricultural produce would tend to lack reliable sources of this vitamin; and the heavy clothing necessitated by the long winter would minimize the amount of skin exposed to those rays of the sun that were available. (Chapter 3 considers more extensively the dietary and cultural practices that relate to rickets and vitamin D deficiency.)

It is generally accepted that the heavy melanin pigmentation producing dark skin acts as a protective barrier, reducing the entry of excess rays from the sun that could have an effect opposite from rickets—the syndrome called hypervitaminosis-D. When this condition is present, calcium deposits are produced beyond the body's metabolic ability to handle them and many serious physiological and neurological problems ensue. But in regions receiving little sun, heavy melanin concentrations in the skin would obviously be disadvantageous. It is possible that the threat of rickets, particularly the symptoms of pelvic distortion that make normal child delivery impossible, would have promoted evolutionary selection for reduced melanin activation, resulting in the pale skins associated with northwestern European populations.

CONCLUSION

The fossil record indicates that disease is and has been an integral part of all life. Survival is possible only when a balance is achieved between the assaults of pathological parasites and the evolutionary selection of appropriate physiological responses that prevent the threatening forces from destroying their hosts. The basic immunological reactions that constitute our inherited, patterned responses are shared by all vertebrate life. Added to this common heritage are species-specific physiological differences that have been selected by evolution to provide extra protection in the presence of certain long-standing diseases. These will be considered in the chapters that follow.

Homo sapiens is the only form of animal life able to complement the arsenal of biological defense mechanisms with the weapons of culture. Throughout the next chapters it will be seen that human societies have been shaped in many significant ways by the particular configurations of diseases present in the environments in which the given societies have evolved. Only humans are able to react to threatening parasitic attacks with sustained nurturing and other attempts to alleviate the impact of sickness; only humans probe for explanations for the mysterious assaults from their unseen enemies; and only humans are driven to conduct their affairs in keeping with the explanations provoked by experiences with diseases.

The uniquely human attributes do not inevitably serve humans best. From the briefly scanned fossil record and the studies that follow, it appears that cultural and social forces occasionally act to favor the parasites over the welfare of the human hosts. As the search for health continues, the social sciences have a vital contribution to make in providing better understanding of the interrelationship of all the forces, both biological and social, at work in the struggle for a full life. As medical anthropology progresses along with the other subdisciplines of anthropological and medical research, much more information will become available on our cultural interactions with the ever-present threat of illness.

2

A COMMON SHARED LEGACY

DISEASE AMONG NONHUMAN PRIMATES

It is popularly assumed that the primate living in the natural state has achieved the idyllic existence portrayed in Genesis before Adam and Eve defected. Although the evidence is far from complete, recent studies of nonhuman primates suggest that quite the opposite is true. In his extensive presentation of the lives of nonhuman primates, Schultz (1972:191) declares, "It can no longer be doubted that perfect health and normality is far from being such a prevailing privilege of living in the natural state."

Some knowledge of the expanding field of nonhuman primate disease provides revealing insights into the human condition. Human beings are found scattered over every possible habitable environment on the earth's surface. Life in many of these areas became feasible only as a result of cultural adaptations that supplement physiological selection. No primates other than humans are found in arctic regions, none at extremely high altitudes, none in desert ecosystems. Scientific evidence strongly suggests that the early evolution of *Homo sapiens* took place in a subtropical environment, near sea level—the same type of environment in which the order Primates evolved some sixty to seventy million years ago.

Today, the majority of nonhuman primates still live in similar habitats; only humans with their technologies and complex societies have ventured abroad with any degree of success. Much useful information for human health has been provided by medical investigations of nonhuman primates. In addition, studies of diseases still shared, as well as parasites that are specific for certain genera within the order Primates, reinforce the theory of a common ancestry and also furnish important clues to the time spans involved in the divergences of various species.

In addition to high rates (up to 33 percent) of fetal wastage from spontaneous abortions, stillbirths, and neonatal deaths, apparently infant primates are subject, according to Schultz (1972), to a "shockingly high incidence" of most of the same viral, bacterial, and protozoan infections that attack humans. Recorded cases of malaria, yellow fever, dysentery, yaws, filariasis, herpes, poliomyelitis, tuberculosis, hepatitis, arthritis, rabies, arteriosclerosis, and many other diseases document a shared legacy of miseries.

Schultz examines the striking fact that no primate other than *Homo sapiens* has experienced a population explosion in spite of the nonhuman primates' comparatively shorter gestation times and extended female reproductive life (menopause apparently does not occur). Other observers have noted the markedly higher number of adult females in simian populations despite a near equal ratio at birth. This skewed distribution is similar to that found amoung adults in many human populations today. The question of whether the uneven sex ratios are results of physiological differences, unexplained social factors, sex-specific diseases, or unknown causes may be answered as research on nonhuman primate populations continues.

The antiquity of tooth decay, subsequent abscesses, and the previously implicated arthritic sequelae is indicated by the prevalence today of all three conditions, particularly among apes living in the wild. The coarse, fibrous diet of the great apes also contributes to the high rates of gum infections that probably are initiated by impacted, tough plant fibers. In one study (Schultz 1972) at least one abscess was found in 14 percent of young adult monkeys and apes examined. The figure rose to a startling 67 percent when examinations concentrated on older adults. The reader who has ever had to endure the pain of an abscessed tooth may wonder how the nonhuman primates manage to consume their rough nourishment and function at all when in such distress.

EVIDENCE OF TRAUMATIC INJURY AND ARTHRITIS

Many of the arboreal monkeys and apes have been studied extensively in recent years through X-ray examinations, which show that surprisingly high numbers of them have endured multiple fractures. Perhaps the epitome of this group is represented by a wild capuchin monkey who, over the course of a short lifetime, sustained three badly broken facial bones, a break and subsequent infection in each of the long leg bones, a fractured breast bone, a broken tail vertebra, and two broken toes (Schultz 1972:196). All of these injuries healed and this brachiating Job, although scarred and deformed, somehow managed to live and fend for himself until he was brought down by a bullet.

Apparently arthritis is no stranger to modern primates. Schultz reports a survey of 233 skeletons of shot wild gibbons in which marked arthritic changes were found in 17 percent of the specimens. Only 2 percent of the young gibbons showed these changes, but, among the older members some 55 percent were affected. Similar studies performed on wild gorillas reveal that chronic arthritis is quite common, affecting chiefly the lumbar vertebrae. On the other hand, studies have not exposed arthritis either in the various prosimians or in the monkeys of the New World. How these members of the same order, committed to similar diets, climates, and environments, escape the crippling pain of arthritis while so many of their "cousins" are affected to the degree indicated is worth serious inquiry.

SHARED EPIDEMIOLOGY

From our own species-oriented perspective we tend to think of epidemics of various diseases as exclusively human phenomena. The facts are quite different. Epidemics affect nonhuman primate populations in nature as well as in captivity. Schultz (1972) reports that in many areas of South America, howler monkeys have been virtually eliminated by yellow fever outbreaks. In Lawick-Goodall's (1971) poignant description of a poliomyelitis epidemic among the chimpanzees she observed, one sees the havoc wrought by disease out of control, with tragedy and pathos no less moving for having occurred in a band of nonhuman primates.

Fiennes and Riopelle (1969) record the first known death from polio in an adolescent mountain gorilla. The knowledge that nonhuman primates do develop the disease has been utilized for human advantage in research on poliomyelitis. In 1909, Karl Landsteiner discovered that polio could be transmitted from humans to apes and monkeys. Thereafter, many nonhuman primates participated in the research that eventually led to effective vaccines and the virtual eradication of that formerly dreaded crippler of the young. At present, most vaccines for polio prevention are produced primarily from fresh kidneys of rhesus monkeys. These vaccines, incidentally, were responsible for checking the epidemic and saving the lives of many of the martyred monkeys' fellow primates when they were administered as oral vaccine hidden in bananas during the above-mentioned outbreak among the chimpanzees described by Lawick-Goodall.

Because many investigations have disclosed that, in one form or another, what happens to humans can happen to nonhuman primates as well—particularly when medical events are involved—many research centers scattered throughout the world utilize nonhuman primates for studies of "human" diseases (Fig. 2–1). Conducting experiments, testing medications, even artificially inducing diseases in these primates in order to study physiological mechanisms, the centers aim

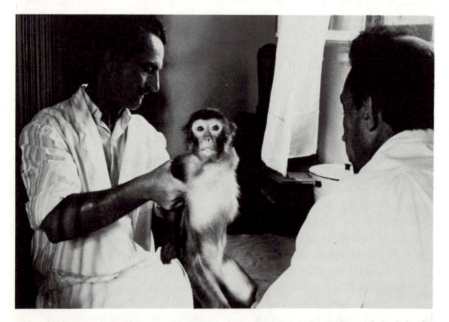

2–1   Laboratory animals are treated with care at all stages of experimental work in the Tirana Institute of Hygiene and Epidemiology. The results of research conducted in such scientific institutions often prove beneficial to both human and nonhuman primates. (Courtesy of World Health Organization. Photo by D. Henrioud.)

to eventually produce vaccines or cures that will be applicable to the whole order Primates.

Knowledge concerning the similarity of parasitic infestations and the physiological responses of the host is also important in establishing the ancestral relationship between any given groups of animals. Indeed, through studies of this nature, as well as recent investigations of serum proteins and hemoglobins that supplement research on primate cytogenetics, biochemical genetics, immunochemistry, and paleontology, Buettner-Janusch (1964) and Miller (1977) propose that material will emerge that will both implicitly and explicitly help bring about a revision and reorganization of the classification of the order Primates.

Hsiung, Black, and Henderson (1964), in an extensive survey of the susceptibility of primates to various viruses, offer many suggestive comparisons in animals' degrees of susceptibility or resistance to the diseases involved. They compared the effects of seventeen viruses on tissue cultures of kidneys from humans, chimpanzees, baboons, patas, capuchins and lemurs, as well as on those of four nonprimate mammals. It was found, as is shown in Fig. 2–2, that human and chimpanzee tissue cultures reacted with striking similarity to all but one of the same viruses. Reactions were alike when baboons were tested with most of these viruses but quantitative differences in susceptibility were noted for several of the diseases. Divergences were marked when the comparisons probed into the lower primates, and became radical when animals such as calves, pigs, dogs, rabbits, and chickens were included.

Other members of the order Primates—the green monkey, *Cercopithecus aethiops*, and another monkey, *Macaca irus*—were also susceptible to many of the same infections but only when much larger doses were administered. All nonhuman primates proved susceptible, for example, to polio virus, although at varying dosages, while all other mammals tested proved resistant to the oral administration of this virus. Similarly, measles viruses infected a wide variety of primates and dogs and some cattle, but could not survive in any of the other mammals tested; smallpox was implicated as an exclusively primate disease, infecting all the primates tested but no other animal except the embryos of chickens; yellow fever thrived in all tested primate cells but was only mildly infective for a few other mammals and then only when the inoculation doses were increased markedly.

Hsiung, Black, and Henderson (1964) point to a relationship

Host range	Virus strains	Primate tissue cultures						Non-primate tissue cultures					INFANT MICE
		MAN	RHESUS	BABOON	PATAS	CAPUCHIN	LEMUR	CALF	PIG	DOG	RABBIT	CHICKEN	
Broad	EEE (ARBO-)	■	■	▦	■	■	■	■	■	■	■	■	■
	HERPES SIMPLEX	■	■	■	■	■	■	■	■	■	■	■	■
	ECHO-IO (REO)	■	■	■	■	■	■	▦	■	■	■	□	▦
Intermediate	MEASLES	■	■	■	■		■	▦	□	■	□	□	□
	ECSO (DS$_3$)		■					□	■		□		□
	ECBO (MOLL)	■	■		■		■	■	■			■	□
	COXSACKIE B3	■	■	■	■	□	□	▦	■	□	□	□	■
	COXSACKIE A9	■	■	■	▦	□	□	□	□	□	□	□	□
Narrow	SV$_{40}$	▦	■	■	■	□	□	□	□	□	□	□	□
	SV$_{16}$	■	■	■	■	□		□	□	□	□	□	□
	SV$_6$	■	■	■	□	□	□	□	□	□	□	□	□
	POLIO − 1	■	■	■	■	▦	□	□	□	□	□	□	□
	ECHO − 7	■	■	■	■	□		□	□	□	□	□	□
	ECHO − 1	■	■	■	▦	□	□	□	□	□	□	□	□
	ECHO − 6	■	■	■	□	□	□	□	□	□	□	□	□
	ECHO − 11 (WB)	■	▦	■	□	□	□	□	□	□	□	□	□
	BRYANT	■	□	□	□	□	□	□	□	□	□	□	□

■ Virus causes cytopathic effect

▦ Irregular or partial cytopathic effect

□ No cytopathic effect

2–2 Susceptibility of primate and nonprimate kidney cell cultures to various viruses. (From Hsiung, Black, and Henderson [1964:18].)

between nonhuman primate susceptibility to the same viruses and similarity in chromosome count. They note that baboons, macaques, and mangabeys each possess forty-two chromosomes and have similar virus susceptibilities. Likewise, within the genus *Cercopithecus*, the monkeys with sixty chromosomes share similar susceptibilities, while the patas monkeys with chromosome counts of fifty-four demonstrate different patterns.

These investigators believe that much of the patterning of viral susceptibilities is determined by inherited cellular components that permit replication by the specific virus. They state (1964:16):

> Doubtless many factors determine the susceptibility of a host cell to a given virus. One of the factors in susceptibility to human enteroviruses has been described as a cell component which adsorbs virus and facilitates the removal of the virus protein coat. . . . This factor apparently must be present before infection of cells with certain viruses can occur.

Studies of this nature prove invaluable adjuncts to paleontological theories. A long and distant separation in evolutionary history, with concomitant differences in subsequent environments, is suggested by the variations found in these virus susceptibilities. The Old World primates and humans share susceptibility to the same viral infections, while the New World monkeys and the lemurs of Madagascar cannot be infected with many of these viruses. These relationships support the claim of a separation of these animals during the Eocene epoch, more than fifty million years ago, when Africa, South America, and Madagascar were splitting apart. Likewise, a longer-lasting relationship or more recent divergence is suggested by the shared susceptibilities among the anthropoid apes and *Homo sapiens*.

Because of this close relationship, the roster of diseases on which research is being conducted on nonhuman primates includes almost all of the infections that afflict human life. The knowledge that chimpanzees are susceptible to infections from the bacteria belonging to the family Spirochete, including *Treponema pallidum*, which causes venereal and endemic syphilis, and *Treponema pertenue*, responsible for yaws, has prompted the use of our next of kin in the study of these widespread diseases. Similarly, the promising development of vaccines for the prevention of human gonorrhea became possible only after extensive research utilizing the chimpanzee.

Simian primates also act as reservoirs for the spirochetes that cause recurrent fever in South America and, as such, have been suggested as the source of human infections. In this instance and in others to be discussed, the close evolutionary relationship between humans and other primates operates to disadvantage the humans involved. In Africa, as an additional example, relapsing fever is caused by a member of the same treponeme family and is thought to be maintained in reservoirs of simian primates. Indeed, Fiennes and Riopelle (1969) suggest that the simian primates are not only the carriers of the treponemal diseases but may have been responsible for their introduction into human communities as yaws in the Old World and as pinta in the New.

Fribourg-Blanc and Mollaret (1969) report a total of 2,272 nonhuman primates tested (including one gorilla from the Congo) in which 267 yielded tests positive for treponemal infections. In lymph glands obtained from baboons, patas monkeys, and chimpanzees, they found a strain with characteristics identical to those that cause syphilis and yaws in humans. They note that the distribution of human yaws coincides with their source of simian treponematosis. The method of contamination among nonhuman primates in nature is not known, nor is the means of spread to humans obvious; but it should be noted that the treponemas responsible for yaws are transmitted nonvenereally.

Some hepatitis antigens found in chimpanzees cannot be immunologically distinguished from the human prototypes. Consequently, the quest for an effective antiserum or vaccine involves extensive research using these relatives of man. On the negative side, monkeys and apes imported for other medical studies, particularly woolly monkeys from South America and chimpanzees from Africa, may contract hepatitis from their human captors in the countries of their origin, and then transfer it to their new handlers in their second homelands. Since the infected nonhuman primates are not patently sick, they present no warning symptoms to their human contacts. Consequently, in recent times, numerous cases of hepatitis have originated from unwary contact with newly imported animals. Within two years after the first reported epidemic of chimpanzee-associated hepatitis in the United States in 1963, the U.S. Communicable Disease Center in Atlanta (Mosley 1965) cited twenty-four cases of hepatitis among handlers, pathologists, veterinarians, and technicians. Investigations indicated that the only common factor among those afflicted was their contact with chimpanzees that had recently been imported but showed no overt symptoms of the disease.

RELATIONSHIP TO HUMAN HEALTH

Apparently nonhuman primates are so susceptible to tuberculosis that most research agencies routinely test every purchased animal before releasing it from quarantine. New World monkeys, while somewhat less susceptible than other primates, do contract tuberculosis in the abdomen, as distinct from Old World monkeys and other primates who are most frequently attacked in the lungs.

Viruses such as "Marburg virus" (see below) and herpes as well as bacterial diseases such as Shigella dysentery and the typhoid-like salmonella infections plague public health officials, veterinarians, and others whose work demands close contact with imported nonhuman primates. The animals can carry all of these diseases for considerable periods without showing any signs of illness. Although humans are phylogenetically very close to other primates, for millions of years they have been ecologically separated. Consequently, human bodies can host many of the pathogens tolerated by our simian cousins, but the separation has prevented or forfeited specific immunological adaptations. As a result, many diseases that are virtually asymptomatic in the free-living nonhuman primates may have devastating effects on humans, and conversely, certain diseases that humans tolerate with only mild reactions have proven fatal to other primates.

A notable example is found in the group of herpes viruses. When Herpes B virus, *Herpes virus simiae*, is present in Asian macaques or several species of monkeys from Africa, their hosts experience mild lesions around the lips and gums, similar to the innocuous "cold sores" caused by related viruses in humans. However, when the Herpes B virus is transmitted to humans, it acquires a deadly virulence, causing a lethal encephalomyelitis. Harrison (1971) records that of the eighteen persons known to have contracted the viral infection from afflicted monkeys, all but two died and only one of the survivors was able to resume a normal life. Another mysterious disease, one with hemorrhagic symptoms, involved the laboratory personnel handling blood and tissues from green monkeys imported into laboratories from Uganda. In West Germany and Yugoslavia, thirty cases, seven of them fatal, were reported in 1967. (The epidemic in the German city of Marburg caused the illness to be called "Marburg disease.") The causative agent has not been positively identified but investigations point to a rickettsia or an unknown virus.

USE OF NONHUMAN PRIMATES FOR HUMAN HEALTH

In spite of the potential risks, the use of nonhuman primates for scientific and medical research continues. Indeed, the demand for these animals has expanded to such an extent that colonies or farms for the planned breeding of nonhuman primates have been established. One of the reasons so many animals are disappearing from their native habitats is that hunters find it easier to capture the desired juvenile by shooting the mother, who is invariably nearby and protective of her young charge. As a result, for each young animal captured, two, including an adult female of reproductive capacity, are removed from their natural state.

Why do research centers continue to import nonhuman primates in spite of the dangers and the ecological disturbances? The answer is that nonhuman primates make the most nearly ideal human surrogates. It is always more difficult to extrapolate results of investigations conducted on animals such as rats, guinea pigs, and hamsters, which are much more phylogenetically distant from the *Homo sapiens* for whom the scientific studies are designed. In the Western world particularly, where arteriosclerosis, heart disease, and cancer dominate medical concerns, the ability to produce and experimentally treat these diseases in nonhuman primates makes them extremely desirable and the risk of handling potentially infected simians secondary.

An additional strong argument for the continued use of nonhuman primates centers on the similarity, particularly between chimpanzees and humans, which permits intrageneric organ transplants. As Goldsmith (1969) points out, the chimpanzee, contrary to prevalent prejudices, is physically and psychologically, as well as immunologically, similar to man. Traeger (1969) reports two kidney transplants from chimpanzees to two men aged thirty-seven and twenty-seven. The older man survived six days beyond the operation and the younger man lived, with a kidney taken from a chimpanzee, for forty-nine days, dying as a result of infections not directly associated with the transplant. Traeger also notes the successful use of chimpanzee kidneys by Reemstma in 1964 on a patient who lived a normal life for nine months after he was given a chimp kidney (cf. Reemstma, McCracken, and Schlegel 1964).

As of 1969, such kidney transplants had been performed with varying degrees of success in Italy, France, and the United States. Goldsmith (1969) argues for continued research on kidney transplants, his conviction being that they can function and provide adequate renal substitutes for human patients who otherwise would be doomed. He also urges "serious breeding programs" since inadequate organ supplies could be a limiting factor in the future, noting also that since only one kidney need be removed from an animal, it too can continue to live.

The space exploration programs of the United States and the U.S.S.R. have employed numerous chimpanzees and other non-human primates in research on many aspects of physiological toleration. Among the unsung heroes and heroines of these studies were twenty-one chimpanzees who served in research to determine the behavior of the body in vacuum conditions, undertaken at New Mexico Aeromedical Research Laboratory preparatory to sending the astronauts aloft. There appears to be widespread agreement among the people dedicated to space exploration that none of the completed programs would have succeeded if the research with non-human primates had not paved the way.

NONHUMAN PRIMATES FOR CARDIOVASCULAR RESEARCH

Research concerned with human arteriosclerosis uses chimpanzees as well as squirrel monkeys, baboons, and other simians because apparently these animals suffer from this in much the same way as humans do. Gresham and Howard (1969) report that baboons captured in Kenya, as well as vervets elsewhere in Africa, were found to have small atherosclerotic plaques, mainly on the aorta, rarely in the coronary arteries. Similarly, 75 percent of 163 free-living baboons that were captured, killed, and autopsied in Kenya were reported by Taylor, Ho, and Liu (1973) to possess arterial lesions. Chawla et al. (1967) studied 150 wild rhesus monkeys, 70 males and 80 females, all aged between one and ten years. They found that five of the monkeys had high blood pressure, five had coronary atherosclerosis, four had aortic fatty streaks, three had small coronary occlusions, and one had atherosclerotic plaques. Other Old World monkeys reveal these conditions very rarely; yet, through laboratory-controlled dietary programs, plaques can almost always be provoked in rhesus monkeys.

Malinow and Maruffo (1966) shattered earlier claims that New World monkeys were relatively free from arterial disease. Examinations of hundreds of howler monkeys captured in northern Argentina disclosed that many of them had naturally occurring atherosclerotic lesions. As is true for their human co-primates, the males of this group suffered the disease more than the females, with greater severity experienced as age increased. Duplicating the human experience, the females began to develop equally severe disease when they reached the ages of the older males.

These studies complicate the generally accepted, perhaps simplistic, origin explanations of atherosclerosis. Etiologies tied exclusively to modern diets, larded with cholesterol-rich, saturated animal fats, falter when the same conditions appear in howler monkeys, as well as other nonhuman primates, which, with rare exceptions, subsist on purely vegetarian diets. However, these findings do not rule out dietary components as important contributors to arterial disease; laboratory experiments demonstrate that, at least in captivity, diet can be a crucial factor.

When Armstrong, Connoe, and Warner (1967) fed rhesus monkeys food containing significant amounts of cholesterol (40 percent of the total calories derived from egg yolks), the animals developed severe atherosclerotic plaques along with high rates of serum cholesterol in less than two years. Various diets, all directed toward high cholesterol and atherogenic levels, have produced severe arterial lesions in rhesus, cebus, stumptail, macaque, and squirrel monkeys as well as baboons and chimpanzees tested in laboratories around the world.

Animals on the special diets were found to develop three times more pathological consequences, including fatty streaks on their aortas, than did their counterparts who were maintained on normal diets. Thus, scientific research makes clear that diet is a factor in the development of cardiovascular disease; but the free-living and control simians who also demonstrate evidence of the disease challenge the proposition that diet is the sole factor.

Inordinate stress, the seemingly unavoidable bugaboo of modern human existence, is also projected as a major antecedent of cardiovascular disease. Here, again, nonhuman primates contribute significantly to our knowledge. Many investigators have studied the relationship of stress and disease in nonhuman primates; they invariably have found significant levels of cardiovascular disease in the wake of such stress-inducing factors as fear, pain, and alienation. One example, among many, is found in the work of St. Clair et al. (1967). Examining thirty squirrel monkeys who had lived on cholesterol-free diets before and after their capture, they found a 67 percent increase in the average levels of serum cholesterol after presumably stressful capture and captivity.

The universal view that life as a zoo animal is stressful tends to be supported by physiological evidence. Stress as a product of zoo life seems particularly implicated in the high levels of arteriosclerosis found in nonhuman primates in zoos. Lindsey and Chaikoff (1966) autopsied sixty-seven primates representing seventeen species, all zoo residents at the time of their deaths. Aortic arteriosclerosis was found in two-thirds of these animals. Interestingly, most had no deposits in their coronary arteries. A similar investigation is reported by Stout and Lemmon (1969), who autopsied ninety-one nonhuman primate zoo inmates, representing thirty-two species. They found parallel results and added that the most severe cerebral disease was manifested in man's closest nonhuman kin, the chimpanzee.

The intimate association between perceived stress, cardiovascular disease, and advanced levels of primates is made more explicit in studies reported by Vastesaeger and Delcourt (1966). In examining the coronary trunks of 210 primates that died at the Antwerp Zoo, they found no coronary changes in the twelve prosimians, and only a slight alteration in one of the thirty-four Cebidae. On the other hand, among the Old World monkeys, there was a 47.5 percent rate of degenerative coronary change in the ninty-five specimens examined, and pathological changes zoomed to almost 96 percent of the sixty-nine specimens of apes studied. Singling out man's closest primate relative, Vastesaeger and Delcourt (ibid.:190) note:

> From the data gathered up until now, it appears that the
> plasma lipids of the chimpanzee are influenced more by
> stress than by the lipid components of their diet. . . .
> Our own experience on chimpanzees showed us that these
> animals very early become hypertensive, under the influence
> of various [kinds of] stress. Figures of 220/120
> [millimeters hemoglobin] . . . are often observed when the
> apes are irritated under various influences.

Deliberately induced stress, of an undisputed nature, was provoked in squirrel monkeys who were placed in restraining cages and taught to press keys to avoid electric shocks that followed warning signals. In addition to transitory blood pressure elevations, many of these monkeys developed high levels of serum cholesterol and increased rates of coronary atherosclerosis. Perhaps more surprising, some of them did not develop any of the expected cardiovascular changes. The legacy from these martyrs of medical research provides cause for reflection for their harried human beneficiaries. One definite by-product of studies of this nature has been a heightened awareness of the myriad stresses in human life and a conscious effort by many to recognize and mitigate or circumvent stressful situations or to train their bodies to relax more readily even under difficult conditions.

As research continues on human surrogates, the catalogue of factors that contribute to cardiovascular diseases also grows. There is little doubt that diet, heredity, age, sex, and physical activity (or its absence) are decisive elements. Nicotine from cigarette smoking and excess vitamin D have also joined the list of contributing agents. Stress is perhaps one of the most difficult factors to evaluate: a set of circumstances physiologically interpreted by some individuals as traumatic, with all the dire ramifications indicated above, may be tolerated by others with no untoward effects. As medical anthropologists investigate methods used by various societies to analyze and deal with stressful situations, the data they accumulate, coupled with some knowledge of the biological background of each population, could contribute significantly to the development of accurate evaluations of stress as a component of human health and disease.

One of the most promising developments resulting from expanded laboratory research is the discovery that atherosclerosis in monkeys is reversible. Armstrong and his co-workers (1967), working with rhesus monkeys, obtained an 80 percent reduction of diet-induced atherosclerotic narrowing of coronary arteries after shifting the subjects to low-fat, cholesterol-free diets for forty months. The close relationship between human and nonhuman primates suggested by all the foregoing studies indicates that there is substantial reason to extend hope for effective symptomatic treatment to the many human victims of this complex of diseases.

MALIGNANT DISEASES IN NONHUMAN PRIMATES

The disease or diseases grouped as cancers are of primary concern to humans living in technologically complex areas of the world. Cancer has been sardonically called a "luxury disease" because it is essentially a disease of advanced age: it is "available" primarily to people who have surmounted all the pathologies that in times past precluded the possibility of surviving to an age when cancer would be most likely to occur. Little evidence of cancers is found in the fossil record and, as noted, the prehistoric human who lived to middle age or beyond was a phenomenon. But in many modern societies where old age is a common expectation and where many environmental carcinogenic agents affect all ages, the threat of malignant diseases is terribly real.

As might be expected, in the field of cancer research, nonhuman primates are making a significant contribution. Naturally occurring spontaneous malignancies among captured animals are infrequent, although not unknown, partly because most captured primates are quite young. But it should be noted that, lacking the necessary statistical information, we know surprisingly little about the true life span of most nonhuman primates. Thus, when we speak of an "old" baboon or chimpanzee, we refer to an animal fifteen to twenty-five years of age, and we may be shortchanging him.

According to O'Conor (1969), as of 1969 approximately three hundred spontaneous tumors, less than one-third of them malignant, had been recorded in the world literature related to nonhuman primates. The malignancies, including leukemia and lymphomas, were distributed anatomically in seventeen organs of the body, suggesting that, as in humans, cancer can affect virtually every primate organ. Tumors in these primates have the same natural history and microscopic appearance as do human tumors, thus favoring these animals as subjects for studies on the effects of environmental factors, particularly in situations where known or suspected carcinogenic agents are being investigated. Studies to date have included investigations of the effects of many chemicals as well as naturally occurring substances, radiation, and specific viruses. Although much of the work is still in its early stages, there has emerged sufficient evidence of a possible early identification to persuade seven different countries to participate in a coordinated study to evaluate a serological test diagnostic of liver carcinoma.

Lapin (1969) reports that in several species of primates, leukemia is caused by a virus. The workers in his laboratory, in Sukhumi in the U.S.S.R., are trying to find out if some human leukemias may also be caused by a virus. Using blood drawn from human patients diagnosed as having leukemia, these researchers transmitted a disease resembling leukemia to several species of monkeys. Although at the time the report was published, they had not positively identified the causative agent, they found both C-types and herpes-like particles in the cells and blood of affected animals. This exciting work gives promise of unraveling the mode of transmission of this dreaded disease and eventually a means of bringing it under control.

CONCLUSION

Comprehensive studies of nonhuman primates have only begun to be included as an important part of anthropology. The primary intent has been to learn more about human behavior and physiology through comparative information gleaned from our fellow primates. In the process, fundamental information on the human evolutionary process has become available. The information concerned with medical problems and adaptations of nonhuman primates, on the other hand, has derived from basic medical research; and the beneficiaries of the scientific studies include the nonhuman estimates as well as their human kin. As interest expands and the many uses of both sources of knowledge receive their proper emphasis from students of the social sciences, this aspect of medical anthropology promises to be well worth the efforts involved in its study.

NUTRITION, ANTHROPOLOGY, AND HUMAN HEALTH

*If you are planning for a year ahead, sow rice;
for ten years, plant trees; for 100 years,
educate the people.*

—Chinese proverb

An anthropological examination of nutrition, reflecting the intimate bond between nutrition and health, must be one of the cornerstones of any consideration of human health and disease. Good nutrition makes possible the robustness of health, the realization of innate capabilities, and a joy of life. Good nutrition does not inevitably guarantee good health; poor nutrition, however, always produces poor health. A major portion of the health problems affecting human populations today and throughout human history can be traced to malnutrition.

Malnutrition is a broad term, encompassing overall food insufficiency, specific nutritional deficiencies, and their opposite, overconsumption. Unquestionably, the primary sources of poor nutrition are economic and environmental. But more often than is commonly acknowledged, the delicate balance between adequate and poor alimentation tilts toward the latter as a result of unfavorable traditional practices. Anthropological research can contribute significantly toward a solution of the overall problems through knowledge of the cultural roots of nutritional beliefs and customs. By pooling their scientific knowledge the disciplines of anthropology and nutrition can enlarge the possibility of resolving the nutrition dilemmas of many populations now doomed to a borderline existence.

THE NEED FOR ANTHROPOLOGICAL CONTRIBUTIONS

Attempts by health agencies to improve nutrition frequently end in frustration or rejection because of insufficient attention to or ignorance of the beliefs, traditions, and customs of the people concerned. An anthropological approach to nutrition embodies an appreciation of the profound relationship between eating practices and the fundamental physiological and psychological needs of a given society. The anthropologist has been trained to respect and sometimes to understand customs often seen as "strange" or deleterious by the untrained observer. Particularly, the anthropologist worthy of the name will strive to ensure that any attempted change in nutrition can function within the framework of the culture's core values.

FOOD BELIEFS AND CUSTOMS

Historically, only exceptional populations have not at some time had to face hunger. In more recent times, undernutrition or nutritional imbalances have been viewed primarily as direct results of poverty (Fig. 3–1). Anthropologists in the course of their field work become acutely aware of this reality. They learn that beliefs, prohibitions, and customs in these same societies not only prevent the use of valuable potential foods but also restrict the consumption of vital nutrients by certain members of the groups because of age or sex discriminations. And occasionally anthropologists have also found that, under certain circumstances, seemingly poor nutritional attitudes can have unexpectedly beneficial aspects.

A further attribute of social attitudes toward food is elaborated in a statement of the Committee on Food Habits of the National Research Council (1945).

> [One] aspect of the way in which edible materials are classified [is] as inedible, edible by animals, edible by human beings, but not my kind of human being, edible by human beings such as self and finally edible by self. These classifications are further reinforced by various sorts of attitudes—that materials which are not eaten are defiling, wicked to eat, coarsening, would alter one's status, etc.

While not defining attitudes toward specific foods, Lee (1968:35) notes that among the !Kung Bushmen of Africa's Kalahari Desert about 90 percent of the vegetable diet is drawn from only 23 species, although some 85 edible species are available in the natural environ-

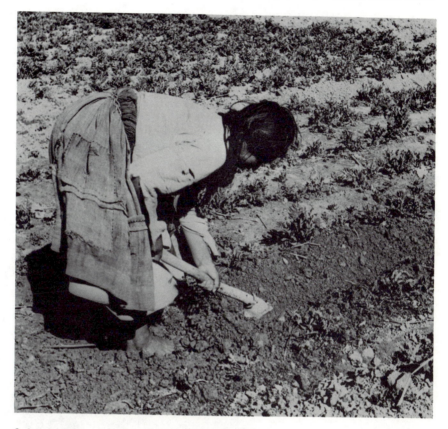

3–1   A woman scratches a meagre existence from the poor soil on a high plateau in Bolivia. Deficiencies in the soil, unremedied by adequate fertilization, lead to some of the nutritional deficiency diseases. In this particular region there is insufficient zinc and iodine. (Courtesy of World Health Organization. Photo by BIT/OMS.)

ment. Further, he records, "Of the 223 local species of animals known and named by the Bushmen, 54 species are classified as edible and of these only 17 species are hunted on a regular basis."

Examples exist at every turn. One of the most familiar is the sacred, woebegone cattle that wander unmolested for most of their lives through areas of India where people perish for lack of food. Similarly, in the United States during World War II, meat supplies were severely rationed while edible horsemeat continued to be used for nonnutritive purposes, except by occasional defiant or hungry individuals, because the society's mores ruled it unacceptable as human food. In recent years, when publicity was given to the surreptitious consumption by many of America's urban poor of products labeled "cat" or "dog" food, the public outcry greatly exceeded that given former disclosures of widespread, albeit genteel, hunger.

Conversely, societies invariably extol some particular staple as a "superfood" without which life is incomplete. Rice fits readily into this category throughout the Orient; yams or cassava (manioc) in parts of South America and Africa (Fig. 3–2); taro in the Pacific Island; wheat throughout much of Europe; and perhaps the myriad forms of "junk food" rampant in the United States.

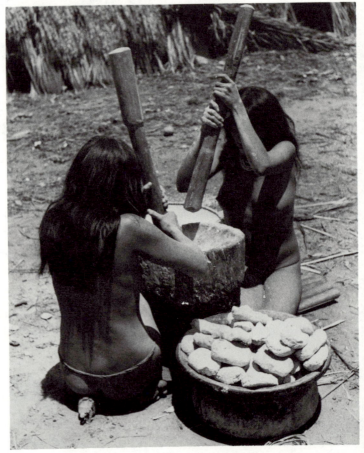

3–2 The preparation of basic foods in many parts of the world often requires intense, time-consuming energy. Here two young women of Upper Zingu in northeastern Mato Grasso, Brazil, pound manioc (cassava) in a wooden mortar. After this processing, the manioc will be pressed through a sieve before being used as flour for bread. (Courtesy of World Health Organization. Photo by Paul Lambert.)

THE LEARNING PROCESS

Through the training of the children, not only all humans but apparently all other primates as well pass on strong convictions of what is proper food and what is not. And a specific food like milk for children is no more highly prized in the United States than grasshoppers or grubs may be in other parts of the world. The lessons learned as part of daily interactions throughout childhood form rigid beliefs and patterns that tend to endure through a lifetime and indeed form a most persistent link between the generations. George Orwell once wrote, "I think it could be plausibly argued that changes of diet are more important than changes of dynasty or even of religion." A thorough appreciation of the potency of nutrition habits, therefore, is a vital prerequisite for a scientific approach to the problems of nutrition and disease anywhere in the world.

To the extent that the environment is able to accommodate more than mere subsistence, eating becomes largely culturally determined. In addition to gustatory pleasure, eating evokes powerful associations of mother-child relationships and often provides group interactions that satisfy deep psychological primate needs. The patterns and beliefs established in early childhood and reinforced every day of life understandably cling tenaciously. Invariably, they are one of the last aspects of life to change, long after clothing, language, economy, and religion have yielded to the pressures of cultural change.

Not only is food itself rigidly tied to the culture; even the question of who eats with whom is often adamantly unyielding to change. In many parts of the world, eating is as private as sexual activity. Throughout much of Melanesia, Polynesia, and parts of Arabia, custom decrees that males and females must never see one another eat. Apparently the patriarchs of the Old Testament followed the same rule. Even unseen presences may constitute a menace to the vulnerable eater. Lowenberg et al. (1974) speculate that the custom of covering one's mouth while chewing derives from the fear in many societies that the open mouth, filled with food, invites entry by one of the evil spirits believed to fill the atmosphere.

EFFECTS OF CONTACT SITUATIONS ON DIET

Although technologically advanced societies can offer an abundance of scientific nutritional knowledge, the sad facts are that when tribal peoples come into contact with industrialized societies and subsequent urbanization, their diets, far from improving, almost invariably deteriorate disastrously (cf. Malcolm 1954; Neubarth 1954). In these situations the old axiom that foods are more important as symbols of status than as carriers of nutrients is proven with tragic consequences.

Bailey (1975:359) notes the changing prestige values of foods accompanying rapid urbanization in Africa:

> The prestige attached to various foods is of very great importance; bread, rice, sugar, canned foods, and soft drinks are generally high-prestige foods. Traditional foods, even the nutritious ones (e.g., green leaves and various insects and other animal foods), tend to have lower prestige and to drop out of the regular diet, especially in urban areas.

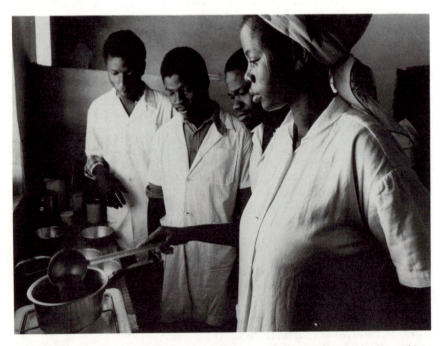

3-3 Utilization of indigeous foods that are rich in nutrients yet ignored by the resident population can often boost the quality of nourishment available. Here nutritionist Georgette Kaboré shows nurses and health workers in a Ouagadougou dispensary in Upper Volta how to prepare protein-rich mixtures from local foods. (Courtesy of World Health Organization. Photo by E. Mandelmann.)

The high status accorded sugar-laden beverages, overrefined white-flour products, and, even more calamitous, the artificial feeding of infants wreaks nutritional havoc wherever tribal peoples are caught up in rapid urbanization. The cultural shock involved in contact situations even without urbanization can be devastating to a balance achieved through centuries of adaptation to a specific environment.

Frequently the contact situation leads to the introduction of a cash crop, heavy tax burdens, and other associated forms of exploitation. This has been the unhappy course of events throughout Africa, India, and much of the New World since the earliest days of exploration and colonization. Disrupted economies and the attendant cultural chaos can be blamed for much of the starvation and malnutrition rampant in these areas in the past as well as today.

Governmental intervention at early stages of urbanization can avoid and even reverse many of the nutritional disasters of the past. Carefully planned publicity extolling the valuable aspects of "native" food of high quality and of the irreplaceable benefits of breast feeding can be critically decisive because it cannot only save countless lives but also ameliorate the trauma of cultural change (Fig. 3–3).

THE PERSISTENCE OF CULTURALLY DERIVED ATTITUDES

Food agencies now considering heroic measures to provide synthetically prepared protein foods for populations experiencing chronic protein deficiencies must expend equal efforts to provide flavors and substances familiar or agreeable to the people for whom the new supplements are destined. The history of food relief bears testimony to the futility of the best intentions that ignore cultural reality. A well-known example occurred in Europe after World War I when corn (maize), a low-status food that many Europeans regarded as fit only for animals, was bestowed upon the starving citizenry. Women did not know, or care to know, how to prepare it. Tragically, the well-intended aid was wasted; hunger and suffering continued unabated because preliminary educational steps had been inadequate.

Lack of attention to seemingly trivial preferences has led to similar rejections of potentially promising aid in more recent times. Amid great accolades, a long-sought new corn, a hybrid variety containing protein of greatly improved nutritive value, was introduced into Latin America in the 1950s. This revolutionary genetic achievement, called Opaque-2 corn, meets 90 percent of a child's daily protein requirement in only 250 grams (about 1.1 cup)—enough to prevent severe protein deficiency in a young child. At the end of a five-year trial period, many farmers refuse to plant the new crop: the texture and flavor of the meal had been rejected by the women. Additional research has resulted in a more acceptable product.

Color alone can determine food choice. For instance, wheat was avoided in many areas of India because its color differed from that of the familiar white rice. And in the United States during World War II, despite strong urging from health and government agencies for households to adopt a new, more nutritious and economical wheat flour, the gray color of the resultant bread made the flour generally unacceptable.

The maze of what, when, and with whom food is eaten is recognized in a statement by the Food and Agriculture Organization (1967):

> What people are willing to eat is determined by a complex
> series of attitudes, ideas and assumptions that form the local
> cultural patterns. They include religious restrictions, taboos,
> ideas pertaining to the merits or demerits of a food and other
> attitudes which are as yet little understood.

Studies utilizing all the expertise and techniques of the social sciences are critical foundations upon which successful nutrition programs must be based. One of the fundamental pillars is a knowledge of the cognitive values held by the members of the involved population.

Each of the leading religions in the world today has prohibited or restricted some food at some time in its history. Anthropological studies of lesser-known religions suggest that they are similarly inclined to circumscribe the diets of their adherents. Significantly, for all religions, the restricted foods are most frequently animal protein.

Among certain groups of Hindus and Buddhists no meat of any kind is permitted; for most Hindus, beef is prohibited. Jews and Muslims are forbidden to consume any product of the pig. Lowenberg et al. (1974) point out that if followers of the Eastern Orthodox Church abide by all the bans against the consumption of meat, fish, and dairy products on certain days, about 38 percent of every year finds these foods absent from the daily diet.

The origins of these religious proscriptions are lost in their very antiquity. Most likely, the explanations offered by religious leaders today are superimposed upon customs much older, with roots in an environment that no longer exists. As de Castro (1952:147) observes in regard to meat:

> These religious prohibitions, of course, simply work a magical sublimation of a hard economic and geographic reality: the scarcity of meat in the region. As a population outgrew the supply of animal products, the religious code sought to relax the tension by setting limits to the consumption of meat—a good example of the hidden connections between the economic and religious life of a people.

Food taboos have not remained the property of religious dogma. Even Homer recorded that all milk should be scorned as a repulsive substance. No population is known that accepts every possible nutriment in its environment as fitting food. And in some societies, the impact of food taboos on nutrition in incalculable. As de Garine (1974) points out, most of the interdicts apply to food of animal origin. In fact, of the 800 interdicts listed by one scholar for West Africa alone, 740 are in that category.

TRADITIONAL EXPLANATIONS OF FOOD TABOOS

When the religious aura is not present, people feel compelled to offer reasons for their proscriptions. Thus, in the Bolivian Highlands it is commonly believed that a child who is permitted to eat animal blood will not learn to speak. In West Pakistan, buffalo milk is thought to make a person physically strong but mentally dull; while lentils, another good protein source, if eaten for forty days will supposedly cause blindness.

Rappaport (1967:79) suggests that in New Guinea the Tsembaga's ban of many kinds of marsupials, snails, catfish, eels, lizards, and frogs in the diet of magic men and warriors is tied to the "cold" label applied to these foods, which would be inimical to the "hotness" of ritual knowledge and ritual experience. Young Tsembaga females who have not yet borne children avoid two of the most common sources of protein consumed by other members of their society: wild pigs and rats. Their culture leads them to believe that the former may result in lice, and the latter will impart a bad odor to the vagina, thus making them less attractive to males. De Garine (1974) reports that in Polynesia in former times all species of fish that were offered to the gods, as well as all meat except poultry, were forbidden to women.

Eggs are blamed for mental retardation in parts of East Africa and for late speech development in Korea. In a number of African countries, eggs are not fed to girls because of fears ranging from infertility to increased fertility and licentiousness. In Bolivia, many people believe that cheese will make a small child mute. In Malawi, fish and chicken are deemed to cause sterility. In East Africa, the nursing mother who eats mutton allegedly harms her baby's vision.

Among the Namoo of Ghana the first-born son may not eat the domestic hen as long as his father is alive. In the traditional Moorish culture, Marabouts and warriors refused to eat hare for fear of incorporating its allegedly cowardly nature. Mutton, pork, and eggs traditionally are shunned by Baganda women in Uganda. The rationale for the rejection of these valuable protein foods is lost in time. However, the reasoning given by the Douala of Cameroon for similar prohibitions may be suggestive: a pregnant woman may not eat bruised bananas lest her child be born with patches of eczema, nor beef lest her child, like the ox, dribble excessively.

SPECIAL FOOD TABOOS DURING PREGNANCY

In many areas of the world there is a widely held belief that an animal's traits, particularly its undesirable ones, are transferred to the child if the pregnant or nursing mother consumes that animal's flesh. One wonders, in confronting so many deleterious beliefs, if desirable traits, such as the strength of the ox, would have been stressed where and when supplies were abundant.

A study of impoverished pregnant women in South Carolina disclosed that nearly half of them held deleterious food beliefs. Included were the convictions that milk drunk during pregnancy causes cancer, pork rots the uterus, eggs harm the baby's brain, fish is poisonous, leafy vegetables mark the child, and cheese causes the head of the fetus to stick to the wall of the uterus, thus preventing a normal delivery.

In many areas where fish is avoided by pregnant and nursing women for fear of poisoning the offspring or causing its skin to become scaly, the same fish are thought to benefit the brains of other members of the society. Many Indian women fear that eggs (and also papaya) lead to miscarriage. The pregnant women say, "There is already an egg in the womb"—and another potential source of good protein is abandoned. Some societies rationalize that avoidance of animal products helps keep the fetus small, thereby making delivery easier. In China, as far back as the Chou dynasty (1122 to 255 B.C.), "pregnant women were warned to be careful of their meat intake. Goat meat would produce a sickly child and turtle meat a shortnecked offspring, while donkey meat would lead to a lengthy pregnancy and difficult labor" (Seifrit 1961:455).

It is perhaps not coincidental that so many of the scientifically erroneous folk beliefs focus on animal protein foods. These are also foods widely associated with totemic images as well as with feasts and ritual occasions. Such taboos, adhered to rigorously, appear to be particularly maladaptive where they are imposed upon women during pregnancy or lactation, the times of particular nutritional stress and need. A cross-cultural inventory of folk beliefs related to food would help clarify some of these questions.

POSSIBILITIES FOR CHANGE IN FOOD BELIEFS

The historical record reveals that many deleterious food beliefs have yielded to change. At one time it was commonly believed through much of Europe that potatoes caused leprosy and fevers. The Presbyterian clergy in Scotland opposed the use of potatoes for food because it could find no mention of them in the Bible. At one time or another, oysters, cucumbers, carrots, pumpkins, apples, peaches, oranges, and lemons have been considered health hazards.

Tomatoes received special attention, and censure, when introduced into Europe from the New World in the sixteenth century, and later when reintroduced in the New World to the European colonists. The French called the tomato *pomme d'amour*, "apple of love," and deemed it a powerful aphrodisiac, while the Germans and English, frightened by its relationship to the same family as the deadly nightshade, pronounced the tomato poisonous. It was shunned by American colonists until, in a heroic public demonstration in 1820 on the courthouse steps in Salem, New Jersey, one Robert G. Johnson publicly consumed a whole tomato before an awestruck crowd of spectators. His unexpected survival did much to shake the near-universal fear of this excellent source of vitamins A and C and other nutrients (Sebrell et al. 1967:149).

A critical factor to be reckoned with in nutrition considerations is the priority list of food allocations when resources are limited. In virtually every society for which information is available, adult males rank first. At the bottom of the list is found the toddler-weanling, with women and older children somewhere in between.

SEVERE OVERALL DEFICIENCIES AND CHILDHOOD DISEASES

Estimates derived from the Food and Agriculture Organization of the United Nations indicate that approximately one half of all children in developing countries suffer in some degree from inadequate nutrition. Closely associated with nutritional inadequacies are the appalling rates of child mortality in much of the world, primarily because the childhood diseases and minor parasitic infestations that are experienced as unpleasant discomforts by healthy, well-nourished children become killers when the malnourished child is affected (Fig. 3–4).

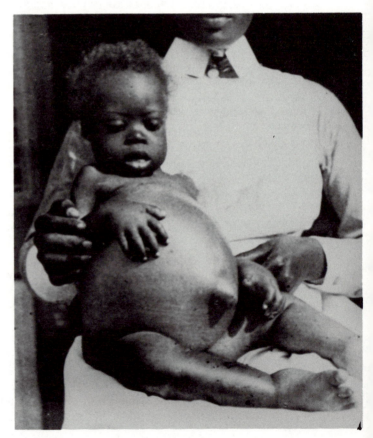

3–4 This African child shows the extremities of swelling and debilitation accompanying severe multiple-worm infestation. In infections of this magnitude, many of the nutrients given to the child are appropriated by the worms, such as hookworms, ascarids, and trichinas, leaving the child undernourished and with acute electrolyte imbalances. (Courtesy of Wellcome Museum of Medical Science, London.)

Berg and Muscat (1973) report that respiratory and gastrointestinal diseases in Nicaragua are responsible for 15 percent of all deaths as compared to 0.4 percent in North America. Schaefer (1966) reports that measles, an especially virulent killer when accompanied by malnutrition, was 325 times more devastating in Guatemala than in the United States or most of Europe. Lowenberg et al. (1974) note that in 1956, in Mexico City, for children without evidence of undernutrition, the fatality rate from infant diarrhea was 14-15 percent while among severely undernourished children the rate reached 52 percent.

MARASMUS, A CHRONIC, EXTREME DEFICIENCY DISEASE

When a daily diet is chronically deficient in both calories and protein, there ensues a syndrome called marasmus, from the Greek word meaning "to waste away." This condition is characterized by gross weight loss, wasting of subcutaneous fat and muscle, diarrhea, severe anemia, jaundice, stupor, and, unless adequate treatment intervenes, death (Fig. 3–5). It responds readily to milk, except in advanced stages, when the electrolyte balance of the body is so disrupted that sudden death often follows initial feeding attempts unless potassium imbalance is first corrected. Apparently adults who are near death from starvation can recover under proper care with little or no permanent damage. But when infants or young children are thus afflicted, permanent loss of growth and learning capacity can be expected (Fig. 3–6).

Schaefer (1966:1092) projects a "permanent mental retardation from 10 to 25 percent below the expected norm." Recent studies indicate that the brain and its associated parts reach 80 percent of their lifelong development before the age of four, thus making the nourishment of the infant and toddler particularly critical in determining the caliber and quality of life for years to come (cf. Ramalingaswami 1975). R. A. Hingson (in Lowenberg et al. 1974:283) poignantly reports:

> I have seen little ones with the tell-tale signs of malnutrition, the distended stomach, sit for hours, as in a stupor, not romping or playing as normal youngsters. And they are marked for life by this lack if they survive disease to which they are prey. They will be as their elders, apathetic, dull and [with] no desire or capacity to work together to improve their lot. Persistent undernutrition indeed leaves its ugly mark, not only in the body, but on the mind and the personality.

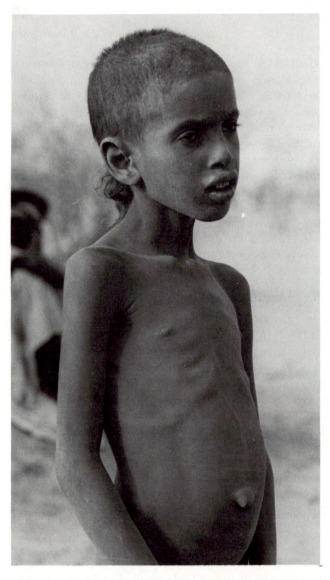

3-5   A victim of the five-year drought that plagued six countries (Mauritania, Mali, Senegal, Upper Volta, Niger, and Chad) in the Sahelian Zone along the southern edge of the Sahara and affected an estimated ten million people, or a third of the area's population. The appalling effect of hunger and malnutrition is evident in the face and body of this nomad child in northern Upper Volta in 1973. His family came from Mali in search of food and water for themselves and their cattle—and found only a wasteland. (Courtesy of Food and Agriculture Organization. Photo by F. Botts.)

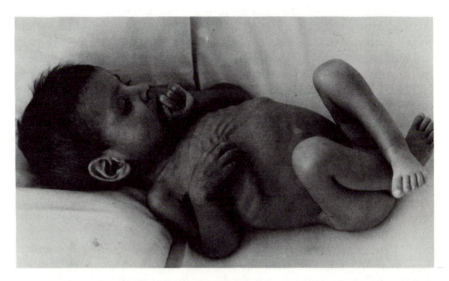

3-6 A young child wasting away from marasmus (severe calorie and protein deficiencies) during the critical period of brain development. The loss of potential brain growth is probably permanent although some research indicates that remedial nourishment and environmental stimulation may repair a portion of the damage done. (Courtesy of World Health Organization. Photo by A. Isaza.)

A National Research Council position paper on nutrition and brain development (Mayer 1973:2, 5) states:

> Malnutrition, reflected in chronic limitation of amounts of food consumed, may result in general stunting of growth accompanied by reduced brain size, decreased brain cell number, and immature or incomplete biochemical organization of the brain....
> ... There are now ample data demonstrating that severe general malnutrition during early postnatal life will affect brain structure and disrupt normal chemical development. Numerous biochemical features have been found to be reduced or altered by early malnutrition. This has been shown by measurements of RNA, DNA, proteins, glycosides, lipids, activity of a variety of enzymes, and neurotransmitters.

The chief factor stressed is that brain growth rate is greatest *in utero*, particularly in the third trimester, and in the first six months of infancy.

The number of children suffering from marasmus is not known. Its incidence is rising most strikingly in areas where traditional cultural patterns are in the process of changing as a result of rapid urbanization. Particularly where breast feeding has been abandoned or drastically reduced in favor of the seemingly more sophisticated artificial bottle feeding, marasmus and other pediatric disasters multiply with calamitous impact.

In addition, where traditional tribal customs of polygamy are being replaced by monogamous relationships, the spacing periods between pregnancies are decreasing and children are being deprived of the traditional long period of nursing. It is this critical time, when the child is no longer given breast milk but is shifted to a nutritionally haphazard diet, that constitutes the danger zone throughout the areas of the world where urbanization pressures are severely disrupting cultural patterns.

Urbanization frequently offers women increased employment opportunities coupled with the need for extra cash income. Unfortunately, job opportunities are rarely accompanied by adequate provisions for child care either by industry or by government. An additional impediment thus is erected to prevent extended breast feeding, and in the process, inadequate and frequently contaminated artificial substitutes are introduced.

Consequently, not only is the nutrition for the infant or growing child insufficient, but his or her body is further burdened by gastrointestinal tract infections, most commonly manifested as infant diarrhea, of which there is a tremendously higher incidence than in the past. Added to the twin problems of poor nourishment and hazardous substitutes for breast milk is the frequent culturally dictated reliance on near-starvation therapy precisely at a time when survival hinges on the maintenance of proper hydration and electrolyte balance (cf. Lozoff, Ramath, and Feldman 1975).

Anthropological research discloses that the mothers of these seriously ill children often do not heed medically crucial advice. A revealing study (ibid.) of beliefs about illness in southern India notes that modern medical practice invariably recommends clear liquids with some source of carbohydrate and salt in order to treat the most common serious complication associated with infant diarrhea: excessive fluid and electrolyte losses. Unfortunately, this Western prescription of "sugar water" conflicts sharply with native concepts.

In southern India, as in many other parts of the world, intrinsic qualities of "hot" and "cold" are incorporated in disease-causation beliefs. The symptoms of infant diarrhea, commonly associated with marasmus and lesser dietary disturbances, are attributed to an excess of "heat in the body." Therefore, logic dictates treatment with "cold" medicines in order to restore the disturbed balance to normal. The sugar water prescribed is considered to be intrinsically "hot." Consequently, it is deemed completely inappropriate by the mothers, and the life-saving liquid may be withheld. When medical personnel become familiar with these native beliefs, they are able to adjust the medication within the framework of acceptable cultural beliefs. Fortunately, honey, which is equally effective as treatment, is deemed "cold" in both Bengal and Tamil Nadu, and therefore is much more likely to be used by the native mother. This is another example of how ignorance of native beliefs can negate the best-intentioned nutritional and medical intervention, whereas anthropological knowledge and respect for cultural differences can become life-saving.

KWASHIORKOR, THE "SECOND-CHILD DISEASE"

Marasmus is apt to occur under conditions of extreme social disruption: profound cultural change, famine, drought, war, or epidemics. On the other hand, it is appallingly common that the deficiency disease kwashiorkor, a Ghanaian word meaning "second-child disease," is found primarily in children who consume insufficient protein for their growth and maintenance needs. This happens particularly to children who have been weaned, generally because another child has arrived or is on the way (which is why some Ghanaian mothers believe the disease is caused by jealousy). The weanling is then shifted to a diet considered appropriate in his culture. Distressingly often, this is a starchy pap based on yams, taro, corn, rice, barley gruel, or any one of the culturally designated diets in which calorie intake is sufficient to satisfy hunger but insufficient to meet the critical protein requirements demanded by the growth phase of the child.

The afflicted child develops the condition that has become familiar to the Western world through the years as a result of pictures such as Fig. 3–7, in which the painfully distended belly, sticklike arms, water-swollen legs, and sorrowful gaze dominate. There is frequently a generalized edema, with water constituting 85 percent of the body's weight rather than the normal 60-65 percent. The skin may develop a "flaky paint" appearance. The hair may become dyspigmented, black hair turning various shades of red or blonde; the

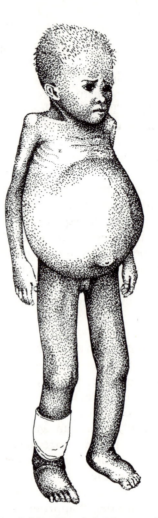

3–7 This young boy, with his painfully distended abdomen, stick-like arms, water-swollen legs, depigmented and patchy hair, and sorrowful gaze, exhibits many of the symptoms of chronic protein deficiency—kwashiorkor. (Adapted from *Time*, November 11, 1974.)

texture may change from thick and curly to lank and so thin that the hair can be plucked out in batches without noticeable discomfort to the child.

Typically, anemia and fatty, enlarged liver are part of the total syndrome, accompanied by distinctive behavior changes, with the victim variously described as "petulant," "apathetic," and "withdrawn"—"a thoroughly wretched child." Evidence is accumulating that the protein starvation responsible for kwashiorkor, like marasmus, prevents complete normal development of the child who is characteristically stricken at a critical time of growth.

The kwashiorkor syndrome was first described in 1906 after studies performed on children in Mexico. By 1918, similar reports began to appear from far-flung areas of the world: first Africa, then Japan in 1923, and France in 1927. In a 1933 article, Dr. Cicely Williams (1933) described a children's disease that she had treated in Ghana (then known as the Gold Coast) and that she associated with a maize diet. In a follow-up article in 1935 she introduced the word "kwashiorkor" (the Ga tribe's name for the disease) into the medical literature (Williams 1935). During the next decades many cases were recognized in Central and South America, the Caribbean, Hungary, Greece, India, and Fiji, and among American Indians in the western United States. In 1964 an International Conference on the Prevention of Malnutrition in the Preschool Child, held in the United States, issued the following statement:

> Malnutrition in the preschool child is one of the world's
> most serious health problems in developing areas. Not
> only is it killing and maiming the children today, but also,
> through physiological, mental and emotional damage, it will
> handicap the society of 1984 and the next generation.

Although anthropologists are generally powerless to relieve the basic poverty that often underlies poor nutrition, a well-founded anthropological understanding of the food habits and beliefs of malnourished people could contribute significantly to attempts to ameliorate those cultural aspects that prevent relief. Under proper circumstances, physiologically erroneous beliefs often will be found to stem from mistaken concepts that will yield to reinterpretation of traditional ideas.

The choice of an inadequate food comes at a particularly traumatic period in the young child's life. This is the time when he loses the constant nurturing that had been his daily expectation prior to the shock of weaning. Frequently this process is interpreted in his immature mind as rejection, particularly under conditions of poverty where the poorly nourished mother is physiologically drained by the recent pregnancy and the nursing needs of a new baby. The denial of the nourishment and comfort of the breast may be abrupt and not only may the substituted food be nutritionally inadequate, but the emotional disturbance experienced by the child may interfere with his appetite, thus further reducing his intake.

It is difficult to determine in all cases why, even when protein foods such as fish and eggs are available, they are denied to the newly weaned child. On this question, cognitive data and anthropological research could help supply answers. Generally, the withheld protein foods are seen as potentially harmful to the young: some undesirable characteristic will be transmitted. The fear of eggs leading to licentious behavior in young girls has already been cited; in Sierra Leone, eggs are not given to children below the age of five because they are thought to cause them to steal; in Rhodesia, it is believed that eggs given to young boys will cause eventual baldness and sterility. In other areas, fish is thought to produce worms or scaly skin in young children, while meat could make them greedy.

There are kwashiorkor victims in societies in which milk, one of the most complete foods, is considered disgusting because it is seen as an animal's body secretion. Among several pastoral peoples of Africa, milk supplies are drastically reduced because social rules dictate that only milk from cows belonging to the mother's family may be consumed by the mother and her children. In African cultures where marriage is patrilocal, this restriction may preclude the possibility of the mother and her growing children consuming any milk unless they are fortunate enough to have received cows from the maternal family in the marriage settlement.

Occasionally a culturally prohibited, but nutritionally valuable food can be successfully introduced in unfamiliar form. For example, in one region in Africa where women and children were deprived of milk because of lineal restrictions, powdered milk—called "powder" rather than "milk"—was deemed permissible. The acceptance of this valuable source of protein was realizable in large part because of the name difference. However, the nutritionists judiciously taught the mothers to add the dry powder to other foods rather than to reconstitute it for consumption in liquid form. As a result, diets of mothers and children improved significantly, additional sources of contamination were minimized, and important cultural foundations remained intact.

In a valuable study of the root crop-dependent Tsembaga of New Guinea, Rappaport (1967:76) points out that the protein intake of adults is adequate simply because they are able to consume large enough quantities of their protein-poor staples to meet their needs. On the other hand, mere size limits the amount their children are able to ingest. Nutritionists generally agree that while the calorie requirement of a young child may be fulfilled by two pounds of tubers, a child would have to eat two to four times that amount to meet the suggested protein allowances.

Noting that the poorest protein diet is furnished by the starchy roots of the cassava and the yam, Lowenberg et al. (1974:335) raise the question of how or why the peoples of coastal West Africa came to depend upon, and to value so highly, these roots that fill but do not nourish. "In former days," they wonder, "did the well-buried roots represent a sure supply of calories when a plague of insects ate all parts of the plants which were above ground?" Historical reconstruction and intensive examination of the legends and mythology of these people might well supply vital information on this point, perhaps disclosing the real basis for the strength of the unfortunate choice and conceivably, in the process, weakening its image as a "superfood."

A similar case in point is found in an examination of the dietary practices of the Masai and the Kikuyu of East Africa. Although these two peoples live in close association, their nutritional histories stand in sharp contrast. The Masai with their dietary reliance on milk, blood, and meat are reported to experience no kwashiorkor among the children. On the other hand, the Kikuyu and their neighbors, the Mbutu, disdain milk and view meat as a gross product, unfit for female and juvenile consumption. As might be anticipated, these people suffer profoundly from protein deficiency, and kwashiorkor-afflicted children are all too common.

It bears repeating at this point that throughout the world and through most of human history, food has been viewed as a means not only of satisfying hunger, but often of obtaining pleasure and of fulfilling ritual functions. Only in recent times has the concept of nutrient requirements begun to gain ground, and that only in extremely circumscribed segments of some populations. For example, Christine Wilson (personal communication) reports that physiological functions are associated with certain foods among the people she investigated in Malaysia. However, it should not be surprising that the association between diet and the manifold symptoms of kwashiorkor is seldom made in the many unschooled sectors of the world where this profound disturbance occurs.

Although the identification of kwashiorkor as a syndrome of protein deficiency has been completely established only in recent years, the symptoms have been part of folk culture in many parts of the world where this condition prevails. From nutrition workers in Africa have come reports of "shame" cast upon village mothers when a child begins to show the tell-tale hair discoloration. Neighborhood gossip is quick to suggest that the child is stigmatized because the parents violated a powerful taboo, particularly some prohibition concerned with postpartum sexual activity. Cases are cited of mothers treating the child's hair with native vegetable dyes to avoid community censure for the devastating changes that appear so mysteriously in the child who only recently thrived at the breast.

Cures for kwashiorkor are dramatic and reliable; quite often the addition of only small quantities of milk over a period of time can reverse the disaster course (Fig. 3–8). But, as in all disease situations, many contradictory factors are in simultaneous interaction. The

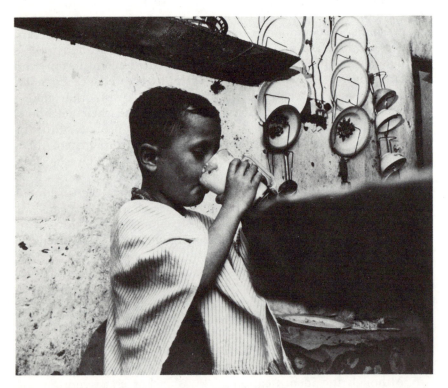

3–8 This Colombian child is drinking a milk mixture that has been provided as part of a supplementary feeding program for mothers and preschool children by the World Food Program. With more than a quarter of the world's population suffering from malnutrition, programs of this type can often mean the difference between life and death. (Courtesy of World Health Organization.)

mother feeding her weanling the protein-deficient pap is doing so because she was schooled by her culture to believe that this is the only appropriate food for her child. In her mind, the addition of potentially dangerous fish or meat to the diet of the child already in serious trouble would not only endanger her child's future well-being but would also add fuel to the smoldering gossip.

The number of children suffering from kwashiorkor is not known, but the present estimated rate of one hundred untreated children for every disclosed and treated child hints at the magnitude of the problem.* At the same time, the permanent damage that results from lack of treatment makes the presence of kwashiorkor in any of today's children an injury to all and a threat to future generations.

Modern science has devised many forms of protein supplementation that can cure or, better, prevent kwashiorkor at comparatively little cost to the governments that must supply them for their people. In addition to the economic and social obstacles that must be overcome, however, experience dictates a judicious approach to the introduction of these nutrients. Any head-on collision between modern scientific knowledge and strongly held cultural values is inevitably self-defeating; the children can be saved to the extent that the mothers can be won over to new ways within the framework of their own cultures.

VITAMIN AND MINERAL DEFICIENCIES

In addition to water and oxygen at least forty-five, and possibly fifty, chemical components are believed to be absolute requirements for human cells to function normally (see Scrimshaw and Young 1976). The conditions considered thus far represent gross undernutrition, combinations of insufficient calories and/or protein deficiencies. These, of course, are usually accompanied by inadequate vitamin and mineral stores. In the cases of marasmus and kwashiorkor,

*Food agencies need an accurate assessment of the nutrition status for many areas in the world, particularly where ages are neither recorded nor attended to with much zeal. In these areas, anthropometric measurements will often reveal deficiencies and undernutrition where none had been suspected. Roche and Falkner (1973) have edited a valuable collection concerning techniques and approaches for conducting such studies.

however, the results of the primary inadequacies are so rapidly catastrophic that they overshadow the symptoms of the more subtle
deficiencies.

It should be borne in mind that many societies have learned
through the years that deficiencies in one food can often be offset by
nutrients in another. Thus, Scrimshaw and Young (1976:59) note:

> Every culture has evolved its own mixtures of complementary
> proteins. In the Middle East wheat bread, which lacks ade-
> quate levels of lysine, is eaten with cheese, which has a high
> lysine content. Mexicans eat beans and rice, Jamaicans eat
> rice and peas, Indians eat wheat and pulses, and Americans
> eat breakfast cereals with milk.

VITAMIN A

Vitamin A (retinol), or its precursor, carotene, occurs naturally in
egg yolks, butter, fish, and many vegetables and fruits, but under
conditions of poverty or social disruption these foods are among the
first to disappear from the diet. An extended period of deficiency of
this vitamin will result in loss of the ability to see in the absence of
sunlight and, in extreme shortages, may progress to irreversible blindness, xerophthalmia (Fig. 3–9). Lack of vitamin A was probably frequently responsible for the large numbers of blind persons recorded
through much of human history.

Historians have depicted the throngs of blind beggars who
formed an integral part of every medieval town in Europe, especially
in the wake of droughts, wars, or crop failures. Soaring rates of the
incidence of blindness were associated with the Irish famine of 1848
and fifty years later with similar conditions in Czarist Russia. In the
time of Hippocrates, nocturnal blindness was not unknown. The prescribed treatment, which may have offered some relief, consisted of
applying slices of fresh liver to the eyes. Perhaps this was the antecedent of the modern Western remedy of applying slabs of beefsteak
to injured eyes.

Large numbers of children in Latin America and in the Middle
East suffer eye damage because of vitamin A deficiency. Even larger
numbers, up to one half of the children, are affected in Ceylon,
Burma, South India, Malaysia, and Indonesia. Acknowledging that
the foods in which vitamin A is found would be unlikely to form
part of the diet in poverty areas, world health agencies are now
investigating the feasibility of supplementing the more commonly

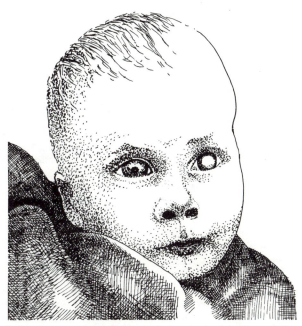

3–9   An extended deficiency of vitamin A causes loss of the ability to see in the absence of sunlight and, in extreme shortages, may progress to the irreversible blindness (xerophthalmia) depicted here. Foods rich in vitamin A are often the first to disappear from diets in time of nutritional stress.

consumed tea with sufficient retinol to avoid the deficiency syndrome. In Bangladesh, UNICEF has since 1973 been engaged in a program that aims at supplying twice every year a small orange capsule containing 200,000 units of high-potency vitamin A to twelve million children up to age six. The cooperation of the well-established, locally accepted antimalaria personnel in distributing the capsule and keeping records apparently has much to do with making this program a success.

VITAMIN B$_1$ AND BERIBERI

Beriberi, a disease caused by lack of vitamin B$_1$ (thiamine), has a recorded history extending back to the third century B.C. in China. An early European description appeared in the writings of a Dutch physician who had worked in Batavia in the beginning of the 1600s. He described a disease whose name, beriberi, he translated as "I can't." This disease produces a loss of sensation in the feet and

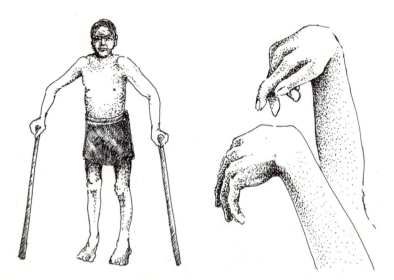

3–10   Beriberi, caused by a deficiency of vitamin B$_1$, is often marked by a loss of sensation in the feet and hands, resulting in a distinctive way of walking and lack of hand mobility. The disease occurs particularly among populations dependent on monotonous diets with disproportionately high amounts of highly refined cereals.

hands, a peculiar and distinctive way of walking, heart symptoms, whole body trembling, and startling levels of psychosis; it frequently terminates in death (Fig. 3–10).

Thiamine is readily available from the germ and outer coating of rice and other cereal grains. It is also found in various legumes such as peas, beans, soybeans, lentils, and peanuts as well as in lesser concentrations in meat, fish, milk, eggs, and liver. Deficiencies are typically associated with monotonous diets that are disproportionately dependent on highly refined cereals such as polished white rice. Because thiamine is a water-soluble substance and is destroyed by high temperatures, deficiencies may occur when large amounts of water are used for cooking and then discarded.

Early in the century it was known that beriberi was in some way associated with rice consumption. Studies of the eating practices of various populations—especially in the Dutch East Indies, Malaysia, and the Philippines—revealed clues that eventually led to an understanding of the etiology of the disease. For instance, in Malaysia, the Malays used crude, home-polished rice and rarely displayed any signs of beriberi. The Tamils, immigrants from southeast India, used parboiled rice, prepared by soaking the rice in the hull, and then drying it in the sun, thus permitting the vitamins to be drawn into the center of the grain. This population also exhibited almost no beriberi. The Chinese in the same area preferred imported, highly polished white rice and had a high incidence of beriberi, while the Europeans living there consumed little rice of any kind and none suffered from the disease.

The evidence suggested that beriberi was caused by some poisonous substance in rice. Many years of intensive research focused on tracking down the suspected toxic agent. Not until the mid-1930s was beriberi proven conclusively to be a deficiency disease. Shortly thereafter, synthetic thiamine became commercially available for food supplementation and is now added to flour, rice, and other foods by legal edict in many parts of the world. Where food fortification has not become a common practice, and poverty deprives populations of thiamine, the people continue to suffer. In 1966, Schaefer estimated that 10 percent of the pregnant women in Thailand had beriberi, and in the Philippines and Vietnam he found that deaths from beriberi among infants exceeded ten thousand and forty thousand respectively in 1959.

A few decades before its true nature had become established, beriberi played an ironic role in association with a sweeping cultural change in the Amazon. From 1870 to 1910, after the development of the vulcanizing process, the price of natural rubber skyrocketed on the world market. Many peoples of the Amazon Basin were diverted from their accustomed way of life to harvest the latex abundant there. Forsaking their traditional diet, which had depended on hunting, fishing, and a "slash and burn" form of agriculture, the people derived their nourishment almost exclusively from imports. The rubber workers' diet, as recorded in plantation accounts, consisted of imported jerky, canned beef, dried beans, manioc meal, polished rice, canned preserves, sugar, chocolate, and alcohol.

Thiamine deficiency moved in its wake; for a time the Brazilian Amazon earned the name "The River of Beriberi." Before long the rubber monopoly collapsed and the artificial prosperity vanished. Imports were no longer possible. The rubber workers had to return to their former way of life and, with the demise of the rubber boom, beriberi disappeared.

NIACIN AND PELLAGRA

Historically, one of the most serious deficiencies experienced by agricultural populations has involved niacin, a member of the B complex of vitamins and sometimes called vitamin B_3 or nicotinic acid. Essentially, pellagra, the disease caused by niacin deficiency, occurs among those dependent on corn (maize). People who are unable to afford meat, fish, or eggs, or other niacin-rich foods such as the whole grain cereals or foods that supply sufficient quantities of the amino acid tryptophan (which the human body can convert into niacin) become victims of this dread disease.

Pellagra was probably first described in 1735 by the "Asturian Hippocrates" Gaspar Casál in northern Spain, where he observed what he thought to be a form of leprosy among the poor peasants who subsisted mainly on corn. During the eighteenth century the disease became common in northern Italy, where it received the name that reflects the initial striking symptom: *pelle*, "skin"; *agra*, "sour" or "rough." Earlier, the syndrome had been called *mal de la rose*, or "rose disease," stressing the scarlet skin, tongue, and oral mucous membrane that supposedly resembled the petals of a fiery rose. In more recent times, medical students, using mnemonic techniques, labeled pellagra the disease of the three D's: diarrhea, dermatitis, and dementia. The victims first suffer from digestive disorders, then ugly red sores begin to cover the skin, and if unchecked, the disease culminates in a characteristic psychosis, marked by hallucinations, delirium and, if not treated, death (Fig. 3–11).

As recently as 1975, 50 percent of subjects in a mental hospital in Africa were able to be discharged after treatment with nicotinic acid. But it was also found, especially among adults in southeastern Africa, that the deficiencies leading to pellagra were a major cause of impaired working efficiency and of psychiatric disorders (Bailey 1975).

The syndrome is found in intimate association with a way of life primarily dependent on a single-crop economy, particularly maize cultivation. During the years following the American Civil War, when poverty and ignorance combined to produce pellagra in epidemic proportions, nutritionists learned to expect the syndrom produced by the typical southern diet known as the three M's: meal (corn), meat (pork, generally fat back), and molasses.

Yet even after its official recognition in 1909 as one disease entity, derived from one specific nutrient deficiency, pellagra continued unabated because its basic antecedent, poverty, did not change. Before World War I, some 100,000 cases were reported in the United States, with an annual death toll of more than 4,000. Until the relative prosperity and full employment associated with World

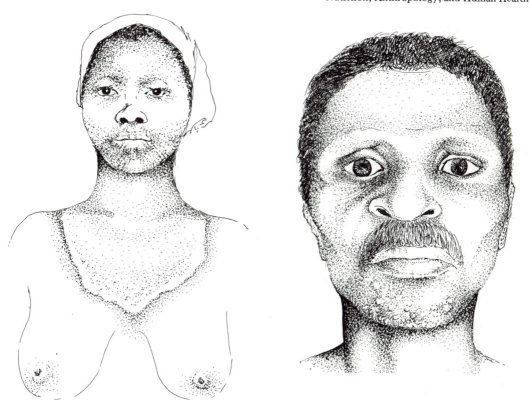

3-11   *Left*: distinctive necklace-like skin disfiguration, sometimes called "Casal's collar," associated with pellagra. *Right*: characteristic facial expression accompanying severe deficiencies of niacin that lead to advanced pellagra and symptoms of dementia.

War II, pellagra continued to leave a trail of misery throughout the American South.

Further demonstrating the close ties between disease and economics is De Castro's (1952) specific correlation of pellagra incidence with the vagaries of the cotton market. He notes the marked increases of pellagra in years following economic depression as well as its diminution during periods of relative prosperity.

Cultural practices may determine whether similar societies, equally poor and dependent on a corn-based diet, may be ravaged by pellagra or escape its woes. Niacin is present in corn, but in a bound form, so it is unavailable when used as meal for cornbread. However,

Mexican populations, strongly dependent on cornmeal for the tortillas that constitute their main staple, treat the cornmeal with limewater before cooking. This releases the niacin and makes it available to body tissues. As a result, pellagra is seldom seen in tortilla-eating regions.

The origins of the practice of soaking the maize kernels in limewater remain shrouded in a distant past. It is generally acknowledged that the grinding and mashing of the kernel is accomplished more easily after the soaking step; nevertheless, one wonders if the practice of utilizing the calcium-containing limewater soak may not have been more than a fortuitous choice.

Ironically, the maize-soaking process may well have been associated with the high incidence of iron-deficiency anemia found among many prehistoric and historic Indian populations (El-Najjar 1977). Although it would seem that a "can't win" situation prevailed, particularly where heavy reliance on maize was the rule, it could be argued that pellagra is inevitably debilitating or fatal, while with a moderate iron-deficiency anemia life is possible, if less than energetic.

Historians have argued whether pellagra was a factor in prehistoric Latin America. Guerra (1964:34) records that the Maya diet consisted almost entirely of maize, but he argues strongly against the presence of pellagra primarily because of the inclusion of protein supplements from domestic fowl and other animal sources in the diet. He adds:

> Beans, squash and other produce, such as cotton, were cultivated, but maize represented more than mere food to the Maya; it was a god—depicted as a young man holding the plant—and the basis of their life. They believed that man had been created by their gods from maize.

It may well be that at some time during the many years of Maya dependency on corn, the custom of soaking the kernels in limewater arose. Eugene Anderson (personal communication) suggests that the custom probably evolved much earlier as a method for softening the hard coating of the Indian corn for grinding on metates—the soft kernels would have been selected out by cutworms and other larvae.

Again we see the fortuitous intervention of a technological innovation when native Americans began the custom of soaking corn in wood ashes, thus exposing the corn kernels to lye, which releases the niacin while producing an American favorite—hominy.

In the American South the traditional backyard plantation practice of soaking cornbread in the "pot likker" from cooking greens acted to capture scarce reserves of the precious nutrients. As a custom practiced by slaves and later by poor freed blacks, it was held in disdain by the equally poor, but biased, southern whites. Under bare subsistence living, whether the nutrients were thrown out with the cooking water or whether they were preserved in the cornbread dipping may have made the difference between who was stricken with pellagra and who was not. The record shows that pellagra struck with higher incidence among poor southern whites.

VITAMIN C, SCURVY, AND CONTROVERSY

Probably no deficiency disease had had a more dramatic impact on recorded human history than scurvy, the disease that results from a deficiency of vitamin C (ascorbic acid). Like the B complex vitamins, ascorbic acid is widely diffused throughout nature. The inclusion in the diet of small amounts of fruits, vegetables, or many of the common root plants readily fulfills the body's requirements. Humans are among the few mammals whose bodies have lost the ability to synthesize this vitamin, perhaps because through most of primate existence the type of diet consumed assured an adequate intake. Only when humans acquire a degree of civilization whereby artificial, preserved, and excessively treated foods become a major part of the diet, or when fruits are not readily available, does scurvy become a critical problem.

De Castro (1952:58) vividly describes the sequence:

> In times of war, on long sea crossings and during economic crises, scurvy has been one of the more vivid of human miseries, gaudy with blood from the hemorrhages of its victims, the strange bruised appearances of their purple skins and the ghastly stench of their rotting gums.

In addition, the vitamin C-deficient body loses the ability to heal its wounds, resulting in open, running, frequently infected sores that add to the overall distress and probably hasten the death that follows untreated cases (Fig. 3–12).

Throughout civilized history—during the Roman wars in the first century A.D., throughout the Crusades, during the Renaissance of the fifteenth and sixteenth centuries, as recently as the frenzied days of the Klondike and California gold rushes—scurvy was one of the afflictions most dreaded by the soldiers, sailors, and adventurers

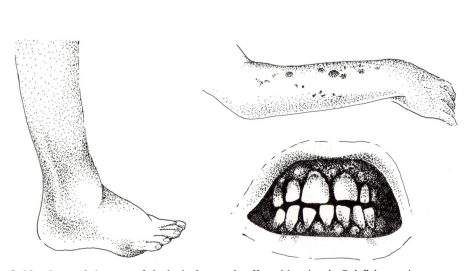

3–12 Some of the areas of the body frequently affected by vitamin C deficiency. Arms and legs show bruised, purpuric markings associated with a subcutaneous bleeding tendency. Gums are often seriously distressed and cartilaginous involvement results in loosening and subsequent loss of teeth.

removed from home and dependent on stored provisions. Fortunately, the body possesses some ability to build up reserves of ascorbic acid, particularly in the liver; after a few months, however, the supply is depleted and must be renewed from external sources. Thus, the stricken individuals were often those who undertook long voyages or expeditions that, in former times, depended on sailing vessels or inefficient means of overland travel.

Stories of ships becalmed and crews cursed may be less legend than historical reconstruction. In 1497, on Vasco de Gama's first expedition to India, more than 100 out of a crew of 160 men died, and the record indicates that during the long voyage, scurvy often struck so severely that only half a dozen sailors on any given day were able to work.

The island of Curaçao was said to have been given its name by the Portuguese sailors on one of Columbus's ships, who, in the final stages of scurvy, were left on the island to die in peace while the rest of the expedition sailed on. Recovering rapidly, thanks to the abundance of vitamin C-rich tropical fruits, the men were able to rejoin their mates and gratefully bestowed the name "cure" on the island where, miraculously, they had been restored to health.

With no means of refrigeration and little ability to preserve foods safely, cooks on sailing ships during the centuries of exploration and colonization were understandably limited in their ability to prepare adequate diets. Ashburn (1947:58–59) reports that when Simón de Alcazaba in 1534 organized an expedition from Europe to Peru through the Straits of Magellan, the "ration provided was ten ounces of biscuits daily for each man, three *azumbres* (about six quarts) of drink for every ten men, the drink consisting of more than half water and the rest cheap wine, and some days less of biscuit but a small bit of salt meat or two or three sardines."

Ignorant of the concept of dietary deficiencies, people looked to mysterious "airs" as explanations for the devastating scourge. Ashburn (ibid.:62–63) quotes Juan de Torquemada, who in 1611 described a disastrous trip of an armada of three ships sent to explore California:

> I wish to give an account of it, for it is the same which commonly affects the sailors in this region who are coming from China to New Spain, and from which most of those aboard the ship usually die. At this latitude there blows a thin and cold air which pierces thin or feeble men, and I understand that it must carry some pestilence. . . .
>   First of all, there is a universal pain in the whole body, and one is so sensitive and touchy that everything which touches him causes such pain that he cries out . . . : and after this his whole body . . . is filled with mulberry colored spots . . . : and after these follow bruises of two-fingers breadth and more, and these are as hard as stones and the legs are embarrassed by them . . . crippled in the state in which this accident catches them, . . . and there are terrible pains in the loins, back and kidneys, so that the miserable body can not be moved except at the cost of pain and groans, which are so cruel that all would think it a very good fate to die rather than suffer them.

More than a century was to pass before James Lind, a physician and surgeon in the Royal Navy, experimented with the diets of British sailors in an effort to cure scurvy. In 1747, on board the *Salisbury*, he carefully noted the typical meals: "water-gruel sweetened with sugar in the morning; fresh mutton-broth often times for dinner; at other times puddings, boiled biscuit with sugar; and for supper, barley and raisins, rice and currants, sago and wine, or the like" (in Lowenberg et al. 1974:179). Lind supplemented this daily fare by giving some of the sailors cider, others vinegar, or sea water, or *elixir vitriol*, or a nutmeg concoction—and still others lemons and oranges. He found the citrus fruits to be "the most effectual remedies for this distemper at sea" (ibid.), and presented this evidence in his book *A Treatise of the Scurvy*, published in 1753. But it then took forty-two years for the Lords of the Admiralty to heed his findings. In 1795, the year after Lind's death, all British ships were required to carry "limes." actually lemons in modern parlance, and throughout the world British sailors became known, somewhat derisively, as "limeys." Subsequently, during the Napoleonic wars, it was said that, because the Royal Navy's fighting forces was free from scurvy, Dr. Lind had contributed as much as Nelson toward the defeat of Napoleon. The introduction of this one dietary item soon made it possible for Europeans to undertake the long voyages that led to the discovery of Australia.

Where fruits are not readily available, native herbalists, particularly in the New World, often use other plants and in the process endow these plants with medicinal, even magical properties. The European attempts to colonize New Foundland in 1535 came close to defeat because of hunger and a specific lack of ascorbic acid in the food available to the colonists. Reportedly, 100 of the 110 men were gravely ill from scurvy and were saved from impending death only by the last-minute intervention by native Indian healers who prepared extracts of the local spruce-tree needles. The identity of the tree used is not certain. According to Lowenberg et al. (1974:178), "Some thought it to be the sassafras tree, others the hemlock. Leaves and twigs of pine, willow, and evergreens have been analyzed and shown to be good sources of vitamin C."

Less fortunate, the colonists of New Plymouth, as reported by Governor William Bradford, were unable to find vitamin C sources during the bitter winter of the first year in the New World. Bradford wrote (in Ashburn 1947:76–77):

> But that which was most sadd and lamentable was, that in 2. or 3. month's time halfe of their company dyed, especially in Jan. and February, being the depth of winter and wanting houses and other comforts, being infected with the scurvie and other diseases, which this long vioage and their inacomodate condition had brought upon them: so as ther dyed sometimes 2. or 3. of a day, in the foresaid time: that of 100. and odd persons, scarce 50 remained. . . . The disease began to fall amongst them [the crew of the *Mayflower*] also, so as

almost half of their company dyed before they went away,
and many of their lustyest men, as the boatson, gunner, 3
quarter maisters, the cooke and others. . . .

The spring now approaching, it pleased God the mor-
talitie began to cease amongst them, and the sick and lame
recovered apace, which put new life into them.

Although scurvy no longer ranks as an important disease in today's world, it is far from unknown. Infants on artificial diets and the
urban aged confined to their rooms and limited in their ability to
purchase fresh fruits are frequently found to be harboring the initial
symptoms of vitamin C deficiency. Scurvy is also frequently encountered in alcoholics, whose diets and damaged livers make for deficiencies that include a lack of ascorbic acid. In addition, in recent years,
mostly in Western countries, mystically oriented movements that
stress dietary "purity" have swept especially through youth groups,
winning converts to grossly inappropriate diets with scurvy as one
likely sequela.

Among many Americans today, vitamin C has assumed an aura
of near-mystical power. The Nobel laureate Linus Pauling (1970)
urges massive daily intake as a means of avoiding the common cold
and other ailments. His recommendation has triggered much controversy, and research on optimum dosage continues in many parts of
the world. At the present stage of the investigations, the leading
nutrition bodies maintain that ascorbic acid is required by the human
body primarily for the prevention of scurvy. They note that this
disease can be prevented through an intake of 10 milligrams daily,
approximately the amount in one quarter of a small orange. The
official recommended daily allowance is 30 milligrams, which allows
for maintaining a body pool of the vitamin and constitutes a com-
promise between United Nations standards and the U. S. Allowance
of 60 milligrams.

THE D VITAMINS AND CALCIUM

Rickets, like other vitamin-related diseases, has many permutations
and contradictions in its interactions with human cultures. This is a
disease intimately tied to various cultural practices and beliefs that
ultimately hinder normal calcium metabolism. The result is painful,
distorted bone growth. A deficiency disease, rickets is nevertheless
not caused by gross malnutrition. If a child does not receive sufficient
nutrients to permit growth, the child does not get rickets. On the

other hand, the poor, slum-dwelling child, living on a diet that permits some growth but lacks a source of the D vitamins (the calciferols), as well as regular exposure to sunshine, grows up with the bowed legs, distorted bones, and contracted pelvis (see Fig. 3–13) characteristic of rickets. For females, in future years the pelvic impairment will preclude the possibility of normal labor and delivery. It is quite likely that the agonizing, extended labor often reported for women of the Victorian era in Europe stemmed from their secluded, overdressed life and consequent lack of vitamin D.

Vitamin D occurs naturally in only a limited number of foods: eggs, cream, liver, butter, and fish oil. Foods of plant origin do not contain it. Fortunately, adequate exposure to sunlight activates the precursors of vitamin D normally present in the human skin, so through most of human history it has not been necessary to obtain vitamin D from foods. Where the human body receives ample exposure to sunlight, there is no rickets.

Under many culturally prescribed restrictions, however, the body is unable to utilize the natural means of manufacturing vitamin D; as a result, the calcium required for normal bone development is unavailable unless the diet chances to be rich in the few vitamin D-containing foods. Bones cannot grow or harden normally and there follows the deformation of legs, chest, spine, and pelvis that constitutes rickets.

An example is found in parts of Nigeria, where custom decrees that infants be completely swaddled or kept indoors. Similarly, in many areas of the world, pale skin is more highly esteemed than darker pigmentation, particularly for future brides, and to prevent heavy tanning, children, especially girls, are restrained from exposure to the sun. Women suffer a high incidence of rickets where class distinctions dictate cumbersome clothing for upper classes or rigid seclusion as well as completely enveloping clothing and veils, as customs of purdah require for women among some Muslim and Hindu sects.

Environmental and economic factors likewise play a significant role in the distribution of rickets. The Pygmies of Congo possess quite deep pigmentation, which would be advantageous for people living under conditions of heavy exposure to intense ultraviolet radiation from the sun. But these people conduct most of their daily life under heavy forest canopy through which few of the sun's rays pierce to the living floor; consequently, the rate of rickets within Pygmy populations is quite high.

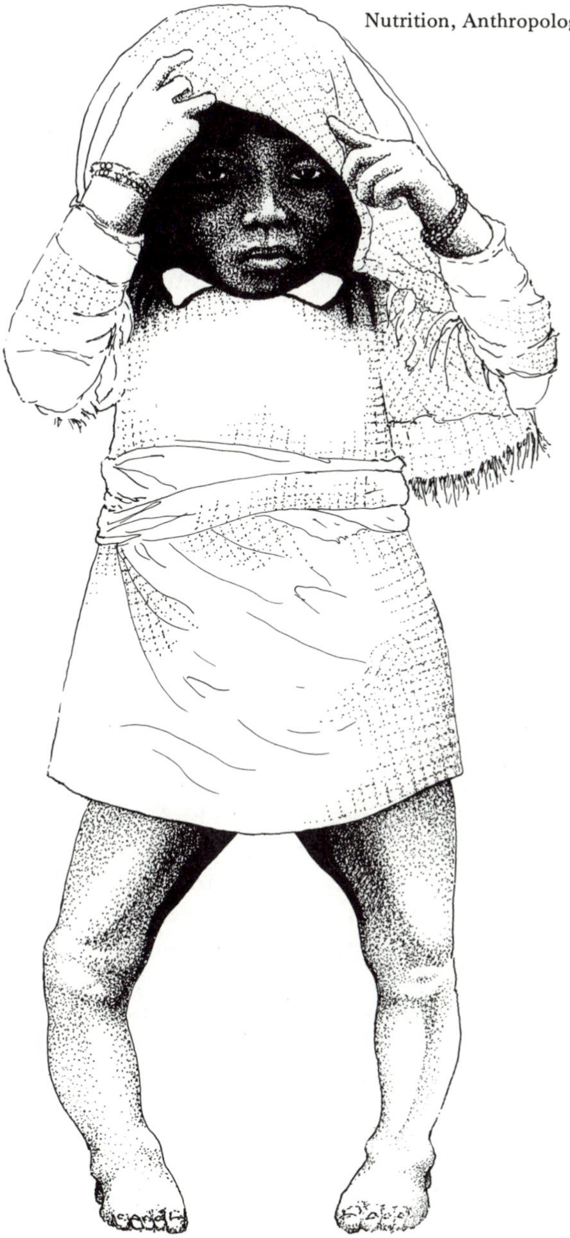

3-13 Distorted bone development typical of rickets, a result of inadequate vitamin D during the critical growth years. The young girl depicted here will undoubtedly have accompanying pelvic bone involvement that could preclude normal child delivery in her later years. (Adapted from Poirier 1977.)

During periods of early industrialization, particularly when the Industrial Revolution spread through much of Europe, work hours for children as well as adults involved virtual imprisonment indoors or underground during all the daylight hours. Wages were miserly; diets were restricted to staples from which vitamin D was absent; and supplementation was unknown. Descriptions of the workers of those days give grim testimony to the appalling numbers of deformed bodies (cf. Engels 1958).

Vitamins D, A, and K constitute the best-studied of the nutrients that cannot be stored in large amounts in the human body. Excessive or inadequate quantities are equally at odds with human well-being. Hypercalcemia, a condition in which calcium levels in the blood are raised, kidney and heart tissue become calcified, and mental retardation and death follow, appeared in parts of Europe during the 1940s and 1950s. The relatively high incidence of this formerly rare syndrome was a result of excessive quantities of vitamin D artificially administered to children. When dosages were returned to lower levels, the incidence of hypercalcemia was proportionately reduced. At present, the National Research Council (Mayer 1973) states, "400 International Units is adequate with an ample margin of safety for normal biological variation. For most infants, 100 I.U. per day in milk would probably suffice."

The metabolism of calcium is closely associated with vitamin D. Calcium is the most prevalent cation in the body. It is involved in bone formation, blood clotting, and normal functioning of the nervous system. Lowered calcium concentration tends to produce increased neuromuscular irritability and has been suggested by several investigators to be the underlying cause of the strange phenomenon of *piblokto,* or Arctic hysteria. It has also been suggested that a combined calcium and vitamin D deficiency was in operation during the late 1800s when epidemic-sized outbreaks of bizarre hysteria were reported among the working classes of numerous European cities.

The predominantly carnivorous diet of the Arctic inhabitants tends to be low in calcium. Studies (Foulks 1972; Wallace 1972; Katz and Foulks 1970) conducted at the end of a long, dark winter when exposure to sunlight was negligible have shown calcium levels to be as much as 75 percent below present National Research Council recommendations. In a comprehensive report on Arctic hysterias, Foulks (1972) tells of his own work among the Innuit Eskimo and examines numerous earlier Arctic studies. He finds that most of the investigators reported a higher incidence among women, an observation that adds weight to an etiology of calcium and vitamin D deficiency because women in the Arctic regions are more likely to be confined within shelters for greater lengths of time.

The most frequent manifestations reported are the hysterical tearing off of clothing and a disturbed manner of speaking, using unintelligible talk (glossalalia) and sounds imitative of animals. The affected person will often run and roll in the snow, jump into freezing water, throw objects wildly, and attempt bizarre behavior such as trying to walk on ceilings or vertical banks of ice. Although it is quite likely that other factors associated with the difficulty of Arctic life are involved in this peculiar syndrome, the evidence points to deficits of calcium and vitamin D as being largely responsible.

Space does not permit an examination of the extensive list of all the minerals that perform vital functions in the body. Iron, iodine, and zinc are among those that have been studied extensively and are intimately related to cultural aspects of life. Examination of the literature devoted to nutrition and minerals will prove rewarding to the serious student.

A WEIGHTY PROBLEM

It is generally assumed that through most of human history, unstable food resources and the necessity for continued high energy expenditures combined to prevent the accumulation of excessive adipose tissue. With the advancement of agriculture, technology, and storage capability, food surpluses became possible and groups of people emerged who were freed from the need to hunt or gather their own food. It was probably at this time that some individuals started putting on extra fat.

OBESITY IN SOCIAL, ECONOMIC, AND EVOLUTIONARY PERSPECTIVE

Eventually, in many societies, obesity became the trademark of the privileged, a sign of wealth, and, for some, the ultimate in beauty. The haughty burghers depicted in the art of the Middle Ages and the buxom beauties painted by Rubens give evidence of the high esteem once accorded to adiposity. Much earlier, the "Venus" figurines associated with Neolithic cultures portrayed gross obesity but the actual context in which they were viewed is not known (Fig. 4–2).

Ironically, extremely high rates of obesity are frequently found today in the United States among the most impoverished segments of the population. Various studies (cf. Wood 1968) reveal degrees of obesity that are almost incapacitating as well as health-threatening. This condition is caused primarily by the poverty that encumbers such groups as Native Americans on isolated reservations and black women in urban ghettos. The cheapest foods offering some degree of hunger satisfaction frequently are the sugar and white-flour products that contain calories and little else. Nevertheless, the consumption of these foods may provide the only solace in an otherwise bleak existence. The consequence is often a vicious circle of empty calories leading to obesity and ill health, which leads to more poverty and continued poor nutrition.

Through much of human evolution, a genetic predisposition toward excess fat-storage cells could have been a characteristic under strong positive selection pressures. Excess stored fat in famine-prone environments could have been a powerful survival factor. This may continue to be a factor in such physiological anomalies as the steatopygia frequently observed among the Hottentots, Bushmen, and Andamanese, particularly the women.

Weiner (1971:121) puts the relationship of food availability and obesity in historical perspective:

> The fluctuation in food supply led to the consumption of very large amounts when food was available. This irregular pattern of food consumption (so different from the continuous foraging of the arboreal primates) is characteristic of hunting people of the present day such as the Eskimo, Bushmen and Australian aborigines. It has been suggested that the hunter's "appetite" has persisted into the modern westernized world where it is now entirely inappropriate; people are apt to overeat in a kind of instinctive anticipation of long periods of dearth, which do not in fact occur. This "overeating" is, of course, the major factor responsible for the obesity, overweight and "endomorphic" physique common in modern western societies but virtually absent in hunting groups.

WHAT IS NORMAL?

The question of body size is a matter of vigorous debate between those who maintain that environment sufficiently accounts for the differences found among populations and those who favor genetic endowments as the primary influence. At present, the bulk of the evidence leans toward the "nurture" theory as most significant, but the genetic limitations of the range of human variation are duly acknowledged. The differences in size between immigrant populations and their children raised in the United States have been extensively examined (Boas 1928). The findings illustrate the tremendous changes possible when positive dietary reforms are introduced. More recently, the alterations in the traditional Japanese diet since World War II, particularly the twentyfold increase in milk consumption (Lowenthal et al. 1974:127), have produced a generation of children who are too large for the school desks used by their parents and who have required government specifications for doorways to be increased by half a foot.

Wherever antibiotics, immunizations, and public health measures have eliminated or reduced the childhood diseases that were formerly thought inescapable, growth has responded in inverse proportion to the former caloric toll extracted by illness and intestinal parasites. Nutrients that are no longer shared with parasites can be utilized by the former host for his or her own growth. This is illustrated by Leff (1953), who estimates that the number of worms living in human beings in the early part of this century equaled the weight of one-half million men and women every year. He speculates that these intestinal parasites can consume a sufficient quantity of food from the bodies of their victims to feed the entire populations of several countries.

Until the disease and parasites can be subdued on a worldwide scale, it is impossible to pose "normal" size or weight for the populations of the world. For the developing countries, no firm figures are available; for the wealthier countries, tables compiled by life insurance companies probably offer the best data obtainable. By convention, a person who weighs from 10 to 19 percent more than the statistical norm for a given population, age, sex, and body build is considered overweight. One who exceeds the norm by 20 percent or more is designated obese. On the basis of these data, it is estimated that almost one-third of all Americans are obese and even more are overweight.

"THREE SQUARE MEALS A DAY" OR FREQUENT SNACKS?

In addition to the quantity of calories consumed, an important factor in the etiology of obesity is the timing of food consumption.

Studies suggest that most nutrients are utilized with increasing inefficiency as the level of intake rises. The venerated ideal "three square meals a day" is found predominantly in societies in which obesity is a problem. Observations of the eating practices of our nonhuman primate relatives, as well as extant hunting-gathering or incipient agricultural societies, disclose an eating pattern quite different.

All nonhuman primates spend a major portion of their waking day ranging through their territories, consuming the available food on the spot. Food is not saved for meal-type consumption and, except for the rare capture of an animal for food by an unusual chimp or baboon, there is no sharing of food. As hominids emerged, with arms and hands freed from locomotion demands they could carry the food they collected, particularly the products of hunting and scavenging, to a home base and share it with other members of the group. In most hunting and gathering societies, the staples of the diet are gathered by the women and children, with protein content ordinarily limited to such nuts, roots, insects, and amphibians as the environments provide. Lush nutritional resources such as the northwestern United States and Canada where meat and fish have abounded are much more the exception than the rule for human habitats. The most frequent pattern observed is one of consuming some of the food as it is obtained and carrying back to the home base whatever requires preparation.

Even today, the most common eating pattern is one of satisfying hunger as it is felt and as the food becomes available. Reports of eating customs generally reveal a daily pattern of several small "meals" augmented by gorging at feasts, the frequency of which depends on such variables as season, custom, and environmental circumstances. This type of consumption is not conducive to the continuous deposition of excess energy in the form of fatty tissue.

As with every other aspect of food, the eating pattern is inextricably interwoven with many other factors in the environment. Daily routines in urbanized societies pivot around the accustomed meal times: households, businesses, industries, and social life are geared to provide time set aside for lunch and dinner, while the consumption of a hearty breakfast has sometimes assumed the trappings of a moral edict. Even individuals whose glucose metabolism is awry or who suffer from an ulcer and are urged by their physicians to eat numerous small meals over the day find innumerable obstacles tied to occupation, as well as custom, foiling the recommended therapy. Of course, some Americans snack on calorie-laden foods all day and part of the night, but true hunger is rarely the reason, and when so many unwarranted calories are added to those consumed at regular meals, the inevitable result is avoirdupois.

NUTRITIONAL QUACKERY, OR "PANACEAS DON'T GROW ON TREES"
By and large, the causes of obesity are well established; nevertheless, medical experience indicates that this syndrome is one of the most difficult to treat successfully. The problem of recidivism dominates this area of human behavior to so great an extent that many individuals can truthfully lament that they have lost hundreds of pounds, particularly through years of "crash" diets, but remain obese. Intense efforts by the medical profession to achieve permanent, sensible solutions have proved generally discouraging.

In their desperate attempts to lose weight, overweight individuals are often attracted to pseudo-scientific fads that regularly sweep through today's urbanized societies. In the United States, nutritional quackery in the past included the sale of reducing pills that contained worm heads (see Fig. 3–14), thyroid hormone, or equally dangerous substances. Although the Pure Food and Drugs Act was passed early in this century largely to outlaw such practices, many persons today continue to rely on potentially dangerous drugs such as amphetamines and phenmetrazine, even injections of gonadotropins, in their attempts to shed the pounds.

Relatively harmless, but perhaps more ridiculous, fads have periodically engulfed those parts of the world where the cultural ideal of a sylphlike figure clashed with contradictory life-styles. In the early 1900s "Fletcherism" swept through the United States and Canada and parts of Europe. Calling attention to the anthropoid attribute of thirty-two teeth, Fletcher and his many distinguished followers derived the edict that every mouthful of food must be masticated thirty-two times and on this seemingly trivial foundation established a widespread cult.

More recently, the fad-based "macrobiotic" diet with its immoderate emphasis on brown rice and other cereals, has resulted in serious illness (including scurvy) and even death among its youthful adherents. Ranging between these extremes have been popular movements approaching cult-status that promise health and beauty through the adoption of low-carbohydrate, "eat all you want of everything else" diets (erroneously attributed to both the Mayo Clinic and the U.S. Air Force). These high-protein, high-fat diets are

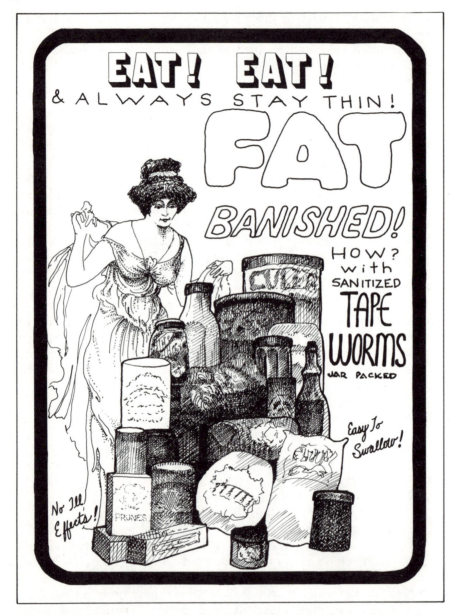

3–14 Fads and fashions lend themselves to the type of exploitation exemplified by this advertisement from the early 1900s. Tapeworm heads were encased in pills and sold on the open market, probably achieving a loss of weight considerably beyond that desired. (Courtesy of J. M. Suchey.)

potentially dangerous because they may reduce carbohydrate consumption to an inadequate level, thus interfering with the metabolism of the fat intake and leading to metabolic disruption and ketosis.

For several years, grapefruit approached magical status and was seen by many as the panacea for the obese. Like the countless other "breakthroughs," the grapefruit cure has had to yield to the unpalatable truth that the only permanent cure for obesity is a sustained reduction of caloric intake coupled with a balanced program of energy expenditure.

CONCLUSION

Nutrition and health are so intimately bound together that every change in one area directly influences the other. Bodies lacking any of the required nutrients are unable to offer maximum resistance to diseases present in their environments. Wherever malaria, bilharzia, trypanosomiasis, and other debilitating diseases continue to ravage human bodies, there weakened workers and disrupted cultures preclude the possibility of food production capable of providing nourishing diets. The reverse side of the coin is that people subsisting on inadequate or deficient diets are physically and psychologically incapable of taking advantage of the optimum technological advances that could provide satisfactory diets.

The present situation—vast numbers of humans suffering from malnutrition while a favored minority wallows in health-threatening overconsumption—creates a world of ugly, inevitably explosive, contrasts. Neither the magnitude of the problem nor the history of past failures should discourage attempts to right the score. In many parts of the world, seemingly overwhelming problems of nutrition and health show heartening promise of yielding to the double-pronged approach of rational economic measures and an educated populace.

Every successful nutrition program has provided a better life for the people involved as well as hope for solutions to many others. A radical change in the nutrition status of malnourished populations is no more beyond the realm of possibility than was flying to the moon a few years ago, but it must be thoroughly appreciated that the accomplishment of the former will take even more knowledge, planning, and concerted effort than was required by the outer-space projects. The result would surely be more profound: an improved quality of life for the many millions who now confront a life of inadequate nourishment, hunger, or starvation. The solutions of their problems lie now in the realm in which the social sciences can make a maximum contribution.

WOMEN AND REPRODUCTION: BIOCULTURAL ENIGMAS

*To the women he said, "I will greatly multiply
your pain in childbearing; in pain you shall
bring forth children."*

—Genesis 3:16

*I also decided that there was something wrong
about God's attitude toward women.*

—Mary Jane Sherfey (1966:11)

The popular myth of carefree childbearing and related reproductive functions among nonindustrialized peoples is rudely shattered when these activities are subjected to thoughtful anthropological examination. The near-ubiquitous proliferation of rituals, taboos, and regulations that surround menstruation, pregnancy, and sexual activity testifies to the overriding concern with these aspects of life in every society where the anthropologist has been permitted to probe. The concern is frequently exaggerated to a degree that indicates fear; indeed an aura of dread all too often hovers around female sexual functions.

WHY FOCUS ON WOMEN?

Unfortunately, as in so many other facets of medical anthropology, most enthnographers have focused elsewhere, leaving gaping lacunas in the data related to these vital phases of human life. With notable exceptions, traditional anthropological studies have concentrated primarily on male activities that commonly occupy the "center of the

103

stage," the public life, and that do not reflect the tensions inherent in sexual investigations. Fortunately, in recent times, under the impetus of militant women's movements, reexaminations of older ethnographies as well as new studies of traditional societies have begun to open new avenues of information about the medical and social aspects of human reproduction.

Today's burgeoning concern with questions of population growth and control makes the study of indigenous attitudes toward every aspect of sexual behavior well-nigh imperative. Recent experience has demonstrated the futility of strenuous efforts to impose population control measures on societies about whose beliefs and customs in the realm of reproduction little is known. Martin and Voorhies (1975:114) echo this basic anthropological tenet:

> The fecundity rate of humans is integrally dependent on cultural factors, because each society has a set of customs that guide individuals in their sexual activity and child- .birth. The closeness between biological and cultural factors makes it necessary to study reproduction in many societies before accurate generalizations can be made about the entire species.

GIRLS ARE DIFFERENT

Human females are unique within the animal kingdom because of the dramatic changes in the young girl when she approaches physiological readiness for childbearing. The distinctly human attributes—conspicuous breasts and copious menstrual flow*—are unmistakable, visible (and in the case of the latter, perhaps olfactory) signals that a being quite different from the child who preceded has arrived on the social scene (cf. Ford 1964; Dobkin de Rios 1978; Strathern 1972). Distinct from the male, who most commonly must "earn his manhood," the female has biological womanhood thrust upon her.

It seems reasonable to state that within the arena under consideration, nature initiates while cultures direct the transition. But even this seemingly elementary proposal is not universally accepted. The fact of biological control over the steps toward womanhood is denied by at least one group of people. Goodale (1971) reports that the

---

*Apes and Old World monkeys also experience menstruation but the amount of flow is considerably less than in humans. New World monkeys and prosimians do not menstruate; the dead cells are reabsorbed (Martin and Voorhies 1975:117).

Tiwi of Northern Australia believe that sexual intercourse is the direct and only cause of breast formation, menarche, and the other accompaniments of puberty. The prepubertal girl moves to the hearth of her prearranged marital partner, and the husband gradually initiates her through a slow process of sexual instruction. Traditionally, her hymen is ruptured early and manually but coitus does not take place until the couple has been married for about a year. Later, when menarche arrives, the young girl says of her husband, "He grew me up; he made me a woman" (ibid.:45).

Whatever the acknowledged explanation for the transition, no society is known in which some cultural recognition does not occur. The notice ranges from severe, traumatic injury to joyful celebration; the one constant is the apparently pancultural necessity to incorporate and acknowledge this "new" creature. As Ford (1964:7) puts it, "The physiological events of menstruation, conception, pregnancy, childbirth and lactation cut across racial, national and cultural boundaries." Nor is social control relaxed after the *rite de passage*: "The culture of each society prescribes recipes for successful behavior during menstruation, conception, pregnancy, childbirth and lactation."

STATUS OF WOMEN: THE RELATIONSHIP TO HEALTH

SEX, GENDER, AND SELF-IMAGE
As Martin and Voorhies (1975:406) observe:

> History teaches us that gender roles have been ubiquitous,
> occurring in every known society extant today and in those
> of the reconstructed past. But history does not teach us
> that these roles are fixed or inevitable.

From sources as divergent as Engels (1972) and Kolata (1974) comes evidence that the social means of production and distribution basically determine not only women's social status but, equally critical, the concomitant treatment of women during one of the most physiologically crucial events of their lives, childbirth.

The status or worth of women and men is established in myriad ways throughout a lifetime by the culture in which they are raised; inevitably each sex comes to accept its society's assessment. A woman's self-image plays an important role in determining the nature of her menses, pregnancy, and parturition, setting the stage for supportive aid where the image is good and, conversely, predisposing her to a traumatic, anxiety-ridden menstruation, pregnancy, and delivery where the self-view is poor.

Kessler (1976:244) proposes an evolutionary basis for the status of women: "There is a real possibility that through the ages, cultural selection has operated in favor of the adaptable, pliable woman as opposed to the aggressive, combative one." But many of the data concerning female productive activities lead one to wonder whether the legendary adaptability and pliability of females may not be products of coercive cultural forces rather than the results of a genetic process.

Most investigators tend to identify social forces as the leavening responsible for conditioning females into roles defined as proper by their culture. Whatever the status accorded females, it is ironic that much of their conditioning is transmitted and perpetuated by mothers who themselves have internalized their society's values. This is seen as well in nonhuman primate societies. Poirier (1975) reports that the rhesus monkey mother threatens and punishes her male infants at an earlier age and with greater frequency than she does her female infants. Her approach toward the female is generally more protective and restraining.

Neuroendocrinologist Ehrhardt (1975:22) acknowledges the vital role of cultural factors in shaping the individual's self-image: "One of the most important variables in determining a person's self-image as a female or male is the sex in which he or she is raised as a child." But she finds "high energy expenditures in outdoor tomboyish activities throughout childhood and a reduced interest in doll play and infant caretaking" among persons who, although genetically female, received high levels of androgen hormones while *in utero* (ibid.:21). This suggests biological factors are also critical behavioral determinants.

INTERACTIONS OF HEALTH AND CULTURAL ATTITUDES

At the bottom of the scale of female status are women like those in the low-income households of India studied by Katona-Apte (1975). Here the female begins life with many strikes against her. Particularly where a woman's parents must present a financially disabling dowry to the family of the groom upon marriage, girl children may be viewed as potential burdens. In days past, female infanticide was a drastic response to these pressures. In more recent times, subtler approaches have been used. Katona-Apte (ibid.:43) notes that female infants are not cared for as well as the male infants: "A female infant is nursed but not as long as the male. She is less likely to have supplements such as powdered milk added to her diet. She will not be taken as quickly to the hospital when ill." It hardly requires adding that she is not likely to grow up with an enviable self-image.

Nutrition studies (see Chapter 3 and Cruickshank 1967) disclose the intimate relationship between successful childbearing and adequate diet. Where bare subsistence is accompanied by prejudicial food distribution based on gender, inevitably the female gets the leavings. These practices are rationalized by statements about the male being the chief breadwinner and are legitimized by beliefs about the unsuitability of certain foods during pregnancy and lactation and even, in some areas, during menstruation (cf. Bullough and Voght 1973). When these factors are compounded by poor health practices in general and inadequate care during childbirth, the outlook for the female is dim indeed. As if recognizing all this, the ancient Chinese are said to have rationalized the practice of female infanticide by saying that killing a girl infant gave her soul another chance to be reborn as a boy (Hammond and Jablow 1976:10). And, not too surprisingly, the traditional Jewish prayer to be recited every day of the male's life includes a passage thanking God for making him a male rather than a lesser being, a female.

In much of "civilized" Europe, early Christianity propagated a distorted view of women as harbingers of evil, particularly in their sexual functions. One of the results was a drastic deterioration in childbirth care that culminated in pre-Renaissance conditions whereby the childbed and the deathbed were all too frequently one and the same (cf. Haggard 1929).

At the happier end of the scale are found attitudes such as reported by Benedict (1934:28):

> Among the Apaches I have seen the priests themselves pass
> on their knees before the now solemn little girls to receive
> from them the blessing of their touch. . . . The adolescent
> girls are not segregated as sources of danger, but court is paid
> to them as to direct sources of supernatural blessing.

Matrilineality among these Native Americans may have determined the difference in attitude, but it could be argued that the attitude of men toward their women and of the women toward themselves may have been requisite for matrilineality to be instituted or maintained.

Attempts to explain the generally inferior position held by women have trailed into so many divergent directions that their very proliferation attests to the lack of consensus. Psychoanalyst Sherfey (1972:138) imagines a somewhat mystical prehistoric era when power that had been held by women was wrested from them over an extended period, so that it took "perhaps 5000 years or longer for the subjugation of women to take place." Brandishing the shield of "objective science," any number of writers have argued that women's "natural inferiority" is related to the supposed debilitation imposed by monthly menstrual cycles (cf. Bullough and Voght 1973). A more recent trend among current investigators (cf. Friedl 1975) is to cite the relative contributions of women to their society's subsistence as the major forgers of gender status.

Friedl compares the status of the Eskimo women, who lived in a society where males furnished close to 100 percent of the food supply, with the position of present-day !Kung women, who gather more than half of the group's food. Among the former, the women were treated as sex objects with "very limited control over their own personal destinies"; male sexual aggression was extreme, and female infanticide common. On the other hand, among the !Kung, "men and women have considerable autonomy and substantial bases of self-esteem (ibid.:39).

THE MYSTERY OF MENSTRUATION

The monthly discharge of some one to five ounces of blood by the unfertilized female probably has evoked cultural responses throughout human existence. Although the physiological mechanisms responsible are more or less charted in modern, industrialized societies, the evolutionary basis remains a puzzle. The extravagant dissipation of valuable iron—some 14 to 28 milligrams each month—and other body stores runs counter to the general efficiency and economy characteristic of animal physiological resources. Why human females have been programmed to excrete rather than recycle the valuable blood supply confounds modern-day scientists (cf. Harrison and Montagna 1973:251) perhaps as much as menstruation disturbs the unschooled hunting and gathering clansmen.

CROSS-CULTURAL SPECTRUM OF PHYSIOLOGICAL THEORIES

The fearful hunter-gatherer and the Western physician have often overlapped with surprising consistency in their desire to exclude or delimit the activities of the menstruating woman. In 1875, the *American Journal of Obstetrics* published an article that argued that menstruation constitutes a pathological condition. As late as 1931, the twenty-second edition of a popular women's "health book" warned that only a minority of women were free from illness during their menstrual period and urged that all rest at least two days, avoid dancing and cycling, and forgo travel during this "treacherous time" (Bullough and Voght 1973:81). By 1972, it was still possible for the physician to the vice president of the United States to proclaim in the public press that women could not fill leadership roles because of the influence of their periodicity (Dr. E. Berman, *Los Angeles Times*, February 21, 1972).

Bullough and Voght (1973) astutely call attention to the less than coincidental reciprocal relationship between the physician "shrill in his emphasis on the instability of the female and the struggles of women and their male allies to challenge the old stereotypes." Nevertheless, the stigmata of a disabling "curse" persist, nor are they negated by data from anthropological studies of attitudes toward the menses among nonindustrialized societies.

Ford (1964:9) reports that of the sixty-four societies he reviewed, less than one-quarter entertain any theory regarding the reason for menstruation. The Choroti, Jivaro, and Toba peoples of South America as well as the Maori of New Zealand postulate a mysterious lunar influence. The Dobuans and Kiwai Papuans of Melanesia believe that a strange sexual relationship occurring between the young girl and the moon results in her first period. The Lepcha of India believe that sexual intercourse is necessary for menstruation to begin and that a divinity peculiar to women makes love to them in their dreams each month and thus maintains the cyclicity. Copulation on an exclusively human plane is given as the cause of menstruation by the Andamanese Islanders, the Murngin of Australia, the Kwoma of New Guinea, and the Apinaye of South America.

Industrialized societies, on the other hand, have in recent years conducted extensive physiological research on the phenomenon of menstruation. In a study of 181 girls in the United States, Frisch and Revelle (1970) determined a spurt in height and weight and a certain amount of stored fat to be necessary for menarche to be initiated and for regular periods to be maintained. They offer as the physiological basis for the onset of menstruation the "attainment of a body weight in the critical range which causes a change in metabolic rate, which in turn reduces the sensitivity of the hypothalamus to estrogen, thus altering the ovarian-hypothalamus feedback" (ibid.:120).

An evolutionary selection factor is postulated by Frisch and McArthur (1974:950) regarding the function of the approximately sixteen kilograms of fat stored by the adequately nourished female between menarche and pregnancy. The function of the extra fat "may be to provide easily mobilized energy. . . . The 144,000 calories would be sufficient for a pregnancy and three months' lactation." As for the cessation of menstrual cycles following chronic undernourishment or rapid weight loss in otherwise normal women:

> If a minimum of stored fat is necessary for normal menstrual
> function, one would expect the women who live on marginal
> diets would have irregular cycles and be less fertile, as has
> been observed, and that poorly nourished lactating women
> would not resume menstrual cycles as early after parturition
> as well-nourished women, as also has been observed.

Earlier support for the effect of nutrition on menarche was offered by Nag (1968:106), who noted that girls on high-protein diets experience menses earlier than those on high-carbohydrate diets. Nag also found that urban and upper-class girls generally begin menarche earlier than those in rural or low-income groups. A related phenomenon occurs among !Kung women (Kolata 1974). The girls among the nomadic hunters and gatherers begin their menstrual periods later than their sister !Kung who have recently shifted to a sedentary, agricultural life and, presumably, to a higher caloric intake.

The wide age range for menarche, can probably not be attributed to nutrition status alone. Frisch and Revelle (1970), working with women from industrialized societies, found a mean age at menarche of 12.9 years, a mean weight of 47.8 kilograms (about 106 pounds), and a mean height of 158.5 centimeters (about 62.4 inches). Nag (1968) reports a range of 13.2 years for East Indian women to nearly 17 years for women of the Asturias region of Spain. He offers 15.17 years as an average of the values for all of 169 nonindustrialized groups studied. On the other hand, Ford (1964) noted that among the Jivaro of South America menarche reportedly occurs at age 10 or even earlier, quite out of keeping with the figures generally found.

MENARCHE AND SOCIETY

There are no rigorous studies available that correlate theories of cause of menstruation with culturally prescribed attitudes toward the menstruating woman. Equally few data are found to explain the frequently virulent treatment accorded the menstruating woman, particularly at menarche. Probably the most traumatic and least understood is the practice of clitoridectomy—excision of the clitoris and often part of the labia as well. This rite is endured by Coniagui girls in Guinea (Gessain 1971) and Bundu girls in Sierra Leone (Hoffer 1975:157), among others. Hoffer reports that the Bundu women told her that excision helped women become prolific bearers of children and "made women clean."

Gray (1958) cites more than forty tribal societies, both ancient and recent, that circumcised young girls of various ages. Their locations range from ancient Egypt to Muslim and non-Muslim Africa, Asia, South America, Australia, and even one sect in Old Russia. An additional female surgery is found among some of the same tribes performing clitoridectomy. This is the practice of infibulation—uniting the labial folds, leaving only a small aperture for the discharge of urine and menstrual blood. Not until marriage is this aperture forcibly widened again, later often being widened still more at parturition. childbirth

The purpose of infibulation seems obvious: no sexual intercourse was possible for the woman until her culture deemed the time proper and reopened the vaginal canal. The reasons for the clitoridectomy are less clear. Gray suggests that in view of the excitability of the clitoris, it was often considered necessary to excise it in cases of "erotomania." Except under the most unusual circumstances this condition was, of necessity, culturally defined. For the most part, the surgery was part of an initiatory process and, though undoubtedly related to sexual mores, led to a much broader set of rationalizations, such as being a necessary step for maturity to begin, being somehow more hygienic, providing an easier passage for childbirth, and so on, all explanations that cannot be substantiated by physiological evidence.

Brown (1963) suggests a relationship between painful female initiation rites and sex-identity conflict. Borrowing from John Whiting's concept, Brown finds a higher number of painful rites when infant-mother sleeping arrangements create a strong mother-identity that conflicts with the patrilocal residence rules at marriage, thus creating a confusion of role identifications. Explanations of this sort,

112

while engaging, particularly to those with Freudian leanings, eventually are found to shed less light than heat.

Less painful, but nonetheless comparable in psychological impact, is the menarche ritual practiced by the Tiwi of Northern Australia, as described by Goodale (1971:48). After removal from the general camp, the *murinaleta*, the girl who has just begun her first menses, makes a new camp in the bush with several older women. They must remain there for five to ten days, during which time the girl is not only forbidden to dig, gather, or cook but is not allowed to touch any food with her hands; she must use a stick or be fed lest she get sick. Likewise, she would presumably become ill if she lifted a container of water to her own lips.

> She cannot scratch herself with her fingers but must use
> a stick because later her arms might break. She cannot make
> a fire for the flames might singe her arm and cause it to
> break at some future time. Breaking a stick in two is taboo
> for her for it would cause her legs to break.

From menarche on she must sleep on the opposite side of the fire from her husband whenever her periods return. The pair are convinced that if they slept together, the husband's eyes would become weak in battle.

Severe psychological trauma has also been observed by Katona-Apte (1975:45), who recounts that the girls she studied in India were given no formal sex education and were only rarely aware of a connection between sexual intercourse and conception. Understandably, "the first menstrual period is often a horrifying and frightening experience to them." The young menstruating girl is isolated and expected not to touch anything nor to sleep near her husband. She is barred from the kitchen and can eat only what is given to her. Apparently not much is given: females in this population have a life expectancy of approximately forty years, their lives cut short, according to Katona-Apte, largely by chronic malnutrition.

FEAR OF POLLUTION
Fear of pollution colors the attitudes toward the menstruating female in many societies. The Gururumba of New Guinea (Friedl 1975:111) provide a striking example. Again we find the girl at menarche a menace not only to men and in this case to the society's treasured pigs as well, but also to herself. She is secluded in her mother's house, where she may not touch her body or eat with her

fingers. During her seclusion, "she is constantly admonished about how dangerous her sexuality is to men and pigs in this period." At the end of her isolation period she is welcomed again into the public domain and for a while is the center of happy attention at a food exchange.

An interesting by-product of the menstrual obsession of the Gururumba is the belief that the contamination extends to the child *in utero*. Thus boys also are affected by the blood they supposedly absorbed while in their mothers' wombs. Consequently, during the male initiation rites bleeding "for purification" is induced by probing bundles of sharp-edged grass into the boys' nostrils. This bleeding is called "male menstruation" but it entails no seclusion or avoidance.

Seclusion is ordained for the WoDaaBe Fulani girls of the Sudan who marry soon after their first menses, following a prescribed ritual isolation of three to five months (Martin and Voorhies 1975). The women of Yap in the Caroline Islands also face a temporary banishment from society. According to Nag (1968), if a woman violates the taboos, the *Kan* or spirit of the menstrual area punishes her by making her periods more frequent.

Because of the Mt. Hagen men's overwhelming fear of pollution from contact with a menstruating woman, females in this New Guinea population also must suspend their normal domestic activities and retire to a menstrual hut (Fig. 4–1). The menstrual discharge is

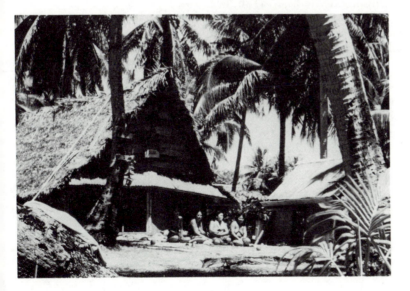

4–1   A menstrual hut in a secluded area of Ulithi, Micronesia. Exclusion of women from the usual routine during their menstrual periods is observed in many traditional societies. (Courtesy of William A. Lessa. From Lessa 1966.)

equated with poison and it is believed that food becomes lethal if contaminated by the most minute amount of blood from a menstruating woman. The discharge is also considered absorbable through the penis; sexual intercourse is therefore prohibited during menses (Martin and Voorhies 1975).

Similarly, the Lele of Central Africa forbid the menstruating woman to pursue her customary daily activities. In particular, she must not enter the forest lest she contaminate it and spoil all hunting or interfere with rituals that depend on forest plants (Hammond and Jablow, 1976). Another tie with concerns about subsistence is found among the Sarakatsani, a pastoral people of Greece, who forbid the menstruating female to approach sheep directly or to cross the path of a flock (Kessler 1976).

On the other side of the world, the Ojibwa Indian girl at menarche, as described by Landes (1971:5), also becomes a menace to herself as well as to most of her society:

> Her proximity blights all young and living things. She
> is hurried by her mother or grandmother out of the family
> lodge into a tiny isolated one built for her in the forest.
> She is dressed poorly, soot is smeared about her eyes, her
> gaze is downwards and she must not look at any living thing.
> She is supplied with a body scratcher that she may not
> poison herself by the touch of her own fingers. She may not
> eat fresh food . . . otherwise, the young growing animals,
> fish and vegetation will be blighted. . . . If she walks
> about she must strew leaves as a warning to men, pregnant
> women and babies. . . . Hers is a conscientious withdrawal
> of her malignant self . . . obsessed and saddened with this
> terror of herself.

For all the rigorous procedures, however, Landes hints that there is perhaps more stress on the ritualized aspects than on a complete internalization of the state of pollution. She describes the rather pleasant visiting back and forth between the "secluded" girls, and notes some unexpected (by the now obsessed anthropologist) violations of the taboos by young men on hunting parties who encounter the menstrual huts containing the young girls and somehow find the courage to defy the taboos and spend the stolen time pleasantly.

Seclusion in menstrual huts is reported by Bock (1967) for six other North American tribes—Cheyenne, Hupa, Kwakiutl, Papago, Sanpoil, and Paiute—with some degree of isolation noted for the Menomini and Winnebago. To this list Ford (1964) adds several more, including the Creek, Crow, and Omaha. Bock (1967:215) comments that "most American Indians seem to have regarded menstruation . . . as producing a state of ritual danger: danger to the subsistence base of the society and to the well-being of the individual." On the other hand, he discerns a male ambivalence toward menstruation and wonders if the restrictions placed on women indicate where the genuine power in a society rests. Others (cf. Sherfey 1972) interpret the customs as evidence of a power struggle in which the losers are periodically banned from normal society.

A purifying bath to remove pollution is found in the *mikva* or ritual bath prescribed for traditional Jewish women at the end of every menstrual period. The Old Testament (Leviticus 15:19) ordains a separation of the catamenial women, who "shall be put apart seven days; and whosoever toucheth her shall be unclean until the evening"—which can be interpreted as a former insistence on seclusion.

Purification rites at menarche are reported by Friedl (1975:39) for !Kung. They believe that menstruation is dangerous to men's hunting weapons, and that coitus during menstruation weakens the husband. Similarly, the Kgatla, a Twana group of the southern Bantu, say that because the woman's blood becomes "hot" during menses, males must avoid her to prevent damage to themselves. The rural West Bengal Indians consider the menstruating woman to be both polluted and polluting, and therefore coitus with her must be rigorously avoided. The abstention extends to six or seven days after the menses for the Muslim women and two to three days for the Hindu.

In all, some 70 percent of the sixty-four societies studied by Ford (1964) were found to have some sexual restrictions during menstrual periods: thirty-three societies forbid coitus and ten others restrict "intimacy." Reasons given by informants range from fear among the Baiga of India that violations will cause worms to attack the man's feet, to the conviction held by the Thonga of Africa that the man will acquire some sort of trembling illness. Beliefs are reinforced to varying degrees: apparently quite lightly by the Ojibwa as illustrated in the account cited above; rigidly by the Ashanti of Ghana who uphold their taboo with threats of execution of violators; and, between these extremes, probably flexibly enough to cover every variation that humans seem gifted at devising. Little concern about violations of sexual relations during menstruation seems aimed at protecting women. Except for the Chukchee of Siberia, who do believe that women can be harmed by cohabiting during their menses, all other societies focus on the possibility of harm to the male from menstrual pollution. Among the societies investigated by Nag (1968), the only exception to the strict taboo was found among the Walapai Indians of the western United States.

In addition to the practices described, Ford (1964) found other restrictions in the sixty-four societies he studied: the menstruating woman must not cook food for men (nineteen societies) she must not consume certain foods (eleven); she must not visit the sick (nine); she must stay away from weapons and hunting equipment (nine); she must keep distant from sacred objects (six); she must stay away from gardens (six), from areas where artifacts are being manufactured (four), and from cattle (four).

GYNECOLOGICAL FINDINGS

Little information exists concerning the degree of actual physical discomfort experienced by the socially beleaguered women. Ford (1964) cites reports of menstrual cramps from women of Lesu and Pukapukans of Oceania, from the Ainu of Japan, and from the Hopi of Arizona. But some Hopi accounts as well as those from the Maori of New Zealand suggest that cramps are exceedingly rare. Indirect evidence of pain and discomfort come from Ford's finding that women in twenty-one societies—one-third the number he studied—employ charms or amulets to protect them from illness and discomfort during their menses. One may reasonably assume that this much attention is based on a real threat.

Although much of the problem no doubt stems from the social opprobrium experienced by the menstruating female, current research reveals fundamental physiological changes accompanying the female cycle that could give substance to complaints. Southam and Gonzaga (1965) conducted an extensive search for documented evidence of physiological factors and record the following changes, among others, during menstruation:

1. Vasoconstriction appears immediately before menstruation;
2. The lowest values of alveolar and arterial carbon dioxide tension are experienced just before menstruation;
3. A measurable weight gain takes place (noted by one-third of the women studied);
4. Changes occur in the distribution of the white blood cells;
5. Anticoagulation factors are present at high levels in plasma and urine;

6.   The level of fasting blood sugar rises.
7.   Numerous cyclic changes in levels of cholesterol, uric acid, bilirubin, calcium, iron, vitamin C and, vitamin E occur.

From numerous studies Southam and Gonzaga found that up to three-quarters of all women in primarily industrialized societies report premenstrual complaints: headaches, gastrointestinal disturbances, nervous tension, irritability, apprehension, anxiety, and fatigue. No general agreement as to etiology can be demonstrated for these symptoms. From other studies, Southam and Gonzaga (ibid.: 154) report that suicides and suicide attempts are more frequent in the immediate premenstrual and the menstrual phases, one-half of the inmates of a woman's prison committed their crimes during menstruation or during the immediate premenstrual stage; and, in England, one-half of all emergency hospital admissions occurred during these same phases of the female cycle. We have as yet no satisfactory method for completely separating the social and physiological factors as they interact upon the menstruating female. It is apparent, however, that social factors are overwhelmingly of a nonsupportive, denigratory nature.

Although there is unquestionably a large psychogenic component in many of the changes described, a "chicken or egg" debate follows attempts to ferret out the sequence of events. Do the physiological changes involved in the cycle produce the symptoms? Or do the anxiety and shame associated with menstruation initiate the physiological responses? Or, as more likely the case, is a feedback process in operation? Answers to these perplexing questions will probably not be found until a culture presents itself for study in which neither shame nor anxiety surrounds the sexual functions of the female. To date, no such society has been documented.

PROFFERED REASONS FOR NEGATIVE ATTITUDES

The universal revulsion against a normal physiological function experienced by one-half of all normal humans after puberty is a source of bewilderment to students of human behavior. Attempts at answers do less to inform than to reflect inadvertently the authors' internalized biases. Coult (1963:33), for example, argues that the taboos and restrictions against the menstruating woman enjoy an empirical and rational basis. He cites investigators who have found that "various secretions from menstruating women produce depressant effects on organic substances, such as inhibiting fermentation by yeast, withering freshly cut flowers and inhibiting the protoplasmic streaming of various plant cells." It is not explained how these factors would have played an important role in the functioning of any of the societies with which we have been concerned.

Ford (1964), who has probably contributed more than anyone else to studies of female cycles and their social interactions, offers a two-edged explanation. He suggests that the sight of blood as a substance associated with wounds and pain is anxiety-producing, and he points to the close genital association of menstrual discharge with feces, both of which produce strong odors and come from the same general body area.

It must be noted, however, that nowhere is a wounded, bleeding individual shunned or thrust out of the group. The wounded warrior or hunter is inevitably accorded great honor and prestige precisely for his shed blood. If, throughout human evolution, the reaction had been revulsion against and exclusion of injured comrades, this would have been an antisurvival tactic indeed.

Further, although rotting, bacteria-ridden blood produces an odor repugnant to most humans, the normal menstrual flow that is discharged before bacterial growth can occur is quite innocuous. Moreover, the same genital area that Ford suggests is shunned because of its proximity to the terminus of the gastrointestinal tract becomes exceedingly inviting to most males for a major part of the female's life. A universal revulsion to association with the reproductive area because it is near the source of fecal material would have precluded the existence not only of the human species but also of most of the animal kingdom as well.

SOCIAL ATTITUDES AND HYGIENE

Postulating an innate panhuman disgust and repugnance for the products of the menses, Ford (1964:17) proposes that the many taboos reported are solutions to the problems of avoiding intimate contact with the menstrual fluid and therefore "it should follow that the more efficient the methods available for collecting, concealing and disposing of her menstrual discharge, the less necessary it will be to isolate [a woman] or paralyze her activities with severe restrictions."

Unfortunately, there are insufficient data to test this ingenious hypothesis. Ford does call attention to the Arunta, of Central Australia, who prescribed complete isolation and whose women supposedly spent their menstruating times sitting over a hole in the ground, which they filled with earth when their periods ended. In New Zealand the less restricted Maori women were reported to use tampons of moss or pads of bark or pounded coconut fiber. They also wore heavy, long skirts made of grass or leaves that, Ford notes, offered additional concealment. But, the one area where native males have openly expressed disgust with the odors of menstruating women is the Yap island group in the far Pacific. Here the women were reported to insert vaginal plugs of spongy moss to collect menstrual discharge. Custom and lack of sanitary knowledge led to insufficient changing of the tampons during the period, and Nag (1968) suggests that this lapse, as well as a high rate of gonorrhea, was responsible for widespread genital infections—which, incidentally, were most likely the source of the unpleasant odors.

The method of dealing with the discharge in modern, industrialized societies undoubtedly reflects the continuing anxious attitude toward this aspect of female life. The use of white, antiseptic "sanitary napkins" resembling nothing so much as surgical wrappings implies a relationship to wounds, injury, and illness. Were contrivances of cheerful colors, gay prints, and so on made available, would women be less likely to associate their menstruation with being "unwell"? The apparent reluctance of commercial enterprises to make such products available acts to perpetuate a psychological association of the menstruating woman with something sick and generally unattractive to herself as well as to other members of her society.

Psychoanalyst Mary Jane Sherfey (1966:11) reflects:

> No matter how much a little girl is prepared intellectually
> for the menses, the first intensely emotional reactions
> she experiences associated with them will remain with her
> throughout life. Contrary to sexual arousal, with the
> menses the experiences are all too frequently unpleasant
> or painful, and almost always carry some note of ostracism
> or taboo.

One wonders if the impact on the young girl at menarche might not be quite different were she joyfully welcomed into her new status of womanhood and presented with beautifully decorated napkins or tampons rather than the stark white "sanitary bandages" that reinforce the sick image (Joan Critchlow, personal communication).

HOW MUCH MENSTRUATION?

Ford (1964:19) and others have also raised the question of an implied power struggle within the societies that ban the menstruating women. Ford proposes, "In a tribe where the woman is regarded as unclean and where she must either remain secluded or strictly curtail her activities for four to five days every month, she is severely handicapped in the struggle for prestige and status." This interesting proposal loses some credence when we consider the relative time that women in traditional societies are likely to experience a monthly period.

The onset of menstruation and, in many societies as well as in nonhuman primate groups, the assumption of an active sex life are followed by an extended period of adolescent sterility (cf. Nag 1968; Kolata 1974). This period generally lasts for several years, dependent, according to Frisch and McArthur (1974), on the girl's nutritional state and subsequent fat accumulation. According to Nag's calculation of a mean age for menarche of somewhat over fifteen years based on values given for 169 societies, it is possible to project several years of menstruation, whose regularity also is a function of general nutrition and other factors during these years of adolescent sterility.

For most of the adult female's subsequent life, however, menstruation tends to be a rare phenomenon: menstruation ceases during pregnancy and is reduced or absent during several years' lactation, which is followed in most nonindustrial societies by a second pregnancy and further lactation, ad infinitum. It could be argued that we have focused inaccurately on menstrual taboos as being generally applicable to all adult women, whereas the focus should probably be reset on the pre-fecund teen-aged girl. In any case, the actual number of menstrual periods experienced by fertile women in traditional societies needs study. The results of such research might engender reevaluations of theories about menstrual taboos.

THE BARREN WOMAN

"MATRESCENCE," A CULTURAL NORM

In most societies, marriage is the social signal for the production of children to get under way. The young girl has been instilled with the social expectation of "matrescence" (Raphael 1975) as her chief function and as the determinant of her future status. At puberty and initiation ceremonies, through prayers and through sacrifices and other magical rites, fertility for the nubile girl is inculcated and reaffirmed as the cultural norm for her.

When a marriage has been consummated and a reasonable length of time has elapsed but no recognizable conception has ensued, a crucial social as well as personal crisis develops. Divorce or the taking of a second wife is a common response. As Albert (1971:204) observed among the Burundi of Africa: "A sterile woman will be retained only in the exceptional case; a man gives the bride-price to have children."

SOCIAL ATTITUDES

Although a few societies acknowledge the possibility of male sterility, the onus for a lack of fecundity is almost universally on the wife. Katona-Apte (1975) shows that the women of India whom she studied considered barrenness the worst affliction that could befall them. Ford (1964), in an effort to categorize social reactions, records that among the Ashanti, Baiga, Pukapukans, and Tiv the nonreproductive woman is the object of social derision, while among the Masai, Kiwai, Mbundu, Nama, and Thonga she is "looked down upon." The response to barrenness among the Kurtatchi, Kwakiutl, Tunala, Tikopia, Venda, and Yakut is one of pity. But the Creek believe in an underlying supernatural revenge for adultery; thus the childless couple, particularly the woman, earns the contempt that is forthcoming.

Similarly, Nag (1968:29) finds that among the rural Sinhalese of Ceylon the sterile woman is treated with disdain. The Kgatla of Africa consider the childless marriage a misfortune and "the childless wife an object of scorn, often tempered with pity." But the Lango of Africa find barrenness so disgraceful that suicide frequently follows continuous failure to conceive (Ford 1964).

An unfortunate circumstance often serves to restate and reinforce culturally specific behavioral expectations. Spencer (1941) notes that a Fijian girl who refuses one man and then marries another invites her society's prediction that she will probably be condemned to a sterile marriage. In like manner, when Losana and Tevita, a young Fijian couple, remained childless after being married two years, an informant observed to Spencer (1941:53) that Tevita has been a less-than-ideal son, continuously disregarding the wishes of his parents, while a second Fijian postulated that the young couple "probably cohabited every night and as a result of such frequency 'the blood came every month.' " When the wife, in desperation, finally consulted a *vuniwai*, a curer and spiritualist, she was told that her husband's ancestors had committed sins that should have been expiated (undoubtedly this was a curer with a heart).

Punishment and vengeance from wrathful gods or ancestral spirits are rationalizations not infrequently encountered. The rural Sinhalese believe that the number of children one has is a reflection of merit achieved in a previous life. Thus the Sinhalese woman's failure to conceive is seen as evidence of a great sin committed in a former time (Nag 1968:45). The marked woman is "considered unlucky to be around and is avoided under many circumstances." Likewise, Coniagui women of Guinea who produce no children are labeled sinners who are being punished by supernatural forces (Gessain 1971).

The search for explanations not only delves into ancestral time but also reflects the belief that the results of the vindictive treatment accorded the sterile woman in her lifetime may produce threats to future generations. Strathern (1972:99) reports that among the Mt. Hageners of New Guinea the childless woman who died was still considered dangerous because she had not fulfilled her life's goals. Hence, her corpse was denied a traditional burial by her husband's kin; her "bones were smashed and her eyes blocked up lest her spirit, frustrated at an unfulfilled life, should plague the living."

TREATMENTS FOR STERILITY

A number of societies are reported by Ford (1964) to regard barrenness as a type of illness that may respond to certain medicines. Medicines may be prescribed to ward off the possibility of sterility or to deal with an acknowledged problem. An extensive pharmacopocia has evolved, relying primarily on homeopathic, magical relationships; substances are utilized from plants or animals that exhibit the desired fecundity. The Andamanese Islanders, for example, have recourse to a special kind of frog, well known for its numerous progeny; the Kiwai woman of Oceania is given spiders or spiders' eggs to eat; the Apinaye woman of Brazil is given a medicine made from the ashes of burnt pigs' teeth.

Within those few societies in which the male is recognized as possibly responsible for the lack of children, the husband without issue is likely to become the object of his society's opprobrium. Nag (1968:73) reports that among the Juang of India it is believed that excessive sexual activity—always a culturally defined concept—will be reproductively counterproductive:

If a man goes daily to his wife, his body turns black and his strength leaves him. He should go once in eight, fifteen or thirty days; then his wife will be pregnant. The man who goes daily never makes his wife pregnant.

Ford (1964) finds only three societies—the Ashanti of Ghana, Bena of Tanzania and Ifugao of the Philippines—that compel the allegedly sterile husband to free his wife from an unproductive marriage. The Ashanti derisively call such a man "wax penis." In Madagascar the Tanala blame his condition on a former or hidden incestuous relationship. Habitual consumption of edible mushrooms is reported as the cause of male sterility among some Iranian peoples.

The rate of sterility in traditional societies is extremely difficult to determine accurately. Those few data that exist include fetal wastage from abortion, miscarriage, and stillbirths as well as sterility. Among the Kgatla, Nag (1968) found 4 percent of 184 ever-married women who had passed menopause and 10 percent of 417 ever-married women of all ages to be childless. Much higher sterility rates are found for the Yapese, whose reproductive rate of 1.1 children per woman was one of the world's lowest. Seen from another approach, this figure means that 34.4 percent of the postpubertal women of Yap reported they had never been pregnant.

Nag's findings reflect the intimate interaction of inadequate diet, health conditions, and childlessness. He suggests a close connection between fertility and total caloric consumption, and notes the correspondence of nutrition within given societies with high child mortality and low fertility rates and, conversely, within low child mortality and high fertility rates. In recent times sterility of women in these societies can be mainly attributed to venereal diseases (ibid.: Table 66) but other diseases and factors such as malnutrition may contribute.

Hammond and Jablow (1976:53) similarly report:

> Bad health and poor hygienic conditions lower the fecundity of women in traditional societies. The prevalence of malnutrition and disease leads to sterility, miscarriage and stillbirths as well as an extremely high rate of infant mortality.

We confront, then, in the barren woman, an ironic set of circumstances: an inability to fulfill her culturally ordained destiny as a result, at least in part, of health and diet conditions over which she has no control, plus an inability to derive any support from family or society precisely because they themselves constitute an integral part of the problem.

HER FINEST HOUR: THE PREGNANT WOMAN

FECUNDITY EQUALS ESTEEM

Throughout known human history, the essential value of a woman has been gauged by her fecundity (Fig. 4–2): "It is a universal cultural idealization that motherhood is the culmination of the woman's hopes, dreams and ambitions" Hammond and Jablow (1976:45). But for the individual woman in any society painful contradictions transform this ideal into a difficult dichotomy of choices. Falade (1971:

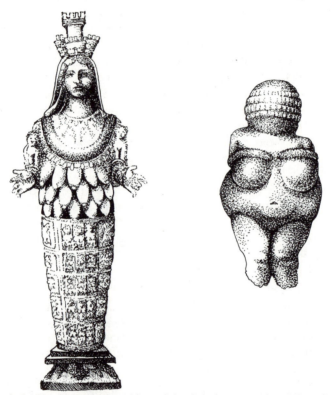

4–2 Female fertility has been the subject of ritual art in many cultures through the ages. *Right*: The Venus of Willendorf, dating back twenty to thirty-five thousand years, is considered by many authorities to represent one of the first artistic representations of the mystery and wonder of the female's role in reproduction. *Left*: The impressive, if exaggerated, nurturing role of women is represented in the form of an ancient Roman goddess from grove Nemi.`

224), in a study of the Wolof and Lebu woman of Dakar in Senegal, writes:

> It would be impossible to overestimate the importance of pregnancy to the Wolof woman. Motherhood is one of the things most ardently desired . . . to be a mother not only ensures the stability of her marriage, but also confers respect upon her as a woman.

Similarly, Kessler (1976:162), describing the Sarakatsani women of Greece, points out, "Only through her children can a woman hope to achieve status of any kind." And Huffman (1931:42) reports of the Nuer of Sudan:

> The greatest desire of a Nuer woman is for children. She realizes that as long as she can bear her husband children he will care for her. Should she fail him in this her position is insecure, and he, no doubt, will try to get another wife who will be able to give him his heart's desire. The mother also realizes that children will care for her in her old age, even if her husband does take younger wives, so her children make her position in old age secure.

Devereux (1955:103) adds somewhat more strongly to this less-than-ideal motivation for childbirth:

> Anthropological data seem to support that, even conservatively speaking, the intensity of the urge toward motherhood is pretty much a function of male attitudes toward fatherhood, the latter being determined in turn partly by the economic usefulness of children and even more profoundly by the role which the fathering of a child plays in the prestige patterns of a given society.

FEAR PRODUCES CONFLICT

Similar themes seem to dominate the attitude toward women and childbirth in virtually every society for which studies are available. On the other hand, ethnographic and medical evidence supports Ford's claim (1964:50, 62) that "fear of a difficult delivery apparently haunts primitive women," for "childbirth is often both prolonged and painful." The difficulties entailed in bringing a living child into the world are formidable: not only physical suffering but an ever-present threat of death seems to overshadow every childbirth.

Given the frequent uncertainty of food supplies, accompanied

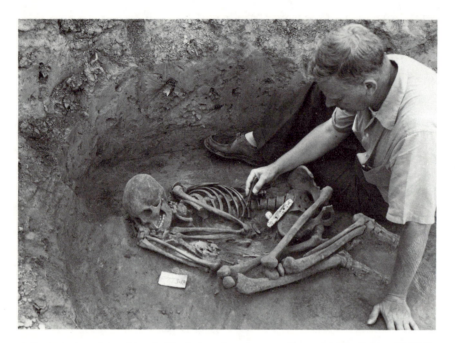

4-3 Remains of a prehistoric North American woman who apparently died in childbirth. The infant lies buried near the mother's arms. Also recovered from the same site was a kidney stone or bladder stone that measured 10 x 8 x 5 mm. The two bodies, found in the Morse Site, have been dated from the Late Archaic. (Courtesy of Illinois State Museum. From Morse, 1969.)

by the near-ubiquitous expectation of parasitic infestations, pregnancy and delivery for many women today, as for all women in former years, are fraught with obstacles and danger (Fig. 4–3). Additionally, the restrictions in physical activities necessitated by the long human gestation period, the reduced self-sufficiency, and resultant dependency on others create significant impediments to "carefree" reproduction. So we see a basic conflict pervading the lives of women: tremendous social pressures pushing toward reproduction, conflicting with powerful legitimate fears, primarily physical, of the actual birth process.

CULTURAL RESOLUTION OF THE CONFLICT
Few would argue with Kessler's statement (1976:14): "Human biology cannot be completely restrained by culture." Nevertheless, since

humans are the only animals known to exercise any choice as to whether or not to become pregnant and particularly whether or not to continue a pregnancy, for human reproduction the cultural milieu is highly significant. Further, it seems that where human societies have perpetuated themselves for a long time, an important factor has been the strength of the cultural value of childbirth.

Indeed the impediments to successful childbirth have been such that only the most powerful cultural drives have made its continuation likely. Ford (1964:86) stresses that the wish for offspring is not innate, not a basic human drive. Rather, it is an acquired desire that has to be culturally implemented and continuously reinforced by social rewards and punishments:

> Promises of security, approval and prestige support the desire
> for children; threats of insecurity, punishment and ridicule
> blocking incipient wishes to escape the pain and cares of
> childbirth and parenthood. . . . If people are to reproduce,
> social life must offer enough rewards for bearing children
> to more than outweigh the punishments involved in
> reproduction.

Reining and Tinker (1975) ask, "What sort of health and medical services must be available so that women may have the number of children they desire and have all of them survive?" (See Fig. 4–4.) The anthropologist aware that the position of women in any given society critically determines their ability and willingness to perform their unique function as childbearers would add: What are the factors within the culture that influence the process? What are the interactions between the roles of women, the beliefs associated with pregnancy and childbirth, and the motivations of the women who bear the children and the men who father them?

An examination of various societies and their views of childbirth as well as a study of the worldwide use of means to limit or prevent pregnancy adds substance to Ford's thesis and in the process offers some answers to the many questions surrounding human reproduction.

THEORIES OF CONCEPTION

With rare exceptions, all human societies recognize the cause-and-effect relationship between heterosexual intercourse and pregnancy. Beyond this basic understanding a great divergence of theories ensues.

For thousands of years the mystery of conception has fired the

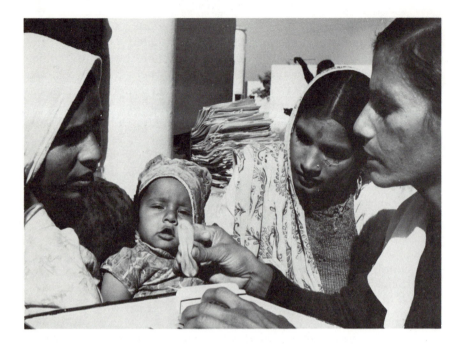

4-4   A family planning expert in India demonstrates a diaphragm. The ability to plan family numbers can mean a healthier life both for mothers and for their offspring rather than unlimited fecundity and eventual "pregnancy fatigue." (Courtesy of World Health Organization. Photo by E. Schwab.)

imagination. As recorded by Ashburn (1947:244), the Talmud, the collection of ancient Rabbinic writings that form the basic authority for traditional Judaism, makes this pronouncement regarding conception:

> Three co-operators are concerned with the making of man [:] God, the father and the mother. The father furnishes the white sperm, from which come the bones and tendons, the nails, the marrow of the head [brain] and the whites of the eyes: the mother furnishes the red sperm, from which come the skin and flesh and blood and hair and the black of the eyes: God gives the life and soul, the shine of the face, the sight of the eyes, the hearing of the ears, the speech of the mouth, the lifting of the hands, the going of the feet, the understanding and insight.

Among the Nzakara women in the eastern part of the Central African Republic (Laurentin 1971:149) a reciprocity between the sexes is theorized and put into practice: every day the woman must prepare food for her husband, keeping him well fed, and, in turn, the semen deposited by him during cohabitation is virtually interpreted as a physiological nutrient. The husband's contribution is considered vital for the well-being of the woman, for without it, "her breasts would sag, her skin dry up and her vitality wane so that she would no longer be able to bear any children." When conception occurs it is the duty of the father to "provide nourishment for the child" until the fourth or fifth month when quickening begins. At this point his job is accomplished and marital relations must cease.

The Azande of Zaire are reported (Ford 1964) also to believe that the growth of the early fetus depends on continuous contributions from the father. Similarly, the Kiwai of Oceania and the Mt. Hageners of New Guinea (Strathern 1972) encourage male participation through sexual relations in the development of the incubating child. The Mt. Hageners postulate that the child is formed as a result of the mingling of the father's semen and the mother's menstrual blood. They believe that after the fifth or sixth month, probably in association with the child's movements, a *min* or spirit is acquired by the fetus and at that time the father's semen is not only no longer required but in fact becomes potentially dangerous.

The Lesu of the Bismarck Archipelago specify that the child's blood comes from the blood of the mother while its flesh is formed from the semen; therefore, frequent coitus is necessary in early pregnancy to strengthen the fetus. The Havasupai and Walapi (Nag 1968), sharing the belief that the fetus is created from a mixture of the father's semen and the mother's blood, consider a single act of intercourse insufficient to produce a viable pregnancy. Thus, all these people believe that conception does not occur from one act of intercourse; rather, the fetus is built up, molded, by the continuous "work" of the parents over an extended period.

Just as the concepts of fertilization vary cross-culturally, so there is little agreement about when conception has taken place. The disparities in pregnancy-recognition are found not only from society to society but probably also from woman to woman. The cessation of one or more menstrual periods is cited as a key by Ford for nineteen tribes, whereas seven others studied pay more attention to breast changes; another seven announce pregnancy at the appearance of morning sickness, while six societies concentrate on behavioral changes such as loss of appetite and decelerated activities as the chief indicators.

CULTURALLY ORDAINED BEHAVIOR DURING PREGNANCY

During the pregnancy every society enjoins culturally prescribed and proscribed behavior for the mother-to-be. Particularly where spirits and sorcery form an important part of life, the pregnant woman is subject to strong intimidation from these sources. Her increased vulnerability is manifest in the many expressed fears of injury from disgruntled kin, living or dead. Among the Mt. Hageners, for example, sorcery from cognatic kin still harboring grievances over the bride-wealth settlements is blamed for reproductive misfortunes that occur during this time. (Strathern 1972).

As Murphree (1968:64) expresses it, "Birth practices and beliefs are valid indices of attitudes not only toward birth but often toward health and life itself." In a few societies, the anxieties attendant on the reproductive process result in the extension of restrictions to the behavior of the father as well. In Central Australia the Arunta husband is forbidden to use a boomerang or spear during his wife's pregnancy. Fear of a deformed child or a stillbirth lead the Hopi to enjoin the husband from injuring any living creature. Even tying a hobbling rope around the neck of any beast is forbidden to the Hopi husband, and to the Sanpoil as well, lest the fetus be choked by the umbilical cord (Ford 1964).

The Ifugao husband also may not cut or kill any living thing during his wife's gestation. Even woodcutting is taboo. Members of the extended family therefore become actively involved by helping the couple and thus caring for the unborn child. It becomes their responsibility to cut the wood, which the husband is then permitted to gather, bundle, and carry. Through this widening circle of participants, the care and responsibility for the expected child also becomes functionally more extensive and effective.

Because of a widespread fear of strangling the fetus with the umbilical cord, the woman is subjected to a multitude of prohibitions. For instance, among the Nama Bushmen-Hottentots (Ford 1964), as well as among the Eastern European Jews (personal communication, Reba Shear), the pregnant woman is constrained from ever raising her arms above her head. One happy by-product of such prohibitions is that the work load of the woman thus becomes somewhat lightened: the Nama woman, for fear of harming her child, can no longer carry water above her head, and the Jewish woman can no longer hang up clothes or perform similar tasks. Again, restraints of this nature have the effect of involving members of the family or clan, who thus begin to take an additional interest in the forthcoming child.

Among the Samoans studied by Mead (1928), manipulative homeopathic or contagious magic was augmented by a belief in a direct alimentary connection between mother and fetus. The pregnant woman was not to drink from a full coconut before someone else had sipped from it or her child would gulp and not be able to swallow its milk well; nor was she to eat the heart of a coconut before it filled its shell or the fetus would loosen in her womb and she would have a miscarriage. If she ate hot food, her child would be blistered. Were she to cut off a piece of meat while holding it between her teeth and lips, a child with a harelip was likely to result. In addition to the alimentary precautions, the mother-to-be was urged to reduce her walking about or her child would turn out to be a runaway.

Studies from the southeastern United States suggest a strong concern with the behavior of pregnant women that Murphree (1968) interprets as cultural statements that reinforce the ascribed status of women. Particularly, "marking the baby," that is, causing birthmarks, is seen as the result of women stepping out of their assigned roles or violating specified norms. Murphree cites a common saying, "Climb a ladder and the baby will be born with a bald spot," and suggests that ladder climbing is considered masculine behavior, unseemly for a woman and therefore producing a masculine "mark," baldness, in the baby. Similarly, attention is given to the craving for particular foods, which in this Bible Belt area might be interpreted as proscribed gluttony. Hence there are reports of birthmarks resulting either from the mother's succumbing to an ardent desire for a particular food or, perhaps more commonly, from craving something that was denied her.

One possible consequence of the eating restrictions and accompanying dietary deficiencies is the practice of geophagy, the eating of clays or soils that continues today among some low-income pregnant women in the American South (Hockstein 1968) and in other areas of the world. The custom is of considerable importance to these women, and although studies have as yet evoked no definite origins or functions, Cruickshank (1967:23) cautions would-be reformers,

"Mineral content of the various earths is not known. These customs should be left alone until they have been studied and their effects are better understood."

"Marking" becomes a matter of concern in many areas of the world and frequently constitutes the substance of folk tales or is associated with unusual natural events that occurred during the pregnancy. In Afghanistan the pregnant woman is warned to avoid touching any part of her body during an eclipse of the moon. Should this precaution be ignored, the child could be born with brown or black spots on that part of its body. The Tanala woman must not touch black-eyed beans, a variety common to her region, lest the child be born with black spots on its skin.

When Songombi, a woman of the Nzakara people described by Laurentin (1971:149), became pregnant all the women in her hut and around the court beseiged her with advice:

> Do not eat the meat of a female animal that is with child, or
> the spirit of fertility will kill your child, and might even turn
> on you; be careful about eating red meat; it has blood in it,
> your child may fall in the blood (miscarry). Avoid animals
> that are harmful to man, especially snakes of all kinds. As for
> fish, choose carefully which ones you eat; the *nzambo* with
> the bulging eyes breathes too heavily, your child would not
> be able to stand it.

In like manner, the pregnant Ashanti woman is urged to keep away from red ants and also never to look at blood. Neither must she look at a monkey during her entire gestation or she might give birth to a child like it (Ford 1964). Lango women are warned never to sleep on the hide of a waterbuck or eat its flesh; nor should they partake of the stomach of a cow, step over the root of a tree, or touch a fig tree or rain dripping from a roof. The pregnant Azande woman must avoid the red pig, waterbuck, and eggs and she may not eat from old pots (Evans-Pritchard 1974).

The Tiv woman and her husband must never look into a grave; accidental abortion is believed certain to follow. The Maricopa woman and her husband must not look at dead animals lest their child become paralyzed; looking at or touching a snake might prevent the child from ever walking. A woman who holds her breath is thought by the Sanpoil to prevent the fetus from breathing and thus produces a stillborn baby. The Tiwi woman must not bathe in the sea or in large bodies of fresh water during her pregnancies for fear of offending the rainbow spirits (Goodale 1971); spitting into a fire or even putting food on the fire will cause the fetus to twist in the womb. Ironically, perhaps tragically, the extensive list of foods forbidden to the pregnant woman includes essentially those that are good sources of protein (see pages 66 and 148).

CONSIDERATIONS OF PREGNANCY TABOOS

Ignorance of physiological laws and a need to seek explanations for reproductive casualties largely account for the avalanche of taboos and injunctions that descend on the pregnant woman. The multiplicity of seemingly trivial and largely disconnected constraints on her behavior must weigh heavily on the already anxious and burdened woman (Fig. 4–5). Among populations living under poor health conditions, deficient diets, and inadequate medical care, total fetal wastage—miscarriage, stillborns, or early infant mortality—is likely to

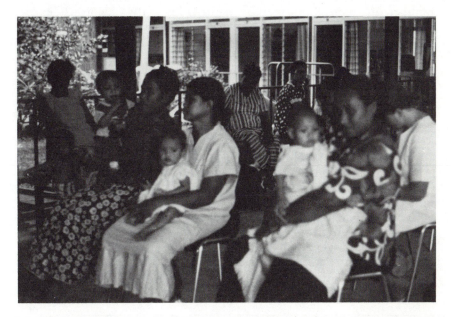

4–5   The introduction of antenatal clinics, exemplified by this Family Welfare Center of the National Hospital in Apia, Western Samoa, constitutes a vital step toward healthful pregnancies and deliveries. In such clinics women can be instructed in proper care for themselves and their children, unfounded fears can be allayed, and medical emergencies can be avoided. (Photo by C. S. Wood.)

approach one-quarter to one-half of all conceptions (Hiraizumi 1964; Reed 1966; Nag 1968; Hogbin 1970). Directing the blame for these misfortunes at the mother for supposedly having violated any of the myriad taboos adds an ill-deserved burden of guilt to an onerous load of miseries.

The combination of biologically irrelevant taboos and the physiological uncertainty of 100 percent success in every pregnancy makes for a "no-win" strategy. Much of the proscribed behavior is unavoidable or may be committed unknowingly. When the pregnancy terminates unproductively, the unfortunate woman must endure not only the sorrow of her loss and considerable physical pain but also guilt for having violated one or more of her society's rules. More often than not her culture imposes an additional sentence of gossip, scorn, and castigation.

In its most cruel form, for example, among the Ashanti of Ghana and the Jukun of Nigeria, a miscarriage is interpreted as supernatural punishment for alleged adultery. Elsewhere violation of any number of other taboos may be blamed. The only "generous" exception is found in those societies that let the woman "off the hook" by ascribing the casualty to venomous acts of revenge or pique on the part of dead kin or malicious spirits. As is demonstrated in the following anecdote from Fiji (Spencer 1941:28), rigid patterns of behavior are required even after a miscarriage has occurred:

> Several years ago Nanewange had a miscarriage. Being an abnormally shy woman, and not wishing perhaps to make a fuss, she wrapped the foetus in a cloth and threw it in a stream without telling anyone about it. She was very ill afterwards and admitted to one of the other women that she had lost her child and disposed of it quietly. When this reached the ears of Teolami, her father-in-law, he was very angry because she had concealed the fact. Sometime later when she was suffering from a series of headaches and was repeatedly indisposed (she was pregnant at the time) she consulted a *vuniwa* and learned her illness was a result of Teolami's anger.

ABORTION—ANOTHER "DOUBLE BIND" IN OPERATION

Most cultures have rigid restrictions concerning when and with whom pregnancy may be initiated. When conception occurs that does not satisfy these requirements, when fear of childbirth or care for existing children weighs too heavily, the only avenue of redress for the woman is the deliberate termination of her pregnancy.

UNIVERSALITY OF ABORTION

According to Devereux (1955:161), "There is every indication that abortion is an absolutely universal phenomenon. . . . It is impossible even to construct an imaginary social system in which no woman would ever feel at least impelled to abort." According to Nag (1968), abortion and infanticide are practiced in almost all societies at least occasionally, with strong social pressures to curb excessive indulgence. In a study of sixty-one nonindustrialized societies Nag found none "in which there is no ostracism as a sanction against abortion" (ibid.:135).

The methods of aborting available to women in traditional societies (see below) are generally so brutal, even life-threatening, that one is moved to wonder at the strength of the forces that motivate these actions.

REASONS FOR ABORTION

Social and/or economic conditions are at the root of the overwhelming majority of the reasons given for abortion. Devereux (1955), in his comprehensive study of abortion in primitive societies, states that anyone familiar with the tremendous burden that primitive women carry and with the great poverty endured by many groups will understand their actions. He and others cite the historical accounts of women of the Antilles, Guam, and Baholoholo as well as those of several tribes of Melanesia who performed mass abortions and mass suicides to save their children, unborn and born, from slavery and abuse when subjected to foreign subjugation.

The women of the Munda Kolh of India, the Payagua of Paraguay, the Nukuoro of Samoa, and other societies have been driven to end their pregnancies when dire poverty threatened the welfare of those children already born. Conditions that are probably impossible for the unaffected to imagine underlie the accounts of the mothers of the Ngali and Yumus of Central Australia who in times of extreme famine are reported to feed the deliberately aborted fetus to starving siblings (Devereux 1955). More than twenty societies reported that the major cause of abortion was the presence of other children and limited means to provide for them.

Ford (1964) lists twenty-seven societies that sanction abortion for the unmarried woman who becomes pregnant and eleven societies that do so when the pregnancy is the result of socially defined (see Devereux 1955:188) adulterous relationships. But adulterous liaisons are not the only grounds for abortion; many societies become feticidal if the father is deemed an improper sire. The definitions of unacceptable fathers range widely. The products of the union are disdained among the Tikopians of the Pacific if the father is unknown; in Korea if he raped the woman; in Fiji if he comes from a lower class; in Gunantana and Sedang Moi if he is too closely related to the woman; among the Cuna of South America and the Tucuna of the Pacific if he is an alien; among the Tupinamba of Brazil and the Toradja of Celebes if he is a prisoner of war or a slave; and among the Pima Indians if the father has died. Under all of these circumstances, social rules have been violated and the price to be paid, by the girl or woman, is termination of her pregnancy.

Gessain (1971) states that, traditionally, among the Coniagui of Guinea a girl is not supposed to have sexual relations before she has undergone clitoridectomy; therefore she will try to induce an abortion, usually with her mother's help, if she becomes pregnant before the proper time. Similarly, if the Suau girl of Melanesia is considered too young, her culture ordains an abrupt termination of her pregnancy, while at the end of the age scale the Chagga woman of Tanzania is constrained to abort if she conceives at an age considered too old.

From this fragmentary survey it becomes apparent that, whereas middle-class women in industrialized nations today may argue legitimately for their right to "control their own bodies" and determine their pregnancies, historically, this right has not generally been accorded to women. As Devereux (1955:135) states:

> Female attitudes toward maternity appear to be largely determined by masculine attitudes toward paternity. . . . The romaticization of the maternal role—the Madonna complex—is conspicuously absent in primitive societies, even where children are ardently desired and where fertile women are much esteemed. We therefore infer—not at all arbitrarily—in our opinion—that even where women abort of their own free will . . . they do so under the impact of a genuine of expected masculine attitude.

Through most of women's history, a "wanted pregnancy" has been one that was defined as such by society and the decision to terminate it likewise has been one in which the individual woman exercised surprisingly little control.

METHODS OF ABORTION IN TRADITIONAL SOCIETIES

Except where modern medical techniques have become available, women driven to terminate their pregnancies have been forced to rely upon magic, emetics, purgatives, and brute force. In the majority of traditional societies, with their serious dietary deficiencies, parasitic infestations, and ineffective prenatal care, women often consider comparatively mild magic and drugs effective enough to produce a required abortion. This delusion is possible because under these living conditions frequently half or more of all conceptions will abort spontaneously: the woman's own tenuous hold on life precludes her ability to support another life. Various other factors such as blood group incompatibilities, venereal disease, and embryological imperfections due to chromosomal defects contribute further to the "natural rate" of fetal wastage (cf. Haga 1959; Reed 1966). It would be reasonable to attribute the success of a sought-for abortion to the use of magical spells or relatively harmless drugs when in fact the responsible agent was one or more of the foregoing.

In addition, most societies maintain a back-up repertoire of mechanical abuses to be used either in conjunction with the medically ineffective but gentler techniques or as final, desperate efforts to expel the fetus. Exclaiming that "abortions in primitive societies often reach the heights of brutality," Ford (1964:51) provides graphic examples of this multifaceted attack that leaves nothing to the gods or to chance:

> Among the Carib skilled old women give the patient an infusion of bush herbs which is said to induce violent abdominal cramps. In addition, they knead the abdomen, occasionally inserting small sharp sticks into the vagina. . . . The Nama Hottentots apparently have several methods of producing an abortion. . . . The principal abortifacient is the inspissated urine and feces of a rock rabbit . . . gathered from the clefts and crannies it inhabits. A decoction of this, boiled and strained is taken in large doses. . . . A certain thorn bush pounded whole and boiled is also used, while still another method is to keep binding the abdomen tightly round with leather straps until delivery is forced.

Similarly, Goodale (1971) notes that all Tiwi women past puberty are familiar with methods of abortion. The initial attempt involves drinking the juice of a milkwood tree or something very hot, or eating strongly seasoned food. This is augmented when necessary by jumping from a tree to the ground or hitting the womb with a stick. In the southeastern United States, Murphree (1968) finds the same pattern, ranging from carrying nutmegs on the person to drinking a mixture of gunpowder in water to jumping from a wagon or shed.

Devereaux's extended compilation (1955) adds to the distressing picture. In former days in Samoa there was reliance on concoctions from the kava shrub plus "expert manipulation by old masseurs but sometimes a boy simply [put] his foot against the girl's side and [applied] pressure rather roughly." The Pima employed heat from the sun, hot stones, drugs, or starvation, or had the woman climb a rope and then fall down, or, leaving no avenue untried, buried her up to her waist. The Aymara of South America administered a strong laxative tea and then rolled a heavy stone over the woman's abdomen until pain was produced, at which point she was violently shaken.

A final example of the tripartite approach—magic, drugs, and mechanical means—is provided by the Yap women. They are reported (Nag 1968) to have used magical manipulation augmented by the drinking of concentrated sea water. This was followed by the introduction of a thin rolled plug of hibiscus leaves into the mouth of the cervix until injury, blood, and eventually, an expelled fetus resulted.

The catalogue of abortifacients often includes substances that suggest homeopathic or magic properties and appear to be specific and traditional for given societies. Camel's sputum, perhaps because of its expulsive association, has been employed by the desert women of Siwah Oasis in Egypt. Hair of the blacktail deer, mixed with bear fat, was swallowed by the Menomini Indian women, who explained that it would act like magic arrows, darting forward in pursuit of the fetus (Devereaux 1955). The use of raw eggs by the Jivaro, vinegar and pineapple in India (Nag 1968), goat dung by the Masai, writing ink with the pulverized heads of matches (ibid.), many species of powdered, cooked, or raw insects—all constitute ingenious albeit bizarre attempts to dislodge a fetus before more drastic means must be employed.

When these drastic means are considered, the list becomes long and numbing in its descriptions of the horrors involved in destroying untold numbers of fetuses—and often the girls and women who

bore them as well. A Mbaya woman of Paraguay is described by
Devereaux (1955) as lying down, having two women belabor her
abdomen with their fists until blood spurted from her vagina and, in
a few hours, the fetus was expelled. A woman of Nufor Island near
New Guinea consumed "a certain beverage," then constrained her
belly with a tightly pulled sash and had someone step on her
(Devereaux 1955). The Bukaua, also of New Guinea, once employed
many herbs and drugs in their preliminary attempts at abortion but
then moved to kneading and sometimes to pulling the woman back
and forth through a tree fork.

Kneading, euphemistically called "deep massage," and pummeling the abdomen, both often accompanied by toxic drugs, have
been resorted to by the women of Dusun of North Borneo (Devereaux 1955), by the Cahita Indian women of Mexico, by the Mt.
Hagen women, who employed pummeling experts (Strathern 1972),
and by the Miriam women from the Torres Straits. The last group
added the refinement of having a long pole placed over the supine
abdomen, held on either end by two men who then pressed down
until the fetus was crushed (Devereaux 1955). Persian, Pukapukan,
White Mountain Apache, Yana-Payagua, Murngin, Kwakiutl, Greenland Eskimo, Assiboine, and Crow women—all are reported to have
resorted to similar means, many, as can be imagined, with results
more tragic than anticipated by the participants.

In a number of societies an equally traumatic method, but one
perhaps closer to modern techniques, is the insertion of foreign
objects into the vaginal canal or beyond the cervix. In both the
present and the distant past, sticks, rolled leaves, stilettos, roots,
papyrus, tobacco, dry sponges, and a wide variety of other objects
have been inserted as a desperate *modus operandi* to dislodge a stub-
born fetus by the Mohave, Fiji Islanders, Chagga, Hawaiians, Japanese, Bataks, Turks, and the ancient Romans and Persians.

Devereaux (1955) calls attention to the curious finding that
in his massive study of 350 groups, with the possible exception of
the Maori women of New Zealand, he could find no examples of
attempted abortion by means of deliberate violation of a taboo for
which the penalty is miscarriage. This finding raises difficult questions in a consideration of primitive abortion. Are the procedures
followed merely empirical efforts to terminate a pregnancy, or do
they incorporate an element of punishment for any of the myriad
social transgressions? And do the many taboos enforced during pregnancy merely constitute safety factors for the mother-to-be, or do

they also contain an element of social reinforcement of roles? If there were only a straightforward belief in violation of taboos producing miscarriage, then surely pragmatic tribal people would employ violation of the taboos to produce a required abortion.

ABORTION AND BEYOND IN MODERN, INDUSTRIALIZED SOCIETIES

Today, abortion continues to be an important, perhaps even the major, method of spacing children or preventing the birth of unwelcome children. Tietze and Lewit (1977) estimate that some thirty to fifty-five million abortions are induced worldwide every year, with about half of these performed legally. Demographic authorities are beginning to view abortion in a more kindly light, as a realistic means of spacing births that would otherwise appear to be subject to little other control. Davis (1975:29) reflects this view:

> Induced abortion is one of the surest means of controlling reproduction, and one that has been proved capable of reducing birth rates rapidly. It seems particularly suited to a threshold stage of a population-control program, the stage when new conditions of life first make large families disadvantageous. It was the principal factor in the halving of the Japanese birth rate, a major factor in the declines in birth rates of Eastern European satellite countries after legalization of abortions in the early 1950's and an important factor in the reduction of fertility in industrializing nations from 1870 to the 1930's . . . probably the foremost method of birth control throughout Latin America.

In most industrialized societies early pregnancies are aborted by evacuating the uterus by suction rather than by the former technique of scraping, while later abortions are frequently accomplished by infusing salt or hormone solutions into the uterus. In the United States, Tietze and Lewit (1977) report a "complications" rate of 0.5 percent for women who have abortions in the first three months of pregnancy and about 2 percent for women who have waited longer. They note an average of 5.7 abortion-related deaths per year per million women for the years 1963–1967, dropping to one death per million by 1974.

Going a significant step beyond abortion in the commonly accepted sense, a new technique is regular, monthly aspiration of uterine contents. This eliminates in one act the possibility of pregnancy and the inconvenience of menstruation and is now practiced by a number of women, particularly in "self-help groups." According to

Nurge (1975:34), at one university in the United States these endometrial aspirations, colloquially called "bobbings," were recently performed on an average of five women per week. Data concerning inadvertent perforations and/or infections or other undesirable sequela are not yet sufficiently available to compile a safety record for this approach. But in light of the shocking record of suffering and abuse experienced by women throughout their known existence and the apparent inability of males to participate in cooperative efforts to regulate fertility, the resort to such approaches should hardly raise too many eyebrows.

CHILDBIRTH TECHNIQUES YESTERDAY AND TODAY IN CROSS-CULTURAL PERSPECTIVE

SPECIAL ASPECTS OF HUMAN CHILDBIRTH

Every human population that has perpetuated itself for any length of time has had to devise some degree of cultural intervention, within the constraints of human physiology, in the delivery of its children. The selection for large brains and a substantial layer of subcutaneous fat that marks human evolutionary history has resulted in an average of six- to eight-pound neonates with heads of a size that strain the dimensions of the circumscribed birth canal. In contrast, recorded weights of newborn gorillas have been in the range of three to four pounds; birth weights of chimpanzees and orangutans, all lacking the layer of fat found in humans, are similarly low (Schultz 1972:230). Thus, all human births require a variable period of labor characterized by tremendous stretching and contracting of musculature in order to expel the comparatively large baby.

EFFECTS OF SOCIETY ON CHILDBIRTH

According to Haggard (1929:1):

> The position of women in any civilization is an index of the advancement of that civilization; the position of women is gauged best by the care given her at the birth of her child. Accordingly, the advances and regressions of civilization are nowhere seen more clearly than in the story of childbirth.

Haggard (ibid.:5) castigates the brutal religious and superstitious forces that dominated medieval Europe and were accompanied by unbelievably poor hygiene in the newly urbanized societies:

> No greater crimes were ever commited in the name of civili-
> zation, religious faith, and smug ignorance than the sacri-
> fice of the lives of countless mothers and children in the first
> fifteen centuries after Christ among civilized mankind.

As Haggard observes, it was typical of the age that intrauterine tubes (see Fig. 4–6) were designed so that an unborn child, trapped by a bad presenting position or some other difficulty, could be baptized and its soul saved; but no efforts to turn the child or relieve the difficulty are recorded.

Indeed, although a procedure for turning and extracting the child, "podalic version," had been introduced by Soranus in ancient Greece, the technique was lost or ignored for some fifteen centuries so that in medieval Europe the incorrectly presenting child was doomed, and generally the mother too, until the practice was reintroduced in the sixteenth century by the French physician Ambroise Paré. Prudery and ignorance ruled to such a degree in the era immediately preceding Paré that when a Dr. Wirtt of Hamburg donned

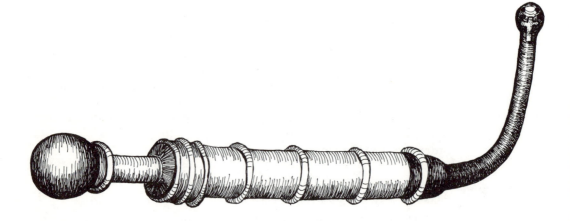

4–6   This baptismal syringe, a relic from medieval Europe, epitomizes a time when the primary concern was the soul of the doomed baby who was presenting incorrectly. When no attempt was made to turn the infant and permit normal birth, this implement was inserted into the uterus, thus baptizing the baby just before it and the mother died. (Adapted from Haggard 1929.)

female attire in order to assist in a delivery and was recognized, he was burned at the stake for his impiety.

It is not surprising that under such conditions, augmented by rampant rickets, tuberculosis, plague, and typhus, legends emerged that primitive women had easy, carefree deliveries. Again, Haggard portrays the process graphically (1929:25–26): "Womankind had indeed fallen into evil days. . . . She paid for the mythical fall of man, under her temptation of him, in the coin of pain and blood and death." So extreme was the suffering of European women during this period that the lot of the primitive female indeed looked good by comparison.

CHILDBIRTH IN TRADITIONAL SOCIETIES

Unfortunately, the record shows that women in traditional societies neither expect nor experience carefree, painless deliveries. With unfailing regularity, these cultures view childbirth as hard work—but not for the mother alone. The unassisted woman, laboring in isolation, is a distorted development of modern, antiseptic Western medicine. Throughout traditional societies, specific relatives, friends, and specialists participate in the birthing, which is commonly considered a community production in which the mother is the chief participant but the attendants play an integral role. As Jordan and Fuller (1974: 7) record for modern Maya villages in Mexico, the attendants "substantially contribute, give the woman mental and physical support, encourage her, always letting her know that she is not alone." Other cultures—for example, the Yukaghir of Siberia—involve the community in the birth process in a more spiritual or homeopathic-magic sense. Ford reports that when labor begins, members of the community untie all knots and unbotton all buttons in a symbolic effort to ease the delivery.

Men are almost universally excluded from the immediate scene, according to Ford (1964), although a few tribes make an exception of the husband, who is always given specific tasks to perform and never permitted to be a mere spectator. Hogbin (1970) reports that among the Wogeo near New Guinea, the husband participates by staying indoors during the wife's labor, opening every box, loosening every bundle, and untying ever knot, in symbolic, homeopathic-magic rituals aimed at facilitating delivery.

Only in modern, industrialized societies does one find a rejection of the services of gravity. In his study of childbirth techniques,

Ford (1964) records customary labor positions assumed in sixty-three societies and finds that none employ the supine position. In sixteen of these societies the woman hangs on to a rope suspended from a ceiling; in fifteen, she ordinarily assumes a sitting position; in eleven she kneels; in another eleven she squats; and in ten there are variations of these positions, all of which accept the help offered by the natural force of gravity (Fig. 4–7). The Nama Hottentots believe that the child would die if the mother were to lie on her back during labor.

Sigerist (1951) notes that ancient Egyptian and Assyrian women maintained a squatting position over ritually blessed bricks after sacrifices were performed to various relevant goddesses such as Nut, Hathor, and Hekate. According to Gann (1918) and Jordan and Fuller (1974), the Maya woman propped herself transversely on a hammock, with her head supported in the lap of a birth assistant.

The Miao women of China (Ling and Ruey 1947) delivered

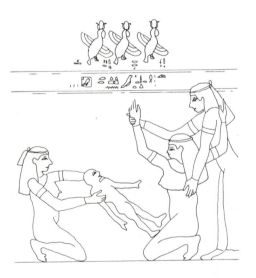
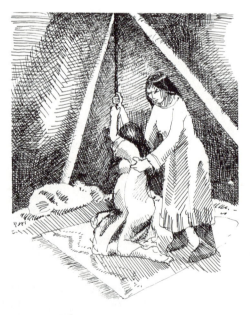

4–7 Various cultural approaches to childbirth. *Left*: an ancient Egyptian tomb drawing of a parturient woman kneeling to deliver her child. This same position is today reported among the Tiwi and other peoples. *Right*: the delivery method traditionally used by many cultures, including the Navajo and other North American Indians.

while standing, with legs apart, body slightly bent, and hands gripping the side of a bed or bench; in case of complications of presentation, an experienced older woman in the village was asked to extract the child with her hands. Similarly, Kessler (1976) reports an account of an "old style" Navajo birth attended by grandparents and many other people. A small hole was dug in the floor and a rope was extended from floor to ceiling. The informant recalls her mother holding the rope, squatting over the hole, and delivering the baby with the assistance of several people.

According to Haggard (1929), until comparatively recently the most common position used by European women was to sit on a stool from which the center of the seat was cut away (Fig. 4–8). He notes that as the midwifery tradition grew, the midwife's trademark became the obstetrical chair she trundled from patient to patient. Not until the seventeenth century was there any mention of the use of beds for childbirth.

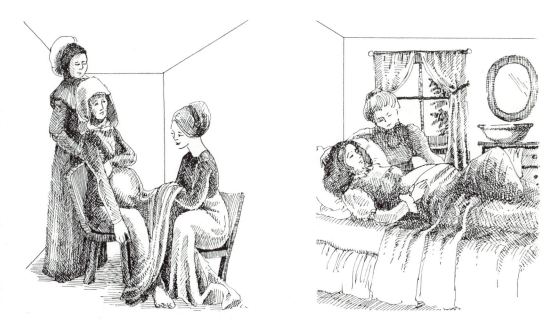

Left: an early European delivery technique, utilizing a midwife's chair and a sitting position. *Right*: the modern Western position with the delivering woman in a supine position. This approach first appears in the literature of seventeenth-century Europe and remains the preferred position by obstetricians in modern hospitals.

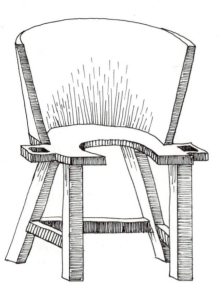

4-8   The symbol of the midwife's trade—the traditional midwife's chair, carried from home to home for child deliveries. (Adapted from Haggard 1929.)

Associated with the modern Western supine position and ob-stetrical customs is the practice of episiotomy, the routine cutting of a section of the woman's perineum in order to widen the birth passage and speed delivery. Newton (1975) finds this practice also among early records of Hottentot and Chagga deliveries but it is quite rare or entirely absent among the overwhelming majority of populations studied. Newton notes that vaginal injury can usually be prevented by the use of relaxation techniques and by support of the physiologic processes that occur during normal childbirth.

A commonly held belief is that labor is a voluntary act on the part of the child who, having achieved a suitable size and age, now wishes to join the rest of his kin and friends on the outside (Hag-gard 1929). Many societies act on this concept and use attendants, music, chants, promises of rewards or threats of punishment, and coaxing sounds to urge the child to emerge. In keeping with this belief, the character of the unborn child frequently is thought to determine the nature of the labor.

Goodale (1971:146) offers a scene of childbirth among the Tiwi in which she participated. The mother knelt with her legs folded under her, one woman sat on a log behind her with legs supporting the mother's back, two other women sat on either side, and a midwife squatted down in front. In all, some one dozen women and children were present for the event of the evening, held outdoors on a hill by the light of a campfire. The children played about, encouraged by the women to increase their noisemaking so that the baby would hear them and want to come out more quickly in order to join their fun. Throughout the labor and delivery, all participated in one way or another, some women supporting the mother physically, others massaging her between contractions, still others heating leaves over the fire to apply to the mother during the various massages, and even the children being assigned an important role in the production of a new tribesperson.

Along with some religious significance the same idea of the child's voluntary emergence was probably associated with the ancient Greek and Hebrew use of specific chants and songs performed by groups of women in attendance during birth. No information has surfaced that would indicate a reliance on any anesthesia for women in labor in traditional societies. Jordan and Fuller (1974:23) note that the hope and expectation are for a speedy delivery but pain is anticipated and endured. They quote their midwife-informant: "The child is born in the center of the pain."

This aspect of childbirth—the presence of pain and the means of dealing with it—affords some revealing insights concerning the position of women in their own culture. Kessler (1976:155), in her discussion of the Sarakatsani women of Greece, observes:

> As might be expected in a society where fortitude is necessary for survival, a woman is expected to bear her pains with dignity and in quiet. During labor she is given a blanket to bite on or to muffle her screams. Other women will talk or laugh or beat tin cans to drown out the noise of the mother.

Paulme (1971:13), writing of tribal women of Africa, is similarly revealing:

> If a woman should happen to have a difficult confinement, her sufferings are usually regarded as a punishment inflicted by her husband's ancestors; she will be accused of adultery and will have to confess the names of her lovers. She herself will be convinced that she is the victim of a spell cast by her husband or by her mother-in-law.

Likewise, Hogbin (1970) reports that among the Wogeo prolonged labor always gives rise to doubts about the woman's honesty and, ironically, she is vindicated only if she appears to be dying and still maintains her innocence of any transgressions. Only at this point will people begin to believe that she must be the victim of evil magic.

A more relaxed and tolerant treatment of women at parturition is indicated in Dupire's (1971) description of the Fulani WoDaaBe of Niger. For the first birth the young woman is permitted to return to her father's camp, where she receives rather solicitous care and is given free rein to cry out when in pain. Even here, however, social expectations toughen as age increases so that at later confinements such behavior is deprecated as cowardly and the woman would lose status for showing such signs of weakness.

Ford (1964) recognizes the universal fear of undue trauma and pain at parturition. He finds that the great majority of societies studied provide the pregnant woman with an ideal of behavior that carries a cultural promise of producing a speedy, easy, normal delivery. Widespread food prohibitions—as usual, almost exclusively animal protein—are rationalized as one method of keeping the fetus small. The Yukaghir of Siberia forbid beef, reindeer fat, larch gum, and fish to the pregnant woman, explaining that their consumption would slow down delivery. The Andamanese of Oceania forbid pork, turtle, and honey, while some pregnant women of the southeastern United States avoid cheese for fear its texture will be transferred to the womb and the baby will "stick" during delivery.

Energetic routines in the pregnant woman's daily life are urged by many cultures, again in the hope of keeping the baby small. But there is also, as Ford notes; a rather widespread belief in the dangers of basket-making by the expectant mother. He suggests that this activity, which apparently symbolizes a difficulty of separation, acts by homeopathic magic to bind the child more securely in the womb, thus delaying the delivery.

The Bena, Fulani, and many other societies consider adultery a cause of difficult childbirth, probably in relation to the concept of "mixing seeds." The woman in labor is thought by the Mt. Hageners to be especially vulnerable to the malevolent actions of ghostly attacks, according to Strathern (1972), whose study presents the many interpersonal and interclan frictions that surface at this stressful time to bedevil the impending delivery.

PARTURITION WITH PROBLEMS
Despite all the precautions taken and all the proscriptions and prescriptions observed, childbirth is nevertheless frequently both pro-

longed and painful; fatal deliveries do occur. Therefore, it is a rare society indeed that does not maintain a stock of malevolent spirits, ghosts, and other forces that become the final explanation for a delivery gone wrong. At this point the mother moves from the center of the stage; her culture intervenes, giving battle to the supernatural forces with the aid of culturally specific experts—shamans, sorcerers, and other specialists (see Chapter 8).

Some peoples do not wait until the evil spirits have moved in; instead, they use their own culturally specific devices to thwart any malevolent emanations. The custom of couvade as practiced by the Charoti of South America is a striking example of this approach to the perceived dangers of childbirth. When his wife's labor begins, the husband seeks to divert the evil spirits by taking to his hammock, mimicking labor, and heroically substituting himself to protect his wife and child. Apparently an ancient custom, couvade was noted by Diodorus and Strabo to have occurred in Corsica and the Pyrenees, and it "has been found by modern observers among [traditional societies] in every quarter of the globe" (Withington 1894:13).

A variation of couvade is reported by Murphree (1968) for the southeastern United States as well as by some Brahmin castes in India. The symbolic presence of the male is incorporated into the birth process through a typical article of the father's clothing. Murphree says that during difficult labor, the father's hat or shirt may be placed on the mother's body with the possible hope of transferring his strength to her or perhaps to divert evil forces.

A more frequent form of magical intervention is the custom of placing a knife, razor, scissors, ax, or other cutting instrument on or under the parturition bed, their customary functions being symbolically employed to cut the labor pains and hasten delivery (ibid.). This practice compares with the above-mentioned Wogeo husband's assigned task of untying all the knots in the vicinity of his wife's labor.

Often accompanying the woman in her confinement, in addition to the purely magic intervention, are prayers, supplications to specific gods of fertility, and culturally ordained sacrifices. The ancient Assyrian prayer intoned at childbirth poignantly reveals the fears and hopes that dominated then, as they dominate now, during this emotionally charged time (Sigerist (1951:399):

> May this woman give birth happily! May she give birth, may she stay alive and may the child in her fare well! May she

walk in health before thy devinity! May she give birth
happily and worship thee!

CULTURAL RESPONSES TO LABOR GONE WRONG

To augment the magical and religious offensives, pragmatic aids are
often employed when difficulties are encountered in childbirth.
Gann (1918) records that among the Maya, when labor persisted too
long, a long coil of hair was thrust down the mother's throat, making
her vomit and thus, it was hoped, speeding up the delivery. Frequently a woman of known exceptional lung power would be summoned to blow into the lungs of the struggling mother in order to
push the child down and out.

Haggard (1929:10) writes that, in many traditional societies,
when labor was not proceeding well, "assistance of the straightforward type might be called into play." The mother might be
picked up by the feet and shaken or rolled or bounced on a blanket.
Certain early American Plains tribes attempted to hasten labor by the
unique practice of "placing the woman on the prairie and having a
horseman ride at her with the apparent intention of trampling her.
Although the rider turned aside at the last moment, the fear inspired
in the woman was sometimes effective in shortening her labor"
(ibid.:11) (Fig. 4–9).

When death in childbirth does occur, it is viewed as particularly unnatural and frightening by the peoples of many societies.
Ford (1964) records that the Ashanti consider it to be shameful;
among the Palaung, horror is expressed and the body is buried in extreme haste; the Ifugao perform special rituals after such a death; and
the Kiwai believe sorcery is responsible for the death and expect the
spirit of the dead woman to return with special vengeance directed at
the men.

Spencer (1966) reports that among the Fiji Islanders, if the
child survives the mother's death, a piece of wood is buried with the
mother in the hope that her spirit will be deceived into thinking the
child is with her and therefore will not be tempted to return to take
the child away. Hogbin (1970) finds that the Wogeo believe the most
malicious and spiteful souls to be those of men murdered during a
raid and those of women lost in childbirth. Normal burial practices
are suspended for such deaths. If the mother dies during childbirth,
she is buried in the bush and the relatives observe no mourning
rituals.

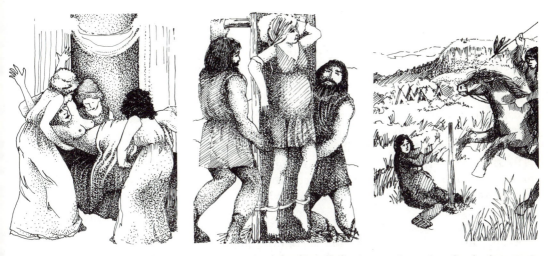

4–9   Three approaches to hastening labor. *Left*: Among the ancient Greeks the woman was sometimes repeatedly lifted and dropped on a couch, in an attempt to shake the baby loose. *Center*: In this variation of the above approach, the woman was tied to the couch, which was then turned on end and pounded against the ground. *Right*: Among some of the prairie Indians of North America a slow delivery was presumably hastened by generating fear, as a skilled horseman rode at breakneck speed toward the woman with the apparent intention of trampling her, then swerved aside at the last moment. (Adapted from Haggard 1929.)

In Samoa, Mead (1928) observed that if the mother died during pregnancy, the fetus was removed after the body had been placed in the grave so that the child might not be born in the grave and return as a ghost to vex its kinsmen. A longitudinal cut was made in the mother's abdomen and the fetus was extracted, wrapped in tapa, and buried beside the mother.

POSTPARTUM PRACTICES

After a successful delivery, Haggard (1929) notes, among most peoples the mother is bathed. In some societies she then returns to her customary routine but, more commonly, a period of isolation and purification follows, often until the cord has dropped off. The purification rituals have frequently evolved into a religious rite.

Whatever form it takes, says Haggard, it serves the purpose of giving the mother a good rest and keeping infections away for awhile.

The high mortality rates of newborns and infants in traditional societies may result in the final cruel irony in a woman's reproductive life (cf. Kaplan 1976). The many perils of early life before effective immunization and resistance take hold, particularly against such diseases as malaria, infant diarrhea, and numerous parasitic infestations, make the survival of the child a most tenuous gamble in a world of no vaccines or antibiotics or proper sanitation. Raphael (1975) suggests that the ever-present danger of losing the neonate may be related to the frequently encountered hesitancy in granting the newborn full human status or awarding the new mother her maternal role.

Not uncommonly, it is believed that envious spirits, jealous of the appealing newborn and the accomplishments of the family, threaten abduction and must be tricked, cajoled, or placated into permitting the child to live. Quimby (1974) describes the Naskapi of the Labrador peninsula and their great fear of the *Katcimedgizu*, spirits who come into the far interior in magical canoes to steal the children. Customs of depreciating the new child, of withholding a name, and of dressing the child in rags probably derive from the fear of losing the fragile being to the evil spirits; thus any means that will fool them into thinking that the baby is not worth stealing may be employed. In our more sophisticated society remnants of these practices can be discerned in the use of depreciating nicknames for young children: "stinker" is one that comes readily to mind. Perhaps the Semitic custom of circumcising the eight-day-old male child is also an attempt to pacify a threatening deity that might be satisfied to permit the child to live on the basis of the sacrifice made.

TRADITIONAL HIGH STATUS AND RESTRICTIONS FOR NURSING WOMEN

As members of the class Mammalia, all human beings are dependent for their early survival on mother's milk or an adequate substitute. Until the relatively recent development of animal domestication, no nourishment other than mother's milk was available and no infant could possibly survive without it. Extended lactation, lasting for several years, as practiced by every society before European contact, probably not only served to nourish the child but, in populations of limited size, ensured a ready availability of wet nurses for children whose mothers had died or were unable to nurse. Moreover, the cessation of ovulation during lactation, particularly in minimally nourished women, has been, and continues to be, one of the most powerful means of pregnancy spacing available for most women.

The nursing mother is universally represented as the ideal of nurturing, benevolent grace. The word "nurture" comes from the Latin *nutrire*, "to suckle." Albert (1971:187) reports that among the Burundi of Africa the best way to thank a benefactress is by means of the formula: "I am a nursing child at your generous breasts," or alternatively "You are to me as a freshened cow." Throughout the world, perhaps one of the strongest, most prescribed taboos is the restriction against sexual intercourse for the mother who has a child at the breast. Frequently the postpartum taboo is therefore nominally in effect for two, three, or occasionally four years, during which time the mother, and sometimes the father as well, must abstain to prevent "spoiling the milk." Particularly, as Strathern (1972) notes for the Mt. Hageners of New Guinea, to become pregnant while nursing a child is cause for ugly scandal.

BELIEFS CONCERNING LACTATION
To produce the milk required to feed an infant, a mother should add approximately eight hundred to a thousand calories to her diet, assuming no excess demands due to infection, preexisting anemias, or parasitic infestations (Cruickshank 1967:13). Nevertheless, scant information is available regarding cultural prescriptions for supplemental nutrients allotted to the lactating mother. Indeed, there seems to be an almost complete disregard for the additional requirement.

Katona-Apte (1975) reports that she found postpartum women in India subsisting on only coffee for three days or more and that for as long as six weeks the new mother was given only one meal instead of the accustomed two per day. Such a meager diet is sorely deficient in foods considered vital by nutritionists, lacking eggs, fish, meat, most vegetables, and milk. Less extreme but similar patterns exist in many societies. The Jivaro mother, for example, is forbidden to eat wild turkey and pigeon for fear the loose stools normally excreted by these animals will be transferred to the nursing child, who would then suffer the dreaded, frequently fatal, infant diarrhea. Likewise, should the mother eat eggs, it is believed that the child will develop yellow feces, another symptom of childhood disease. The Kiwai nursing mother avoids any large fish, believing that the smell will go into the milk and kill the baby (Ford 1964). In India, among the Lepcha of Sikkim, if the baby does get sick, the mother abstains from salt, meat, and butter (Ford 1964).

154

THE CLASH BETWEEN PHYSIOLOGICAL REQUIREMENTS AND CULTURAL PRACTICES

As discussed in Chapter 3, the third trimester of pregnancy and the first year of an infant's life are the most critical periods for the brain's development, a development that is highly dependent on adequate nutrition. Further, the body of the child whose mother suffers from a deficient diet is hampered in its attempts to establish immunological barriers against the myriad parasites and diseases encountered in early life. Dumond (1975) reports that at least a third of the children in nonindustrialized societies who survive gestation, childbirth, and early infancy die from various diseases before puberty. Likewise, Hogbin (1970:141) reports: "The infant mortality is high in Wogeo and only about one-half of the babies survive to reach puberty. A common assumption is that an envious ghost has snatched the child's soul and that the immature body is unable to withstand the shock." Nag (1968: Table 77), comparing thirty-six societies for child mortality rates, finds rates ranging from 4.4 percent among the Hutterites of North America to 48 percent among the Alorese of Indonesia and 50 percent among the Mende of West Africa.

The most critical component required for immunological response is adequate protein. Yet repeatedly, we have found taboos, superstitions, and prohibitions that serve to eliminate or reduce potential sources of protein from the diet of the menstruating, pregnant or lactating woman. At first glance this counterselective, culturally derived behavior might seem explainable simply on the basis of shortage or inaccessibility, particularly of animal protein in societies without domesticated animals. But closer examination reveals that many of the prohibited protein foods are, in fact, rather readily available in the given ecosystems. The denial to women of various sources of protein could well be merely part of the overall configuration of their society's requirement that the symbols of higher status, such as meat, must be awarded to those members who are not biologically programmed to be periodically completely dependent or unproductive.

To an extent not fully known, the generally inferior diets and medical treatment prescribed for women, particularly during the crisis periods of their reproductive life, have the effect of multiplying not only fetal wastage and infant mortality, but also female mortality. The maternal deaths from what Alfin-Slater and Jelliffe (1977) term severe "maternal-depletion" frequently occur among women in their thirties who have had too many closely spaced pregnancies (Fig. 4–10). Indeed, as Dunn (1968) shows, life expectancy among hunters and gatherers is consistently lower for females than for males because of maternal deaths during childbirth, the stresses of multiple pregnancies and deliveries, and, in some cultures, dietary disparities between males and females.

One may indulge in far-flung speculations regarding the seemingly contradictory or at least nonfunctional aspects of the apparent dilemma: the demographically oriented may see a cruel, but effective form of population control at work; the psychoanalytically-minded may point to male envy of the female's dramatic role in reproduction; and, with equal justification, ardent feminists may perceive a centuries-old conspiracy in operation to suppress the status and welfare of women. The explanations are probably as numerous and varied as the points of view from which problems of this nature are

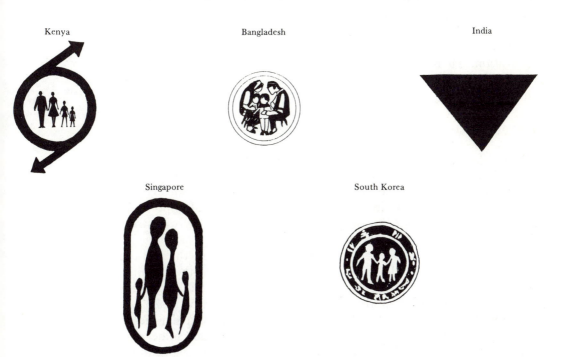

Kenya

Bangladesh

India

Singapore

South Korea

4–10 Representative emblems of planned-parenthood services from various countries. These agencies seek to improve the parents' ability to care for their children as well as to prevent "maternal depletion" resulting from uncontrolled fecundity.

approached. Perhaps the most reasonable position at this point in our fragmentary knowledge of women's reproductive life, with all its medical and social ramifications, is to acknowledge the many puzzling aspects and await more definitive findings.

CONCLUSION

Recent scientific findings as well as popular literature reflect a mounting concern over many of the problems raised in this chapter. In industrialized nations, the move into nontraditional job markets by many young women represents a sharp break with a restrictive past. Many women categorize this past as one that did not permit them the full expression of their potential. In numerous acculturating areas of the world, women are also moving in large numbers from the traditional village environments to urban milieus where they must compete with men for education, jobs, advancement, and self-realization. Their struggle can be cushioned by accessibility of improved health care and social responsibility for them and their children.

The much-heralded advances of women into important decision-making posts in government and production have been accompanied by realistic attempts to ease women's reproductive role through free medical care and extensive infant and child care facilities. These efforts, which stem from the realization that sound maternal and child care are beneficial to all members of society and therefore eminently within the province of governmental responsibility, have characterized those nations that have radically restructured their societies in this century.

Responding to the rapidly changing situation, the United Nations in 1967 passed a momentous "Declaration on the Elimination of Discrimination against Women." Health and child care constituted a critical part of the declaration. More recently, 1979 was declared "The Year of the Child." Slogans may play a significant role in loosening the hold of the past; but slogans alone can become echoes of their own futility. Studies of the past teach us nothing if not that old ways, old neglects, and old prejudices are deeply embedded in all cultures.

Medical anthropology and indeed all the social sciences confront a profound challenge in discerning the cultural impediments to good health as well as the culturally acceptable means of surmounting them. Through an approach that involves a sound anthropological understanding of the beliefs and practices of a given society, the social scientist can help provide the crucial knowledge that could make more widely available many of the technical advances and resources that are now underutilized by the majority of women and their offspring in much of the world.

5

THE NEW WORLD– A DIFFERENT PERSPECTIVE

People were never sick in those days. They did not get sick until they commenced wearing White clothes and the men began to cut their hair.

—Ruth Landes (1971:125)

THE TRUE CONQUERORS

The anthropologist who studies the indigenous inhabitants of the Americas and their past is ultimately forced to focus his or her attention on their medical histories. In many ways the American continents can be viewed as a gigantic laboratory in which were conducted medical experiments on a scale more massive and cruel than the world has known for any other human habitat. The true conquerors were invisible but unrelenting; before the battle had ended, the vast American lands had witnessed what Dobyns (1963:514) calls "in all likelihood the most severe single loss of aboriginal people that ever occurred."

The familiar portrayal of a New World conquered through the overwhelming technological supremacy of European invaders loses credibility when one examines the medical side of the story. In fact, it is not unjustified to claim that the sneeze, the cough, indeed, the ordinary respiratory activities of the Conquistadores, were the true agents of conquest.

In the New World, apparently, diseases such as smallpox, measles, influenza, and later, malaria and yellow fever had been given no opportunity to evolve the truce achieved in the Old World through

159

generations of human exposure to the causative agents. This "working relationship" between populations and the organisms that parasitize them depends on a continuous selection for some degree of resistance to endemic diseases so that a measure of immunological response is acquired. No such process was at work for the native populations of the New World, judging from the catastrophic impact the common Old World diseases had on them. Consequently, in their early years of contact with Europeans and Africans, the indigenous Americans were ensnared in epidemics of such devastating proportions that effective resistance was out of the question.

In addition, and perhaps more mysterious, there is some indication that health conditions in parts of the New World had declined even before the Spaniards arrived. One of the chief protagonists of this view is Dobyns (1963:494) who claims that "aboriginal times terminated somewhat prior to conquest, at least in biological terms. The Inca Empire conquered by Pizarro's few hundred adventurers probably numbered less than half as many subjects then as it had a decade earlier."

THE COLD FILTER

The final word is far from having been written concerning who the first human inhabitants of the New World were, how they got there, and where they came from. Most geological and archaeological evidence points to the shallow Bering Strait, a small expanse of water today separating Siberia and Alaska, as the main area of entry. During the most recent glaciation of the Ice Ages, so much water was bound in the mountainous glaciers that a land bridge hundreds of miles wide was exposed between Eurasia and North America. There is little doubt that thousands of years ago some of the hunters who depended for their food on the mammoth animals living on both continents followed the herds that led them to the New World.

During the climatically unsettled millennia that followed the Ice Ages, much of the formerly frozen water was released, submerging the land bridge and effectively closing that means of entry for any animals, including humans, who depended on foot transportation. Some investigators (cf. Sherburne F. Cook, in Jarcho 1966) believe that there were immigrants from the Eurasian continent as well as from various sites in the Pacific who navigated their way across the ocean. Cook (ibid:114) projects "a very sporadic, casual movement of a few individuals of European or Asiatic origin into untouched areas . . . the recurrent landings of Japanese on the northwest coast of this continent, the Norsemen in Greenland and New England, the very early Spaniards in Central and South America, the voyages of Cabrillo and Drake up the Pacific coast."

Without denying the possibility of multiple "mini-entries" into the New World through much of historic times, one can make an equally strong case for the proposal that the earliest populations walked to the humanly uninhabited continent. Moving with the herds they followed, they would have been unaware of leaving one continent and entering another. In time, when sufficient ice had melted and the strait was once more under water, the populations in the Americas became completely isolated in the New World.

According to Steward (1960:264):

> The peopling of America can be described as the filling of a humanly uninhabited and generally attractive cul-de-sac through a relatively inaccessible northern entrance. In other words, the American aborigine constitutes a major isolate. . . . Obviously, the only mixture that took place here for many thousands of years was that between groups of much the same genetic make-up.

The small bands traversing the icy reaches at the edges of the glaciers would have journeyed through environs inhospitable to the many respiratory, viral diseases so common in temperate and tropical settled communities. In a sense, many generations passed through a "cold filter" during which time innumerable temperature-labile pathogens were strained out. It is also most likely that the populations during the long periods of migration were too small to maintain transmission of many of these diseases.

As a result, when Old World contact was reestablished in historic times, the native American populations were immunologically virginal to many Old World diseases. The thousands of years of life in the isolated American continents had never presented the indigenes with the need to select for resistance to many of the diseases that had existed for much of human history in the Old World. Thus, the sixteenth-century invaders needed neither guns nor military skills for their takeover; the viruses and protozoa they unwittingly carried with them were all the armaments required to conquer the biologically defenseless populace.

There is much to be learned from the fossil remains, the archaeological record, and early accounts regarding the original inhabitants. Dubos (1968:68), like many other writers, records the glowing commentaries of the early travelers and missionaries regarding the physical attributes of the first Americans: "In the account of his travels, Christopher Columbus expressed great admiration for the beautiful physical state of the Carib Indians he had discovered." Dubos compares these people with the Eskimo tribes, who "constitute examples of such isolated groups reputed to have enjoyed glowing health and great vigor despite the harshness of their environment and the primitiveness of the ways of life." And Behar (1968:116) quotes Friar Diego de Landa's moving description, written in 1560, of the radiant health of the children of Yucatan at the time of the conquest:

> They grew wonderfully handsome and fat during the first two
> years. Later their skin waxed dark with continuous bathing
> by mothers and many suns; they were nonetheless bonny and
> mischievous throughout childhood, never ceasing to wander
> about carrying bows and arrows and frolicking among
> themselves, and thus they grew.

In addition to the probable loss of many pathological parasites in the prehistoric long trek across the frigid North, another reason for the reputed healthful conditions of the early Americans was their way of life for most of their existence. Until comparatively recent times, New World populations depended on following herds of animals in order to survive, occasionally settling for varying periods in those areas where a balance could be achieved with what nature was able to supply, and thus gradually peopling distinctly different types of environments.

So long as human populations remained more or less nomadic, the only efficient interacting size was the band, a group ranging in size from fifty to several hundred persons. In such groups births must be widely spaced in order that infants and young children born into a nonsedentary way of life can receive the additional care they require. Under these conditions, population size tends to remain stable partly as a result of the relative sterility that accompanies extended lactation and partly because of the frequently documented tendency for small groups to fission off when the band approaches a size that the immediate environment will not support (cf. Chagnon 1968). From studies of tribal groups living under similar conditions today, it is found that the precarious existence and the difficulties of caring for infants and small children lead to the adoption of such population control measures as infanticide and abortion when new pregnancies threaten the mother's ability to care for her existing children who still need intensive care (cf. Devereux 1955).

The transmission of diseases familiar to the majority of settled populations today or in recent history (smallpox, measles, mumps, whooping cough, influenza, cholera, and bubonic plague) has been shown by epidemiological studies to require large numbers of people in close, continuous contact. As a result of the long trek across the Arctic lands, the nomadic way of life, and the isolation of the American landmass, it is quite likely that the indigenous populations would have had no experience with any of these diseases until contact was established in comparatively recent, historic times (Fig. 5–1).

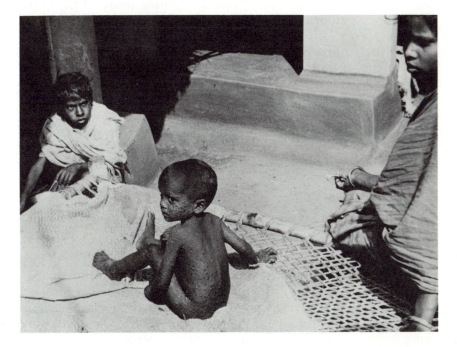

5–1   This child with widespread smallpox pustules lives in the Santhal area of Bihar State in India. Before the days of smallpox eradication this disfiguring disease was a common expectation of childhood in most areas of the world. The children who recovered acquired lifelong immunity to the disease. Lacking any exposure before the arrival of the Europeans, the indigenous Americans had acquired no immunological resistance and consequently suffered devastating losses. (Courtesy of World Health Organization. Photo by Nedd Willard.)

Moreover, Cockburn (1967) postulates that many of the most common diseases probably gained access to humans as hosts during the times when people lived in close contact with the original animal hosts. Thus, he cites the human smallpox virus, which is similar to the cowpox found in domestic animals; the human measles virus, which belongs to a group that causes dog distemper and contains the cattle rinderpest agents as well; and the influenza virus, which has close relatives among domestic animal viruses, particularly that of the hog. Cockburn (ibid.:97) succinctly sums up the relationship: "Man and cow living side by side would share their pathogens."

Except for some use of llamas in Bolivia and Peru, however, early American populations did not tend to domesticate animals on a scale likely to introduce animal disease that could affect humans. The inferential evidence thus points away from many of the upper respiratory viral diseases, particularly those with which we are familiar from present or historical experience, as having been relevant in the lives of prehistoric New World populations.

Nevertheless, from the evidence available, we know that the New World was scarcely a Garden of Eden. As more medical historians and anthropologists focus their research on health and disease conditions of indigenous populations of the pre-Columbian Americas, some of the luster of the earlier accounts begins to fade. Well before the advent of the Old World invaders and their diseases, the indigenous populations already had a wide range of troubles.

PREHISTORIC INDIANS OF NORTH AMERICA

When the Europeans and Africans came to the New World, agriculture had been the mainstay of life for thousands of years in many scattered areas of the Americas. Vast civilizations had risen, persisted for centuries, and then faded. Villages and cities were the habitats of many Indian populations, whose accomplishments rivaled or, some think, exceeded any of those of the Old World peoples. With the advances of agriculture and sedentary living, burials became regulated and today provide valuable sources of information regarding the physical conditions, as well as the way of life, of the ancient Americans (Fig. 5–2).

Lacking translatable records, we do not know what epidemic-

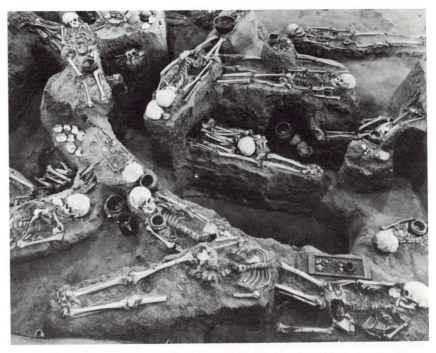

5-2 Extensive section of the Dickson Mound in Illinois where skeletal remains have been preserved in the same setting and positions in which they were found. Note bowls, shells, and other personal implements indicative of ritual burials and belief in an existence after death. (Courtesy of Illinois State Museum. From Morse 1969.)

type diseases, if any, existed. But from medical examinations of burial material, from funerary art and artifacts, and from archaeological reconstructions, we are able to gain many insights into the lives of these people and, importantly for our purposes, to rebuild a convincing picture of the interactions of the various disease states with which they had to contend.

Cockburn (1971:53) reports that eggs of the pinworm *Enterobius vermicularis* "in which the larvae inside were still clearly visible" were found in human coprolites from the Wetherill Mesa cliff dwellings in southwestern Colorado. In Utah such parasites as this pinworm and the thorny-headed worm *Acanthocephala* (the latter native in some of the wild animals of America) have been identified in specimens of desiccated fecal remains found in caves occupied by humans more than ten thousand years ago. These parasites would not necessarily have constituted a grave problem; on the other hand, they never have made a positive contribution to the quality of life.

PREVALENCE OF EAR PROBLEMS

A distressingly common source of pain and subsequent disability is disclosed by the frequent appearance of bony growths on the mastoid processes, a condition called "ear exostoses" (Fig. 5–3). Generally, these are thought to derive from tumors or inflammatory processes. Impressed by the frequency of their occurrence in the New World bones he uncovered, anthropologist Hrdlička (Goldstein 1957) suggested a widespread hereditary predisposition for this condition among American populations.

The same bony growths were often found, especially among males, by Goldstein (1957) in his examination of 348 skeletons

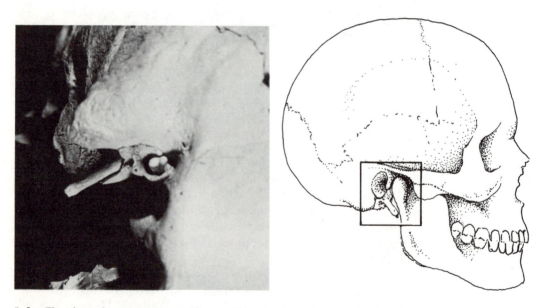

5–3   The photo shows an ear exostosis on a skull from an ancient Peruvian burial. Such bony growths, found with unusual frequency among ancient New World remains, are thought to have derived from tumors or chronic inflammations and undoubtedly affected hearing ability. The drawing shows the positioning and location of the growth. (Courtesy of San Diego Museum of Man. Photo by Mary Edgecomb.)

from populations that lived between 800 and 1700 A.D. in a region of present-day Texas. Ear specialists Gregg, Steele, and Holzheuter (1965:51), using X-rays and morphological techniques, examined 417 temporal bones of skeletons from Arikara burials, from a Plains, Middle Woodland people and from a Sioux population and other indigenous American tribes. Almost half these groups demonstrated changes that suggested to the investigators "a significant amount of infectious middle ear disease during the period of the development of their mastoids."

A similar "startling" incidence of otitis media and hearing loss was reported by Reed, Struve, and Maynard (1967), who observed that this is today the most commonly reported disease for Indians in the United States. Working with another contemporary tribal American population, Foulks (1972) found a high rate of chronic middle-ear disease among the Alaskan Eskimo. He tested the hearing ability of his patients and found "severely impaired hearing" in many of the children brought to his attention.

Foulks attributed the syndrome to the dry, overheated traditional Eskimo homes where nasal passages become irritated and minor respiratory infections degenerate into chronic conditions that eventually involve the auditory system. Apparently the hearing loss is so gradual and insidious that the victim is unaware of it. In their acculturating society, the affected children were distinctly disadvantaged, particularly in school, where teachers frequently labeled them uncooperative or unable to learn. Here again, one wonders how the adaptation achieved under former, more primitive living conditions would have compared.

In light of the observed bone changes, the early Indians almost surely suffered intense pain and marked hearing loss. They would have been at a considerable disadvantage as hunters though probably capable of performing satisfactorily in any agricultural or gathering endeavors. We may never know how these people adapted to their disability or, equally provocative, what adjustments their cultures made to integrate so large a number of partially deaf members. Were there special tasks for these people for which acute hearing was irrevelant? Do the heavily pounding rhythms of the traditional Indian dances and chants reflect an accommodation to a common infirmity? Some insights may be gleaned in a future time from the archaeological record or anthropological studies; at present we confront the dilemma of one body of information pointing to a larger assemblage of questions.

SHORT LIFE SPAN AND POSSIBLE CONTRIBUTING FACTORS

As with so many ancient people, the average life span of the prehistoric inhabitants of North America was quite short. Roney (in Jarcho 1966) describes the remains of forty-four individuals who lived between 600 and 300 B.C. in the Sonoma region of California. Almost 40 percent of this group died before reaching the age of twenty. The oldest person for whom an age could be determined was forty-five to fifty years old when he died. Roney notes that no gross pathological conditions were found in those dead before the age of twenty, nor does he find any indications of nutritional deficiency. He surmises that they died from some acute process such as trauma or infection.

Arthritis appears frequently among the Indians who once lived in the Sonoma region. Roney notes the occasional association with healed fractures and suggests that the disease was provoked by the Indians' rugged life. Ten of the individuals examined had alveolar abscesses. These may have been related to the marked attrition of the teeth, which, in turn, was probably due to a diet heavily dependent on shellfish and other foods cooked by methods that caused ashes and other abrasives to be chewed along with the food. In addition, the distribution and characteristics of periostitis usually associated with untreated syphilis were seen by Roney in nine of the skeletons he examined.

Morse (1969a) examined bones from more than a thousand individuals found in excavations of ancient populations of Illinois. He reports a rather frequent generalized periostitis, which comes from an extension into the bone from an adjacent soft-tissue infection. In related sites were discovered many kidney stones, suggestive of further disease in organs that do not persist in the fossil record. Morse (ibid.:70) found that accidents and infections were numerous, arthritis and bone disease fairly frequent (Fig. 5–4). Teeth, on the average, were good but by no means perfect: "There were examples of most of the dental diseases and anomalies encountered today: pyorrhea, caries, impactions and abscesses affecting both the teeth and surrounding bone."

From the Dickson Mound, Morse determined that the occupants of the site had a short life expectancy and a high infant death rate. Ashburn (1947) cites the large proportion of skeletons of young women in Indian burials as suggesting that childbirth was a relatively common cause of death (see Fig. 4–3 p. 126).

Some insight into the daily life of these ancient Americans

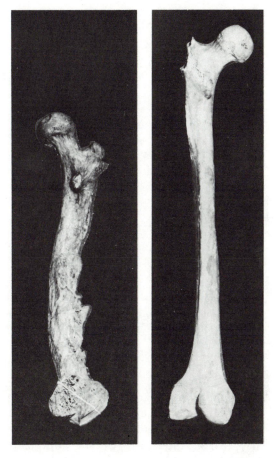

5–4   Two femurs from an adult who lived in Illinois (Crable Site) during the period known as the Mississippian culture. The bone on the right is normal; the one on the left shows severe deformity as a result of osteomyelitis that started before the growth period was completed. The disease process was still active at the time of death. (Courtesy of Illinois State Museum. From Morse 1969.)

comes from the frequent finding of "squatting facets" (see Fig. 5–5). The habit of squatting with the feet flat on the ground and buttocks resting on the heels causes the formation of facets owing to persistent overextension of joints, which brings surfaces in apposition (Morse 1969a.:37). These facets commonly occur in hip, knee, and ankle bones. Snow (1948) found 95 percent of the adult skeletons from Indian Knolls to have squatting facets at the ankles, and Harris

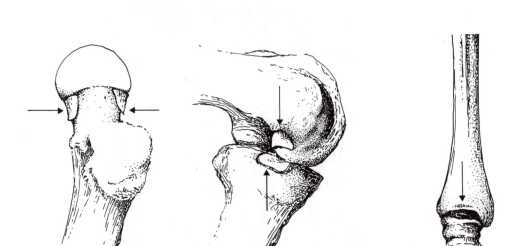

5–5 Years of squatting with feet flat on the ground and buttocks resting on the heels produce "squatting facets" (indicated by arrows), particularly on such stressed areas as hips, knees, and ankles. These facets have been found in abundance among prehistoric American populations. (Adapted from Morse 1969.)

(1949) found the same type of facets among nearly 50 percent of the skeletons of Huron Indians he examined. The physiological strains involved in maintaining the squatting position—evidently a common one among early North Americans—can be appreciated only if the unaccustomed reader tries it for several minutes!

Reporting on skeletal remains excavated in Oklahoma, Alice Brues (in Jarcho 1966) says she found that one-third to one-half of the adults in this population had suffered from severe bone disease. T. D. Stewart (in ibid.) states that an "immense amount of arthritis" was found in a series of 177 adult Eskimo remains, the arthritic deformation being particularly evident in the lumbar region. On the other hand, in a study of eighty-three Pueblo Indians, though the same arthritic pattern was observed, the neck was more frequently involved. Apparently the site of arthritic deformation is in some way, related to specific stresses of a given society or environment, but without firm knowledge of the disease's etiology, no definite statements seem justifiable.

From a large number of burials at Mesa Verde, Colorado, Miles (1966) studied some forty thousand bones from people who had lived there from A.D. 600 to the late 1200s. He found a striking incidence of degenerative arthritis, particularly of the spine, with numerous instances of fused vertebral bodies, even in many of the younger bones. All but one of the individuals estimated to be older than thirty-five years at death had apparently been crippled with arthritis for a significant part of their lives.

For the Texas population examined by Goldstein (1957) the estimated average life span is given as approximately thirty years. Accompanying the premature deaths Goldstein found manifestations of gross pathology or defects among a startling 30 percent of the adult crania and 18 percent of the seventy-three skulls belonging to juveniles who had died before reaching the age of eighteen. Some of the skulls showed evidence of osteoporosis, abscesses of the palate, questionable syphilitic damage, and occasional fractures. The second most common skeletal pathology involved lesions inflicted by various kinds of weapons and/or possibly injuries from falls.

HINTS OF CULTURAL RESPONSES TO HEALTH PROBLEMS

To what extent were these afflictions derived from living conditions? And equally tantalizing, how did these cultures integrate their everyday activities amid the heavy burden of painful ailments? Do the encompassing clan ties and kinship relations, so typical of primitive societies, become an unexplored but critical survival mechanism when disabling illnesses pervade everyday life? The answers to these questions will remain in the realm of conjecture unless future investigations by social scientists put an end to the guesswork. And until medical science unravels the etiology of arthritis, we can merely speculate about associations with arduous living conditions, periodontal origins, or "predispositions."

We do know that during the period investigated, someone living in Mesa Verde made a pair of crutches suitable for a child. The support area of these crutches indicates long, continuous use. In the same area were found two corset-type appliances, fashioned from aspen bark, that presumably were used to alleviate back pain.

In the societies for which we have any information were many individuals who suffered much pain, but we also know that there were people present who attempted to ease their burdens. Much in the record substantiates the concept proposed by Sigerist (1951:198):

If anywhere, then certainly among the primitives disease was not considered a private matter of the individual. It never is, but primitives were quite outspoken in looking at disease not only as a social sanction but also as a social responsibility. When a tribesman was stricken with severe illness, it was a misfortune that concerned the whole social group, and the family and sometimes the community joined in order to readjust the sick to his environment by common action.

Occasionally, perhaps during periods of extreme stress from famines or epidemics, the "common action" may have consisted of ritual activity that also left a legacy disturbing to present-day students. Fowler (1975) cites a pre-Columbian urban-center burial mound on the banks of the Mississippi River, near today's St. Louis, where archaeologists found the bodies of four men whose heads and hands were missing. Below them, lying side by side, were the remains of more than fifty young women, all between the ages of eighteen and twenty-three. Fowler reasons that the pattern of the burial and, particularly, the closeness in age of the women argue strongly against the probability that they died from disease or in a common disaster. He concludes that the four mutilated men and the young women were sacrificed as part of an unknown ritual.

The pre-Columbian record of the northern New World tells us, then, of a population considerably burdened with medical disabilities. Many of the conditions found must have been doubly onerous where survival depended on hunting prowess and a nomadic way of life. Their apparent chronicity would favor the selection of a more sedentary life style, one permitting the rest and care required for existence with arthritis, mastoid infection, kidney disease, and other ailments. It is tempting to speculate that some of the impetus toward settled agriculture derived from these and other medical conditions that conflict with the vigorous requirements of most hunting economies.

More positively, it is equally tempting to stress the evidence of the caring and succoring manifested directly and indirectly by this ancient record. Once again we see that the survival of a given human population was strongly favored by the human ability to cooperate and share. From the medical record it becomes evident that these modes of behavior would have been critical under the stressful conditions that existed. It may also be written in the record, in language we are not yet able to decipher, that humans are quite capable of reacting to such situations in ways that are intelligible only when the true extent of the pressures confronting them are appreciated.

PREHISTORIC SOUTH AND MIDDLE AMERICA: THE INCA AND THE MAYA

INCA MEDICAL PROBLEMS AND CULTURAL RESPONSES

After examination of Inca burials found by Hrdlička in 1913, Courville and Abbot (1942:108) wrote:

> Physical combat seemed to figure largely as a way of life and judging from the evidence of the healed wounds, traumatism to the head must have been common and often survived! Death too was often a consequence of assault and combat, taking place in scenes of violence in which women as well as men played their role.

They note that many of the injuries undoubtedly resulted in severe neurological damage, causing such conditions as paralysis, epilepsy, or loss of speech. Nevertheless, means were found in the ancient societies to fit these people in—no small achievement in view of the prolonged nursing and care that would have been required to survive extensive skull injuries, and considering the injured victims' reduced contributions to the group.

Courville and Abbott find the incidence of recovery from extensive wounds impressive. In addition, they call attention to the scarcity of evidence of infections following injury (Fig. 5–6). They speculate that the Incas may not only have had a natural resistance to the microorganisms responsible for posttrauma injury, but also perhaps great skill in treating these scalp wounds. Similarly, Wells (1964:49) describes a surprising number of well-healed slingshot wounds found in the remains of ancient Peruvians. He also notes a "peculiar double or triple depressed fracture of the cranial vault which can be explained by their use of 'star-headed maces' as a favourite weapon" and which produced a more severe injury.

Perhaps a direct sequel to the frequent use of weapons designed to injure the head was the practice of trepanation, which reached incredible proportions—probably the highest in the world—among the ancient Peruvians. As noted in Chapter 1, many crania of these

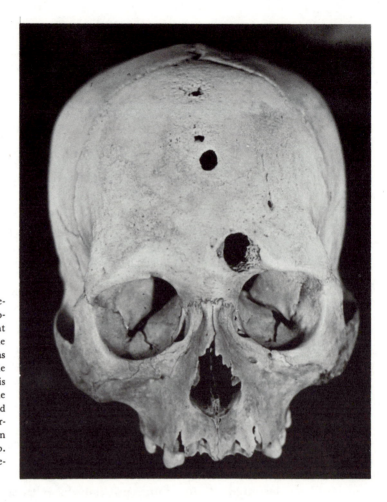

5–6 Cranium from pre-Columbian Peru showing probable wound and subsequent infection that perforated the frontal region of the head as well as the top of the skull. The individual who suffered this trauma most likely lost the vision of at least the left eye and was immobilized for a considerable period. (Courtesy of San Diego Museum of Man, cat. no. 709. Photo by Mary Edgecomb.)

people show evidence of several holes cut and healed over extended periods. Since many trepanned skulls show no sign of prior injury, it is obvious that other factors, probably motivations of a magic or religious nature, were involved. In any case, there is no question that many ancient Peruvians made repeated visits to their local trepanners. The skill and extent of the surgical practice among the pre-Columbians and, particularly, the high rate of recovery from this traumatic operation continue to evoke amazement (cf. Moodie 1923:278; Mason 1971:226) (see Figs. 1–15, 1–16, and 1–17).

It is quite likely that the soporific effects of the coca plant (*Erythroxylon coca*) helped make the trepanations bearable. The coca leaves in the little bags found tied to the necks of many of the pre-Columbian Peruvian mummies attest to the important role this drug played in the Inca survival kit. Less beneficial adjuncts to the use of coca are proposed by Wells (1964:126), who speculates that the "appalling level" of loss of teeth from alveolar osteitis is related to the use of the coca plant. He notes that the anesthetic effect would have reduced sensitivity to sharp spicules of food or other matter that might initiate infections (Fig. 5–7). At the same time, the pain of the resultant abscesses would have driven the sufferer to stronger dependency on the analgesic effect derived from the cocaine alkaloid.

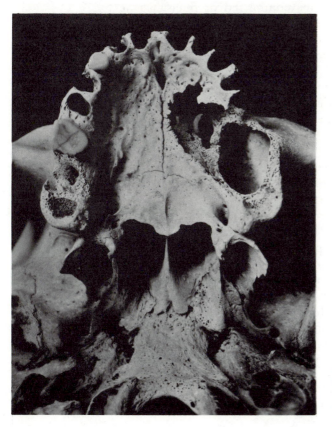

5–7 Underside of the palate of an ancient Peruvian, exhibiting the effects of an extensive tumor. (Courtesy of Field Museum of Natural History, Chicago.)

Like many early Americans, the Inca of Peru attributed the cause of specific illnesses to be some foreign object maliciously placed in the body by an evil sorcerer (Mason 1971). Supernaturally caused, the object could be removed only by magical and religious techniques. Although an extensive pharmacopeia existed, the medications were probably viewed as beneficial for the magical power they provided rather than for their purely therapeutic value. Human sacrifice was deemed necessary to appease angry gods only in extreme situations such as plagues, epidemics, or the illness of a ruler, and in the Maya and Peruvian cultures never reached the fantastic proportions associated with the ancient Aztecs.

Among the Inca, as in many other cultures, frightening infirmities led to a strong dependence on and an awesome attitude toward the priestly class. The priests were deemed capable not only of intervening successfully in a health crisis but of evoking the same traumas from the gods in retribution for sins committed or obeisance neglected. According to Mason (1971), diagnosing and curing were among the priests' most important functions. They prescribed sacrifice, prayer, penance, fasting, confession, bathing, and other treatment. With the generally accepted belief that sin or external malevolence was the underlying cause of illness, any naturally occurring recovery—which all humans experience for most illnesses except the final one—served to maintain and perpetuate the system.

THE MYSTERY OF THE MAYA

The ancient Maya civilization was one of the most magnificent achievements of all time. Long before any contact with Old World civilizations, the Maya Empire arose mysteriously in one of the world's most unlikely environments and disappeared—for reasons that will probably continue to be debated for years. Nevertheless, by using a medical anthropological approach, it may be possible to unravel some of the mystery of the "collapse."

So many contradictions and incongruities are associated with the ancient Maya that the name itself conjures an air of the mysterious. Why would a society choose to erect splendid cities, containing a vast complex of awe-inspiring temples, in one of the world's most inhospitable habitats—the lowland, steamy jungles of Middle America? What were the origins of these people? Why, after almost fifteen hundred years of highly advanced, structured, and productive life, did the Maya culture disintegrate just prior to the tenth century A.D., leaving only tantalizing ruins? (See Fig. 5–8.)

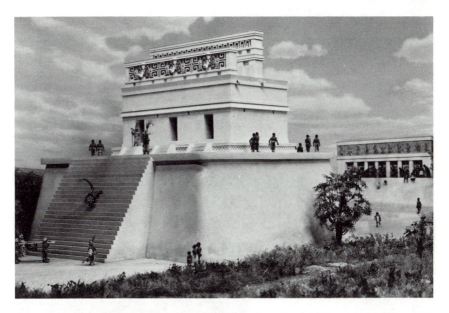

5–8   An artistic reconstruction of part of Chichen Itza, the magnificent ancient Maya city, suggesting some of the splendor of the Maya culture at its height. (Courtesy of Field Museum of Natural History, Chicago.)

Peopled possibly as early as the third millennium B.C. in what today constitutes Guatemala, Belize, part of Honduras, and the Yucatan Peninsula, the Maya area covered some 200,000 square miles. Here a highly developed, complex society emerged, with a flourishing agricultural economy and hieroglyphic writing. Little is known concerning the diseases that afflicted the Maya. As will be shown, much of the medical evidence is hotly disputed by present-day authorities. Nevertheless, from the dominant role given by the Maya to the gods in their pantheon responsible for disease, historians (cf. Guerra 1964) reason that illness and its treatment assumed a substantial role in Maya life. Particularly, from the biographies written in the bones that remain, it is clear that health problems were of decisive importance in the fate of the Maya culture.

THE EVIDENCE IN THE BONES—MORE MYSTERY

As humans seem disposed to do, the Maya were great hands in "improving" on their natural physical forms. Belonging to a naturally round-headed population, they valued long, distorted head styles. They induced cranial deformities among selected infants by forcibly flattening the frontal and occipital lobes between two flat pieces of wood, producing the retracted profile so characteristic of their archaeological paintings and bas-reliefs (Figs. 5–9 and 5–10). Courville and Abbott (1942:126) call attention to Dr. Malcolm Roger's observation that these deformed skulls lack the otherwise frequent lesions. This absence suggests that the distorted crania may have belonged to specially privileged personages—priests, nobility, or other high-ranking individuals. The selection of the heads to be molded must have occurred at or very shortly after birth since the pliability required for the transformation is present only in the extremely young (Fig. 5–11).

Wells (1964:167) notes that the practice of cranial deformation was widespread in the New World, with many variations in the techniques of shaping the skull toward a desired ideal. Evidence of the

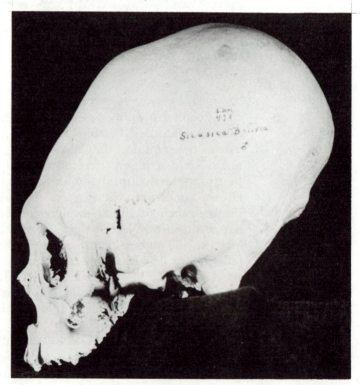

5–9 Ancient Maya cranial deformation. Deliberately deformed skulls are found in many areas of the New World but are particularly noted among the prehistoric Maya. The drastic reshaping of the skull's contours may have been reserved for selected infants who were destined for elevated positions, since such skulls rarely show evidence of any of the wounds found in so many other ancient crania. (Courtesy of San Diego Museum of Man. Photo by Mary Edgecomb.)

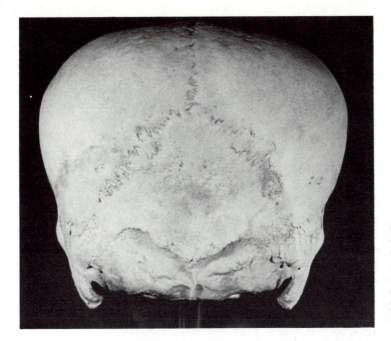

5–10   A pre-Columbian frontal occipital deformation that contrasts with the deformation in Fig. 5-9. The reasons for the particular types of reshaping are unknown. (Courtesy of San Diego Museum of Man. Photo by Mary Edgecomb.)

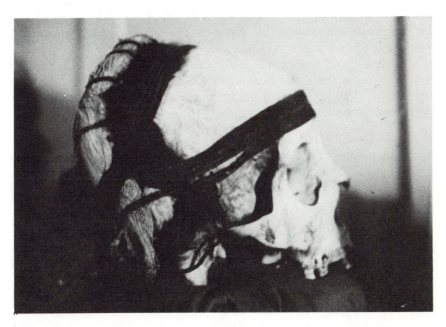

5–11   Ancient Peruvian headdress, probably associated with the coveted skull shape seen in the cranial deformations. Although little deformation is evident here, the headdress was probably intended to emphasize the desired shape. (Courtesy of San Diego Museum of Man. Photo by Mary Edgecomb.)

custom has been found among the Iroquois of the Northeast, the Adena people of Ohio and Kentucky, the Natchez of the lower Mississippi, and the Nootka and Kwakiutl of the Northwest Pacific Coast, but the practice was rejected by most of the Plains Indians of North America. Again the deformations generally appeared to be associated with high rank.

From idealized paintings as well as actual cradle boards, it is clear that the Maya considered crossed eyes a sign of beauty, or at least desirable. This effect was achieved by hanging an object from the forehead of the selected child until cross vision resulted. Teeth were also selected as part of the anatomy to be altered. Jade, turquoise, and pyrites were apparently deemed the most desirable substances to inlay into incisors and canines (Fig. 5–12). And many burials reveal teeth that had been filed in particular patterns, presumably to beautify or to indicate a particular status.

Other depicted rituals or mutilations include bloodletting from the ear or limbs, and passing a cord through a hole in the tongue or through the body of the penis by certain priestly personages. Since all these surgeries required considerable expertise to avoid infection or hemorrhaging, it can be assumed that highly skilled personnel were maintained to perform them.

Our primary concern is the cause of the collapse, even though the answers to the other puzzles raised by examination of the Maya remains undoubtedly are intimately related. The archæological and historical literature bulges with the writings of champions of favored

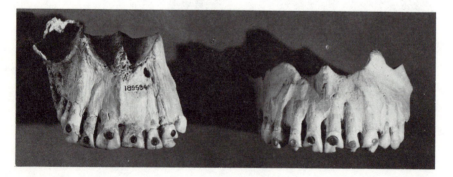

5–12 Maya teeth inlaid with jade. These teeth were "beautified" or "sanctified" during the late Classic period for someone who undoubtedly was a very special person in what today is British Honduras (Belize). Note also the ritual filing of the edges of the incisors. (Courtesy of Field Museum of Natural History, Chicago.)

explanations, which include soil depletion, epidemics, overstratification of classes leading to social upheaval, invasions from the North, and, of course, outer-space connections.

In the view of Guerra (1964:33), "the sudden spread of epidemics—yellow fever in particular—has more foundation in fact [than agricultural exhaustion], and this supports the statement that Maya civilization was destroyed by a mosquito." On the other hand, others (cf. Carter 1931; Ashburn 1947) argue that yellow fever did not exist in the New World until it was imported from Africa in the sixteenth century.

Saul (1972:29), after examination of the remains of ninety Maya skeletons found at Altar de Sacrificios in Guatemala, notes that "the most striking features of the data presented are the decline in the male stature over time at Altar itself and the tallness of both the male and female Altarians as compared with modern Maya." Was this striking, continuous reduction in stature, Saul asks, a consequence of climate, nutrition, or disease, or of their interaction?

EVIDENCE FAVORING THE PRESENCE OF IRON-DEFICIENCY ANEMIA

Perhaps closely associated with the decrease in the size of the Maya is the strange "hair-on-end" X-ray appearance, or, more accurately, porotic hyperostosis, found with uncommon frequency in the skulls of the ancient Indians, particularly in the southern hemisphere (Fig. 5–13). This condition is described by Holvey (1972:1237) as "decreased bone mass, involving loss of both mineral and protein matrix components" and by Moseley (1965:135) "sieve-like porosity involving the outer surface of the skull or parts of it."*

Speculations regarding the controversial bone pathology are offered by Hrdlička, (1914), Hooton (1930), Sigerist (1959), Moseley (1965, 1966), and others. Recently Saul (1972) found the spongy lesions in thirty-two crania of the ninety individuals he examined from Altar de Sacrificios and was able to differentiate the pathology into an "active" and a "healed" form.** In a sacred well in

*For a more recent, comprehensive monograph on the subject, see Mensforth et al. (1978).

**"Active: spongy or corallike appearance of portions of the outer table of various cranial bones and thickening of the associated diploe or cancellous tissue with which the openings in the outer table communicate.... Four showed similar lesions in the vicinity of the metaphysial or growing end of the shaft of various long bones. Healed: smaller porosities, in the outer table of various cranial bones and by thickening of the associated diploe or cancellous tissue ... no involvement of post-cranial bones." (Saul 1972:38.)

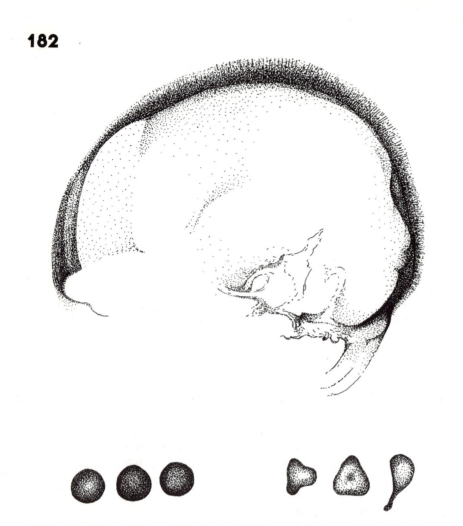

5–13   Cranial bones from a child whose probable age at death was about ten years. These fragmentary bones show lesions of active spongy hyperostosis of probable anemia and were found in a burial at Altar de Sacrificios in Guatemala. (Adapted from Saul 1972.)

The drawing also shows the "hair-on-end" appearance of the bones as revealed by X-ray. Skulls like this one are unusually frequent among ancient Maya and other early New World burials. Much of the evidence associated with these finds suggests nutritional and iron-deficiency anemias. Inserts below depict normal red blood cells (left) and distorted cells resulting from a diet deficient in iron (right).

Yucatán, Hooton (1930) found the same condition in skulls of four-teen out of twenty-one children who had died before reaching ado-lescence.

Sigerist (1951:47) notes that this "strange" condition is not limited to American material, but has been observed in skulls from

Neolithic France, from Egypt (especially Nubia), and a few other regions, although "never to the extent in which it occurred in America and notably in Peru." According to Moseley (1965:141), this bone abnormality "seen so frequently in the ancient skulls of Peru and Yucatan may, in fact, be the result of iron deficiency anemia." This diagnosis is reinforced by comparisons of X-rays of some of these ancient skulls with X-rays of skulls of present-day individuals afflicted with this anemia (ibid.; Moseley 1966).

One of the basic causes of an iron-deficiency anemia, a critical one in relationship to the ancient Maya, is revealed in a common alternate name, "nutritional, hypochromic anemia." According to the hematologist Wintrobe (1951:642):

> A number of factors are concerned in the production of iron deficiency and the consequent hypochromic microcytic anemia. These include chronic blood loss, disorders of the alimentary tract (including achlorhydria, chronic diarrhea and hookworm infestation) and faulty diet. This type of anemia is encountered particularly in infants and in females.

He notes further (ibid.:643) that "hypochromic anemia is common in regions where the soil is deficient in iron and the vegetables grown are low in iron content." Moseley, (1965,1966) on the other hand, stresses the frequency of this type of anemia among young patients maintained on milk, a food containing little iron. But he does not discount the likelihood of anemia resulting from chronic blood loss due to hookworm infestations.

Although several factors often interact to produce anemia, the higher incidence in females is generally considered to be directly associated with a history of numerous pregnancies, repeated at frequent intervals or terminating in miscarriages in which excessive bleeding occurs. Nutritionists are particularly aware of the special biological needs of women, including the normal loss of blood by females during menstruation. Consequently, iron requirements for women are generally given as two to four times those for men. In addition, people who live in the tropics are almost inevitably burdened with intestinal parasites and therefore require a proportionally higher iron intake to compensate for the chronic blood loss caused by the "worm factor."

When the blood stream lacks sufficient iron, hemoglobin stores drop to a level incompatible with health. The affected individual experiences chronic weakness, irritability, fatigue—an "ever-present feeling of 'dead-tiredness'" (Wintrobe 1951:647). Along with the persistent state of poor health, 28 to 39 percent of cases reported by Wintrobe had sore tongues (papillary atrophy) or sore mouths. One may speculate about the seeming coincidence of this type of tongue pathology and the Maya practice of piercing the tongue (Fig. 5–14).

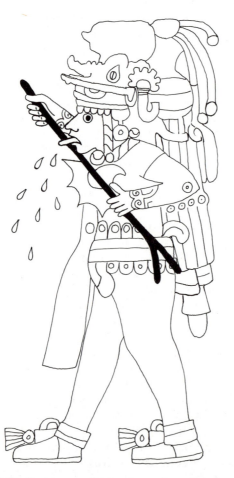

5–14 Depiction of ritualized tongue piercing, from a bas-relief of a Huaxtec sculpture of Quetzalcoatl-Huilocinth. Was the preoccupation with the tongue among ancient Maya peoples a carry-over of possible iron-deficiency anemia and its associated tongue pathologies? (Adapted from F. D. Petersen 1959. Original in Museo Nacional de Antropologie, Mexico.)

In addition to the evidence suggestive of iron-deficiency among the Maya, Saul (1972) and Hooton (1930) find indications of vitamin C deficiencies. They note the unusually large numbers of periodontal pathologies, particularly those found in combination with signs of superiosteal hemorrhages of the bones. From the skeletal remains at Altar de Sacrificios (Saul 1972), only two of the forty adults whose dentition was studied were found to be free of caries or tooth loss. In the less fortunate adults the remaining teeth and the location of the lesions indicate that the pathologies occurred in early childhood, probably beginning at age three or four, thus strongly suggesting deficiencies and/or illnesses during the critical weaning stage. El-Majjar (1977) reports the same condition in 397 (11.8 percent) of 3,361 crania examined from eleven prehistoric and historic indigenous American populations. He links its occurrence to a dependency on maize, noting in particular the traditional presoaking of the kernels in lime solutions (see page 86).

CONTRIBUTING ECOLOGICAL AND SOCIAL FACTORS

Summing up the startling findings—spongy porosities in the crania, suggestive of anemia; widespread caries and periodontal distress, indicating nutritional deficiencies; and the marked decrease in stature from pre-Classic to post-Classic times, probably related to nutrition and health stress—Saul (1972:73) comments: "All this suggests that the Maya at Altar de Sacrificios and perhaps elsewhere, were exposed to an essentially unhealthy ecological setting within whose confines survival was difficult and decline was always a possibility." In fact, (ibid:75), "One might wonder, not *why* they declinded, but rather, *how* they managed to survive for so long."

Apparently the stress was not shared on an equal basis by all members of the rigidly stratified Maya society. Willey and Shimkin (1971) report that the skeletal remains of the elite found in the ceremonial centers do not reveal the same signs of poor health as those of the Maya buried in the outlying domestic-quarter districts. This suggests that the high-ranking Maya continued to obtain adequate nutrition (most likely through imports of animal protein from coastal regions) and thus maintained their health and vigor, while the malnourished peasantry and working masses acquired anemias and associated diseases, surviving, when survival was possible, by forces of natural selection that included less robust growth.

The process outlined was not, of course, an overnight phenomenon. It followed a steadily deteriorating course for well over a century, from approximately A.D. 790 to 950. The unusual abundance of rich soil (cf. Sanders 1973) invited, and made possible for centuries, a highly advanced, densely populated, sedentary society. But the susceptibility of this soil to erosion plus the population growth eventually probably compelled the beleaguered Maya to devise, minimally, a three-pronged strategy: exploitation of new areas for agriculture; more intensive cultivation of those areas already in use; and increased reliance on crops such as manioc and sweet potatoes that yielded five to six times more calories to the hectare than did the traditional maize but were even more grossly lacking in critical protein.

Agricultural intrusion into new and probably vector-infested forest areas, plus adjacent congested and ill-nourished human populations, could create circumstances ideal for initiating epidemics of yellow fever or other diseases derived from formerly undisturbed primate hosts and transmitted by the mosquitos that would multiply prodigiously in the disturbed conditions. Pictures left by the Maya and interpretations of their hieroglyphics depict individuals vomiting blood and displaying other behavior symptomatic of such epidemic diseases (Guerra 1964).

In addition, under these conditions, the triatomid bugs which carry Chagas' disease (a form of trypanosomiasis) could also have been introduced and would have thrived in the thatched shelters of the poorer Maya citizens. This disease continues today to decimate young people living in poverty in Latin America and would have been equally debilitating to individuals suffering nutritional inadequacies in earlier times.

To this dismal picture Willey and Shimkin (1971:110) add the probability of a concurrent increase in maternal and infant mortality resulting from the effects of any or all of the factors projected. Any of the stress situations described could be critical; the addition of the others would serve only to intensify the crisis.

One sees here, in this brief examination of an age-old mystery, a model of the interaction of ecology, economics, culture, health conditions, and social structure, wherein the interdependence of all factors constitutes a delicate balance. The maintenance of this balance ultimately determines the fate of any given society. In the case of the ancient Maya, discordant conditions skewed the balance unfavorably and culminated inevitably in disaster.

THE CONQUEST OF THE NEW WORLD

PRE-COLUMBIAN POPULATIONS

By the time the European period of exploration and conquest had begun at the close of the fifteenth century, many peoples of the Americas were evidently thriving; indeed, numerous areas were quite densely populated. As Dobyns (1963:494) remarks:

> Whosoever gazes upon the massive and extensive systems of agricultural terraces lying unused today on the Andean [slopes] . . . , must perceive that human pressure on land resources has never been so great during historic times as it was prior to Spanish conquest and the introduction of Old World diseases.

The writings of the explorers and of those who accompanied them support this view. For example, the Spanish historian and missionary Bartolomé de las Casas saw Nicaragua in the early 1500s as "the happiest country of the world, a veritable nursery of men" (in Ashburn 1947:15). The same author wrote of Hispaniola, "It is impossible to conceive of a land more thickly populated," and of Tierra Firme (the mainland), "That country is a beehive of men and it seems that God has made choice of it especially as a place for the multiplication of the human species" (ibid.:14).

In 1602, Captain Bartholomew Gosnold (ibid.:16) explored the northeastern American coast and described its inhabitants as "people of a perfect constitution of body, active, strong, healthful and very witty." Similarly, Gabriel Soares de Souza (ibid.:17) had written of the coastal region near the mouth of the Amazon in 1587, "The people call this river the Fresh Water Sea . . . and it is thickly populated with settled and well-conditioned people."

These descriptions were of conditions that were to be short-lived. With the Europeans, and later with the Africans, came what Asburn (1947:xviii–xix) calls

> A secret, unknown army of unconscious mercenaries fighting with equal vigor for either side—an army that walked in darkness but struck in the noonday. . . . And this mortal invisible army of disease killed more white men than the Indians did and more Indians than the white men did and, as time went on, more black men than either of the others. . . .

... It is a rather appalling thought that even (the white men's) sicknesses were more terrible than the red man's and in the end prevailed.

INTRODUCTION OF SMALLPOX

As discussed earlier, the isolation of the Americas, coupled with the human passage through the "cold filter" of the northern passage, had served for many millennia to insulate the populations from the diseases that were common throughout the Old World. Whereas the individual raised in medieval Europe could scarcely arrive at adulthood without having contracted or been exposed to smallpox, influenza, measles, and other "common childhood diseases," the American aboriginal population apparently had experienced no such exposure and therefore no process of natural selection for an immunological response to these viruses had occurred.

There appears to be no doubt that smallpox was completely unknown to the American populations until the time of the European invasions. On the other hand, hundreds of years of continuous exposure had given Old World inhabitants a degree of tolerance so that, although smallpox was always considered a serious disease and dreaded because of the disfiguring scars left in its wake, it was an expected part of medieval life and left more recoveries than deaths when it struck (Fig. 5–15).

Indeed, smallpox was so common as a childhood disease for Europeans that Cockburn (1971:52) cites a notation from Ruy Díaz de Isla, a sixteenth century Spanish physician and writer, who considered it sufficiently unusual to be worth recording that he was acquainted with a man who had not contracted smallpox until he was more than twenty years old! Díaz de Isla, writing in 1539 (in Ashburn 1947:86), offered an explanation that had been given over five hundred years earlier but was probably still accepted in the Old World of his day:

> Smallpox is caused by residual blood in the veins which we bring from the wombs of our mothers, of the menstrual blood in which we are engendered, and . . . each of us according to his nature finds himself strong enough to cast out and get rid of these remains at the age of two or four or ten years.

For the original Americans, however, smallpox was a wholly new terror. They knew no way to avoid it, no way to treat it and within a century following its introduction it had annihilated mil-

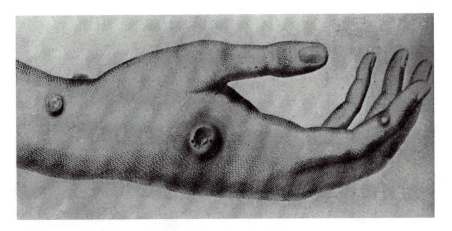

5-15   Cowpox sores on the hand of an eighteenth-century milkmaid. Relatively mild infections of this sort prevented the victims from acquiring the much more serious smallpox that was endemic throughout Europe for many centuries. The relation between minor cowpox infections and subsequent resistance to smallpox was observed and used by Edward Jenner in his work to provide immunity to smallpox. Neither the protection of cowpox nor other exposures to smallpox viruses were available to the native Americans before the arrival of the first Europeans. (Courtesy of World Health Organization. Original drawing in Wellcome Museum of Medical Science, London.)

lions (Fig. 5-16). In Peru alone, the population under Inca rule before the epidemics struck is believed to have exceeded ten million. A census performed by the Spaniards from 1548 to 1553 showed 8,285,000 inhabitants; a census taken in 1791 reported 1,076,122—a loss of more than seven million people (Ashburn 1947:20). The decrease was attributed primarily to disease, notably smallpox. Dobyns (1963) documents seventeen massive epidemics, including smallpox, in the Andean region alone in eighty years of the sixteenth century, with little reprieve in the century that followed. As early as 1563, the six colonies founded by the Spanish Jesuits in the New World were no more.

From the time that smallpox was brought to the American shores until the waves of virulent epidemics subsided (primarily because the subsequent reduction of population made geographic isolation an effective barrier) the loss of life in the Americas constituted the most devastating loss of aboriginal people the world had ever seen. As pointed out by Cook (in Jarcho 1966:115), demographic studies of recent origin indicate a much larger original population in

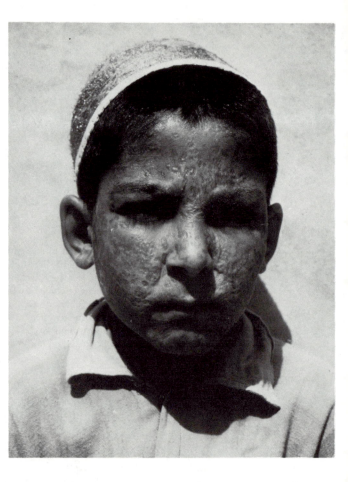

5-16 Smallpox has been virtually eradicated by world health agencies through the appropriate use of medical technology and the social sciences. This Afghan boy, who was not immunized, will remain scarred for life but he is one of the last victims of smallpox. The indigenous Americans, who had had no exposure to this disease before European contact, suffered even more severely. (Courtesy of World Health Organization. Photo by P. Almasv.)

the New World prior to European contact than earlier scholars had projected. Figures range from 100 to 150 million original inhabitants, with at least 300,000 in California and 25 million in central Mexico. The depletion eventually reached the catastrophic order of 90–95 percent.

Brought first to the Caribbean Islands, smallpox appeared in Santo Domingo during December 1518. By late May of the following year, according to Dobyns (1963:494), it had killed the majority of the population there. Early in 1519 it spread to Puerto Rico, with the same terrible impact. By 1520 smallpox had reached Mexico, where it figured critically in breaking the Aztec military resistance and undermining Aztec leadership. Included among the smallpox victims was Montezuma's successor, Cuitlahuac, who died from the infection four months after taking reign.

In short order, Vera Cruz was stricken, then Guatemala, where it killed half the population of Cakchiquel, including two rulers. The epidemic then moved to the northern interior of the Yucatán Peninsula, where the formerly dense population virtually disappeared. By 1524, 1525, or 1526, smallpox had advanced on the Inca Empire, where unknown numbers of people succumbed. Included among them were the reigning emperor, Huayna Capac, then his heir, his brother, his sister, his uncle, and several lesser-ranking nobles, as well as generals and other officers (ibid.:496).

Almost certainly from all accounts of its effects on its victims, the smallpox virus in the New World was of the deadly hemorrhagic type. From today's perspective, it may also be assumed that many of the deaths occurred because of the accompanying breakdown of society. All ordinary functions that maintain life, particularly in urban societies, would be disrupted as the numbers of the stricken mounted. In addition, the inevitable panic must have led to flights from the afflicted areas, thereby adding to the geographical magnitude of the epidemics.

It must have been cruelly apparent to the American indigenes that despite any extremes of sacrifice and ritual employed in appealing to native gods, no intervention by these gods could match the power of the weapons wielded by the gods of the invaders. Under the impact of successive disease attacks, the hold of allegiance to the old gods may have become quite tenuous. The conversion to the Catholicism of the disease-bearers was therefore accomplished with dispatch—so much so that many of the indigenous customs and practices were never discarded but tagged along, producing a blend of Catholicism and native American religion that persists today. At the same time, the driving force of overwhelming distress among the survivors implanted a depth of reverence, with overtones of fear, that remains scarcely equalled in other parts of the world.

The onslaught was no less severe in the Northern Colonies. An account written in 1634 by Governor William Bradford of Massachusetts (1908:312–313) depicts the horror experienced by the Indians when smallpox swept through their settlements and at the same time reveals the immunological protection the Europeans enjoyed:

> This spring, also, those Indians that lived aboute their
> trading house there fell sick of ye small poxe, and dyed most
> miserably: for a sorer disease can not befall them: they feare

it more than ye plague: for usually they that have this disease have them in abundance, and for wants of bedding and lining and other helps they fall into a lamentable condition as they lye on their hard matts; ye poxe breaking the mattering, and running one into another, their skin cleaving (by reason thereof) to the matts they lye on; when they turn them, a whole side will flea of at once . . . and they will be all of a gore blood, most fearfull to behold; and they being very sore, what with could and other distempers, they dye like rotten sheep. The condition of this people was so lamentable and they fell downe so generally of his disease, as they were (in ye end) not able to help one another; no, not to make a fire, not to fetch a little water to drinke, nor any to burie ye dead; . . . The cheefe Sachem his selfe now dyed, and allmost all his friends and kindred. But by ye marvelous goodness and providens of God not one of ye English was so much as sicke, or in ye least measure tainted with this disease.

A less compassionate account is found in clergyman Increase Mather's interpretation of the smallpox epidemics among the Indians in contact with the British colonies (Mather 1864:110):

About this time [around 1630] the Indians began to be quarrelsome . . . but God ended the Controversy by sending the Smallpox amongst the Indians of Saugast, who were before that time exceeding numerous. Whole Towns of them were swept away, in some not so much as one soul escaping the Destruction.

In like manner, another Puritan wrote that "by this means Christ made room for his people to plant" (in Ashburn 1947:22). Similarly, Gonzalo Fernández de Oviedo y Valdés, a Spanish chronicler who had been governor of Santo Domingo, reported to his masters in Spain that Columbus "found here, when he discovered the islands, a million or more Indians . . . of all of whom and of those born later there are not now believed to be in this year of 1548 five hundred people" (ibid.:21). He continues in the same vein but concludes that the reason for the epidemics was that "God repented having made such ugly, vile, and sinful people and that it was His will that they should die" (ibid.:22).

THE IMPACT OF MEASLES

To those who had somehow survived the smallpox attacks, it must indeed have seemed that a curse had fallen on their lands for within a decade after smallpox began its predations, a new scourge appeared. In 1529, measles swept through the island entrances to the Americas. Dobyns records that two-thirds of the Indians left alive in Cuba died in that year; and by 1531 one-half of the population of Honduras succumbed as the virus began its murderous pathway through Central America.

Tracing the probable route of the disease, Dobyns shows how measles was spread southward among the Incas by the European conquerers, particularly the messengers, troops, and colonists, and the missionaries who accompanied them in their constant movement among the Andean people. He pinpoints the travels of the Dominican and Franciscan friars who had gone from infected Nicaragua to Peru in the beginning stages of Pizarro's conquest, returning to Panama in early 1532. They could well have borne the virus directly from Nicaragua to the coastal hinterland of the Andes.

It cannot be determined if the particular strain of measles that struck at that time was entirely responsible for the profound impact of the disease or whether the lack of former immunizing exposure alone was the decisive factor. Undoubtedly, the onslaught of smallpox that preceded and the subsequent social disruption fostered by each of these diseases contributed critically to turning this generally inconsequential disease into a mass killer.

NEW EPIDEMICS

More horror was to come. In 1557 a severe epidemic of influenza swept through Europe and was carried from Spain to the West, adding to the other catastrophes that besieged the natives of the New World. Like the measles and smallpox varieties, the virus responsible for the influenza seemed to acquire increased virulence when it encountered the new population.

Threading its way through the other onslaughts of disease that threatened to extirpate the entire New World population was a disease as yet unidentified by modern epidemiologists. So intense was its impact in Peru in 1546 that, according to contemporary reports, countless people died and even the llamas and sheep were stricken (Dobyns 1963:499). The Aztecs called the disease *matlazahuatl,* a name that implies a rash similar to, but different from, smallpox or measles. Additional symptoms included raging fevers and hemorrhaging from the nose. Zinsser (1934:257–258) theorizes that typhus may have been the disease responsible while Ashburn (1947:95–96) argues that, because of the conditions of filth, crowding, and lice vectors required for its transmission, typhus would have been "almost un-known in the low, hot, moist coastal regions, where little clothing is worn and where that which is used is often washed, and the bodies are bathed daily." Asburn's argument, however, does not take into account the chaotic conditions produced by the epidemics that must have preceded *matlazahuatl*.

A contemporary historian of Arequipa, as reported in Dobyns (1963:507), thought a similar contagion in 1589 was "at the same time smallpox, scarlet fever and measles with such a revolution of the bile that they were complicated by furious fevers." The description by Dobyns of this syndrome reveals the terror that must have gripped the populace:

> The onset of the disease brought severe headaches and kidney pains. A few days later, patients became stupefied, then delirious, and ran naked through the streets shouting. . . . Ulcerated throats killed many. Fetuses died in the uterus. Even patients who broke out in a rash might lose chunks of flesh by too-sudden movement.

It was common, Dobyns notes, to lose the facial skin, including the lips or the nose, so that only the bone-work remained. Victims, of whom no count was possible, were interred in open ditches during the three-month episode. When the epidemic reached Peru, a Jesuit Provincial recorded (in ibid.), "Virulent pustules broke out on the entire body that deformed the miserable sick persons to the point that they could not be recognized except by name." By 1590, Chile began to experience the same horror, and it was reported that the epidemic eventually destroyed three-quarters of that land's Arau-canian Indians.

It is quite likely that the true agent involved may never be known. The elements that created the near annihilation—an immuno-logically defenseless population brought into sudden contact with diseases for which no effective prevention or treatment were avail-able—no longer exist in any degree remotely comparable to that at the time of the conquest. This was, as Ashburn (1947:5) puts it, "medical history writ large," for "this was the greatest mobilization of disease, of its introduction to new and susceptible peoples, the most strking example of the influence of disease upon history, of which we can speak with any certainty." And he writes of the incal-culable impact of smallpox, typhus, and measles:

> More terrible than the conquistadores on horseback, more
> deadly than sword and gunpowder, they made the conquest
> by the whites a walkover as compared with what it would
> have been without their aid. They were the forerunners of
> civilization, the companions of Christianity, the friends of
> the invader. (Ibid.: 98.)

Although the picture with all its horror is known, the toll was
nevertheless so overwhelming that many still question why isolated
or primitive groups have such appallingly high mortality rates when
first exposed to diseases like smallpox, measles, and influenza. Cockburn (1971:59) asks:

> Is this high mortality due to a basic susceptibility of genetic
> origin, or to cultural factors, or simply to the collapse of a
> precarious economy when all become ill at one time? If it is
> the latter two, then death occurs from starvation, thirst,
> or lack of care.

It is probably futile to attempt to separate the factors involved.
Even today, a death certificate that implicates one specific disease
agent oversimplifies by ignoring a background of poor nutrition, poverty, and poor nursing care. Undoubtedly, a resistance based on
many generations of selection for immunological response to a particular disease, coupled with a strong, well-organized society, provides the best defense against any disease. Under the conditions outlined for the New World at the time of the invasions, the initiating
factor was lack of immunological preparation; the other elements
quickly became relevant and, perhaps, at some points became the
major contributors to the irreversible cycle of disease and tragedy
that followed.

In historical perspective, because of the catastrophic confluence
of all the factors described, the world will never know what heights
the civilizations of the aboriginal populations of the Americas might
have attained. Unlike the Maya civilization that had waned by the
time the Europeans arrived, other cultures throughout the New
World were struck down at their pinnacle. To an unknown extent,
the roots of much of the poverty, sickness, and demoralization in the
Latin American world today can be traced to the encounters with
overwhelming disease, the true agents of conquest, almost five hundred years ago.

SLAVERY AND DISEASE

On first inspection, it may appear a gross overstatement to suggest that the roots of African slavery in the New World stemmed from relative resistance to disease. Yet on closer examination this proposal does acquire considerable substance: the record shows that enslavement of the Africans brought in chains to the Americas was lucrative largely because of their ability to survive the diseases that destroyed other populations. The natives of the New World could not be profitably enslaved because they succumbed to the diseases brought by the foreigners; the Europeans could not be counted on to perform labor worth exploiting since they too were destroyed by the disease conditions they brought with them in the form of captives from the tropics. Only the African populations who had emerged through centuries of selection for resistance to the diseases of both continents could survive in sufficient numbers and with enough strength to make the plantations of the New World worth the investments of Europe's royalty and rising entrepreneurial class.

IMMUNOLOGICAL DIFFERENCES CONTRIBUTING TO AFRICAN ENSLAVEMENT

Slavery was introduced into the West Indies in 1501 or earlier, according to Ashburn (1947:30). In 1501 a royal edict permitted slaves to be transported to Hispaniola, and within a few years many of the first settlers were taking full advantage of that edict. Ironically, the vast trade in human cargo—numbering some ten million persons before the institution of slavery was abolished—was not the initial strategy employed by the European colonizers. As outlined by Curtin (1968:193):

> The Europeans experimented with a number of alternative locations and forms of development between 1500 and the middle of the seventeenth century. . . . The solution of the early planners was thus empirical; trial and error showed that the expedient of importing labor from Africa to the American plantations succeeded, while other alternatives failed.

The other alternatives included attempts to establish plantations along the Gulf of Guinea and efforts (by the Portuguese) to exploit the Congo. In the New World, the Spanish and Portuguese set up plantations in Brazil and Hispaniola, where labor was based on enslaved Indians. France and England made similar efforts in the Americas, using convict or contract European labor.

The enterprises in Africa failed because the European managers and missionaries could not survive the tropical diseases, particularly malaria, sleeping sickness, and other parasitic infestations from which they had no protection. Mannix and Cowley (1962:13) state:

> It was chiefly mosquitoes and malaria dengue and yellow fever, that protected the vast continent from conquest and even exploitation. One portion after another of the African coast—first Senegambia, then Sierra Leone, then the Bight of Benin—was called "the white man's grave."

But the English undeterred,

> kept sending out new recruits, with no consideration for the risks they ran. Some of them died on the day of the arrival, and half of them were dead in two years, which was regarded as the average term of life for an Englishman on the Guinea Coast. (Ibid.:79.)

Statistics derived from later British military personnel illustrate the obstacles encountered by the colonial powers as they attempted to exploit new territories. Whereas the civilian mortality rate among males of military age in England from 1817 to 1936 was 11.5 per 1,000, in the African Gold Coast it was 668 per 1,000. And during the same period the mortality rate among African troops in Sierra Leone was 2.5 per 1,000. Obviously no permanent exploitation could succeed if based on the transplantation of European colonists to Africa.

ECONOMIC RELATIONSHIPS

Curtin (1968) states that, despite the terrible conditions of the notorious middle passage and subsequent ill-treatment, the Africans transported to the New World, nevertheless outlived a comparable group of Europeans by a ratio of 3.2:1. From a purely economic point of view, assuming that the cost of maintaining an indentured white worker or an African slave was the same, "the slave was profitable at anything up to three times the price of the European" (ibid.: 207). Thus, acceptable profits would not be forthcoming if they depended on Europeans laboring on the New World plantations.

And profit was the name of the game, the primary goal toward which the slave trade was directed. At first, the trade was in the hands of pirates and privateers, but it quickly became too lucrative not to develop into an organized business, endorsed by government and blessed by church authorities. After his initial slaving voyage in 1562, Sir John Hawkins, the first English systematic slave trader, became the wealthiest man in Plymouth; after his second trip, he was the richest man in England (Langdon-Davies 1965). In the treaty that ended the War of Spanish Succession, signed at Utrecht in 1713, England secured the monopoly for supplying the Spanish colonies of the New World, with one-quarter of the profits to revert to the British Crown.

Before the slave trade, the native Americans were already dying in numbers that threatened annihilation, from diseases such as small-pox, measles, and influenza, all introduced by the very people who wished to exploit their labor. Then when African labor began to be introduced into the New World, the diseases that accompanied the slaves—malaria, sleeping sickness, and perhaps, yellow fever—provided the *coup de grâce* that killed or enervated most of those Indians who remained. Hence, the third alternative, native American labor, became unsuitable for the financial returns demanded by the Royal Companies.

INTERRELATIONSHIPS OF MALARIA AND SLAVERY

As will be shown in Chapter 7, after the devastation caused by the first-introduced viral agents had subsided, the most critical agent, so far as establishing plantations in the New World was concerned, was the protozoa responsible for malaria, especially the most virulent form, *Plasmodium falciparum*. Immunological resistance to this disease is achieved only by continual exposure from infancy through childhood. For populations lacking early exposure, falciparum malaria kills vast numbers of people and periodically debilitates those who survive.

Under the epidemic conditions that prevailed once malaria had obtained a foothold in the Americas, virtually no one was spared. Only the Africans who had grown up in endemic areas possessed the biological and genetic mechanisms to withstand its onslaughts. For example, only those populations in long contact with malaria possess sickle-cell heterozygosity, as well as other hemoglobin variations such as hemoglobin C and E, all of which have been shown to enhance the powers of resistance to the virulent protozoa. Consequently and trag-ically, the Africans became the only people capable of performing the labor and surviving under the conditions prevailing in the New World after the conquest.

HEALTH CONDITIONS AND SLAVERY

Even though the Africans "succeeded" to their unenviable position as the only population that could survive under slavery in the Americas, this proposal should in no way be interpreted as minimizing the conditions of cruelty and degradation that accompanied the "peculiar institution" (Fig. 5–17). Almost from the first days there were revolts: at the sites of origin, aboard the ships of transport, and at the final destination. At no time were the conditions of slavery such that the slave population could or would reproduce sufficiently to sustain an enslaved corps. Those who sought to profit from enslaved labor had to maintain slave numbers by continuing the trade in humans. Because the slave traders realized a higher profit from the sale of male slaves, the population remained out of balance. Perhaps more important, enslaved women chose, whenever possible, not to bring forth children under conditions of slavery; and, as might be predicted, those infants and children who were born suffered an exceedingly high mortality rate. Complete figures are not available for the excess of deaths over births but the death rate in general was notoriously high. For example, in one year on the island of St.

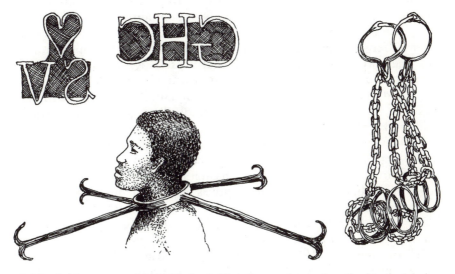

5–17 Implements associated with the traffic in human slaves: a branding iron for burning the owner's initials into the flesh of the slave; a neck halter that linked slaves together during transport and was sometimes used to punish rebellious slaves. (Adapted from Clarkson 1808.)

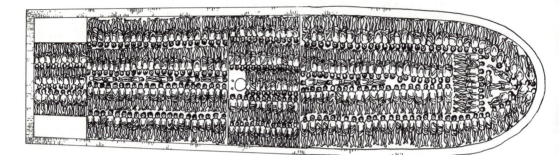

5-18   Conditions of the "Middle Passage" are typified by this diagram, which a slave owner submitted to an insurance company to indicate the "efficient" packing of the human cargo by using every available inch of space on the slaving ship *Brooks*. Under such conditions disease was rampant and 25 to 40 percent of the slaves died before reaching the New World market. (Adapted from Clarkson 1808.)

Vincent there were 2,656 births but 4,205 deaths. A comparison of population figures with the number of slaves continuously imported is equally suggestive of a nonsustaining population.

The incredible crowding, miserable food, and deplorable sanitation suffered in passage provided almost unparalleled opportunities for the spread of any infection that arose (Fig. 5-18). Dysentery (then called "the bloody flux"), hookworm, sleeping sickness, smallpox, and, most dreaded, scurvy, were rampant. As described by Mannix and Cowley (1962:121): "The Middle Passage was a crossroads and marketplace of diseases."

The crude attempts to save the costly cargo, such as dosing with white lead to treat the hookworm infections and forced exercise to cure scurvy, often served only to hasten the end. Figures from ships' logs reveal that the loss of the captives making the infamous passage exceeded 25-40 percent. Mannix and Cowley state that only one slave was added to the New World labor force for every two purchased on the Guinea Coast. DuBois (1947) estimates that from 1713 on, between 40,000 and 100,000 Africans were exported for enslavement every year. The practice lasted almost four centuries, during which time, according to Mannix and Cowley (1962:287), "it had involved, by a conservative estimate, the forced migration of fifteen million Negroes, besides causing the death of perhaps thirty or forty million others."

Exceeding even the high death toll during passage was the toll among the captured people who perished either in the inhuman caravans and camps that preceded the ocean crossing or from the treatment encountered after arrival in the New World. According to Ashburn (1947:32), it is doubtful if one-quarter of all captured Africans survived for the purpose for which they were enslaved.

Still the plantations of the New World clamored for more and more slaves. One of the chief sources was Angola, then governed by the Portuguese throne. The government endorsed the trade with one stipulation (in addition to the demand for sizable return of the profits to the government): the Africans sold into slavery must be baptized immediately before being shipped or else immediately after being unloaded. In recognition of the odds against survival, it was advocated that the former was more judicious.

In keeping with the tortuous rationalization that accompanied the traffic in humans, the colonies were ready to deal with the dilemma that arose regarding the enslavement of those survivors who had been baptized and, thereby, were Christians. In 1667, Virginia colony ruled that baptism provided for freedom in heaven; it did not confer freedom on this earth. Maryland followed suit four years later, then New York and other colonies. Baptized or not, however, those Africans who did survive represented the end product of a selection for disease resistance and pure physical endurance that few, if any, populations had ever been called upon to withstand.

HEALTH CONDITIONS OF SOME PRESENT-DAY INDIANS

The evidence examined thus far was derived primarily from bones and histories of individuals long dead. Attempts to reconstruct aspects of the culture and state of health of the people examined have depended largely on circumstantial and retrospective information. But a major part of anthropology is concerned with living populations, particularly those remaining few—the hunters and gatherers— whose conditions of life most closely approximate those that prevailed during the first 99 percent of human existence. It is estimated (Neel 1971) that approximately two million unacculturated Indians survive in the New World today. Yet there is a deplorable dearth of information concerning the health or diseases of such people. Opportunities to study their societies are rapidly disappearing as these people vanish or become assimilated into the agricultural or urban worlds that engulf them.

STUDIES OF GE-SPEAKERS OF SOUTH AMERICA
Several investigators have made an invaluable contribution to science in general and anthropology in particular by conducting in-depth studies of a number of villages of the Ge-speaking Indians of southern Venezuela and northern Brazil in which live the Xavante, Yanomamo, and a few Makiritare (Chagnon 1968; Chagnon et al. 1968; Neel 1971; Neel and Chagnon 1968; Neel and Salzano 1967; Neel et al. 1964, 1968; Salzano, Neel and Maybury-Lewis 1967; Weinstein, Neel, and Salzano 1967). These villagers represent some of the few surviving unacculturated populations of the New World, and possibly are descendents of peoples who were among the earliest inhabitants of the South American continent.

Over the past decade the leaders of the investigations have brought together anthropologists, physicians, dentists, epidemiologists, geneticists, immunologists, virologists, and other experts in various fields concerned with human biology. They have ventured again and again into the tropical forests in order to study the inhabitants. Each expedition has amassed information that offers important insights into our human ancestry, and, as might be expected, each has raised almost as many problems. Coincidentally, the groups of scientists have also been frequently called on to provide life-saving aid during medical emergencies.

Except for a brief period of peaceful contact with Brazilian soldiers and colonizers in the late eighteenth century, followed by more than a century of enmity—which resulted incidentally, from an epidemic of measles in the wake of the initial contact—no sustained contact with non-Indians was experienced by these Ge-speakers until 1950. Neel and Chagnon (1968) report that most of the villagers they studied had had no prior encounter with non-Indians.

The villages are composed of beehive-shaped huts that are used for only a few years. The majority of the villagers do not stay in the compounds. For most of the year the villages are essentially deserted as the Indians travel in a wide arc within their territory, gathering and hunting as they move, and returning to the base after several months. Illness and death are viewed as results of malevolent sorcery and frequently are the basis for disputes that lead to factions hiving off to join other villages or to establish their own new base.

The long isolation of this population is emphasized by the complete homogeneity of various aspects of their physiology. Everyone tested was found to be blood group 0 and Rh-positive (D+); all have a uniformly round, broad facial structure, normal color vision, and copper-brown skin pigmentation. Although the fertility rate was not found to be notably high, all but one of the women of reproductive age had given birth to at least one child.

"SUPERB PHYSICAL SPECIMENS"
Every investigator was struck by the "exuberant health and vitality" exhibited by both children and adults. Neel and Salzano were led to exclaim (1967:566):

> The young Xavante is a surperb physical specimen. Health is more than freedom from disease. An American population is healthy but fails to project the sense of vitality and physical resilience of the Xavante. There are differences by the more objective criteria we attempt tu use—specifically, the musculature, the keen vision, the lack of dental caries, the slow pulses, and the low blood pressure—but these tell only a fraction of the story.

Unfortunately, the picture of glowing health was marred by at least three factors. First, the exuberance was not shared equally by both sexes—the females fared much more poorly. Second, despite the stated practice of killing malformed children at birth, an unduly high number of congenital birth defects were observed. Finally, elders were almost nonexistent; as in so many of the cultures we have examined, life span on the average is almost one-half that expected by humans in much of today's world.

THE DIFFERENT HEALTH WORLDS OF THE MEN AND THE WOMEN
Some of the studies have furnished partial answers to these enigmas. Neel et al. (1964:110) write, "Indeed, one of the most striking impressions of this study was of different medical worlds of men and women." Particular attention was drawn by all investigators to the women's early aged appearance and premature loss of youthful vitality. Weinstein, Neel, and Salzano note (1967:540): "On the basis of a number of observations, the women are less healthy and obviously under greater biological pressures."

Palpable spleens, a common stigma of chronic malarial infestation, were found in fifteen of seventy-eight persons examined.

Twelve of these fifteen were female. This may be because women remained longer in one place to care for the children or the sick, thus exposing themselves to the mosquito vectors of malaria that generally favor settled areas. Carious teeth were found in some women, none in the men. Is this a factor of dietary differences that act in favor of the males? No cardiac murmurs were detected in the males; they were relatively frequent, although not severely pathological, among the women. It was more often the women who were unable to perform the visual acuity tests.

Unfortunately, many of the data that would be relevant to the apparent health differential between the sexes of these seminomadic Indians are not available because the field work was conducted primarily by males. The fact that virtually every woman had borne one or more children indicates an unusually high fertility rate. At the same time, the rather low number of children per woman—approximately three living children for females who had completed their reproductive life—was in part a result of the high loss of young children. The Xavante reported a 33 percent loss and the Yanomamo, 16 percent; both groups acknowledge a culturally accepted practice of infanticide.

The low number of children may also, however, suggest recourse to abortion practiced on a rather extensive scale. In this quite primitive existence, abortions would necessarily be conducted under unfavorable conditions. Neel and Salzano (1967) report the use of herbs to prevent conception and of herbs and "trauma" to induce abortion. The exact meaning of "trauma" is left to the imagination but it is not likely to involve mechanisms conducive to exuberant health.

In other studies (Neel et al. 1964) found that the average hemoglobin levels among the Xavante were surprisingly low, particularly in light of the robust health reported. The average level among the women was 10.9 grams per 100 milliliters of whole blood, which is in a range associated with anemia by universal medical standards. In addition, microscopic examinations of blood specimens revealed red blood cell morphology typical of moderate to severe anemia. Male hemoglobin levels averaged 12.35 gm./100 ml. blood, approximately 3–4 grams or 25 percent lower than would be expected for healthy males in the United States.

These findings, coupled with indications of intestinal parasitic infestations and poor sanitation in the home bases, may in part account for the deleterious condition of the women as compared with the health of the men. It might be most rewarding to include medically trained and anthropologically skilled women in future expeditions in order to obtain more detailed information about these Indian women, whose conditions of life may most nearly approximate those for women through most of human history.

APPEARANCE VERSUS REALITY

The consensus of the descriptions by experienced medical personnel of "exuberant health" were such as would lead to expectations of reasonable old age among the Indians studied. Instead, as Neel (1971:571) expresses it: "In view of this picture of health among the children and young adults, the relative paucity of older persons in these villages constitutes an enigma." The average age of the villagers was about twenty years, and less than 20 percent were thought to be older than thirty.

Several explanations are offered but no single cause is likely to constitute the complete answer. Recent measles and whooping cough outbreaks may have disproportionately extinguished the lives of the older members of the groups. Parasitic infestations, as noted above, are perhaps sufficiently prevalent to lower resistance to other diseases, particularly insofar as the parasites may be responsible for the generally low hemoglobin levels.

The culture of the Yanomamo, who call themselves "the fierce people," suggests that traumatic death is quite commonplace, especially among the young adult males. Although warfare, raiding, and deaths following accusations of sorcery are fairly frequent occurrences, as are brutal wife-beatings, the majority of violent encounters seem to contain built-in cultural mechanisms that serve to terminate most confrontations somewhat short of fatal injury. On the other hand, the Yanomamo studied by Chagnon (1968) were found to lose 24 percent of their males through internecine conflict.

But the trauma factor, while important, does not completely explain the paucity of elders, particularly female elders. Another contributing factor is suggested by the attitudes toward illness expressed by the members of these cultures. This was noted several decades ago among the Maya descendants studied by the physician Gann. He observed (1918:36):

> Indian men and women of all ages and classes, when attacked by any serious malady, are found to be lacking in vitality and stamina; they relinquish hope and relax their grip on life very easily, seeming to hold it lightly and as not worth a fight to

retain. An elderly man or woman will sometimes take to a hammock without apparent physical symptoms of disease beyond the anemia and splenitis from which nearly all suffer, and merely announce *Ile in cimli,* "I am going to die." They refuse to eat, drink, or talk, wrap themselves in a sheet from head to foot, and finally do succumb in a very short time apparently from sheet lack of vitality and absence of desire to continue living.

More than half a century later, the same phenomenon is recorded by Neel (1971:577): "Whereas in an epidemic, most of us would expect to survive until proven otherwise, the Indian seems to expect to die, an attitude which in some obvious ways but in other ways we still do not understand, probably influences his probability of survival."

The relationship of expectations of life and resignation to death is beyond the scope of this discussion. The attitude of the sick individual is well known to be critical in the prognosis of an illness. But rather than view passive resignation as typical of the Indians, it would appear more scientifically valid to seek the cause of this defeatism in the anemias, parasites, and other molestations that are likely to sap the resiliency and spirit of their victims.

The investigations by Neel and his associates probably constitute the most comprehensive medical study ever performed on a tribal people. The expeditions were conducted so as to make possible quite sophisticated tests to determine the population's degree of exposure to or infection from many representative human diseases. These tests revealed an unexpectedly heavy burden of disease borne by the Indians.

It was found that more than half (an average of 62 percent) of the inhabitants of several villages had experienced malaria attacks. In one Yanomamo village, virtually all the people had acute malaria when encountered by the investigators. Fifty-eight percent of the Indians studied had been exposed to whooping cough. Measles antibodies were found in 89 percent of one group. Between 30 and 80 percent of the villagers had been in contact with salmonella infections, whose symptoms range from moderate distress to severe dysentery; and almost half the population had positive tests for histoplasmin, a disease that may produce serious pulmonary symptoms or may be indistinguishable from grippe-like illness.

Antibodies to various types of poliomyelitis were found in 71 to 95 percent of the subjects and extensive exposure to various members of the Arbovirus group of infections, including yellow fever, was noted. Every person tested showed prior encounters with toxoplasmosis, leading Neel et al. (1968:488) to state, "This is, in fact, the highest prevalence of positive serologic reactivity yet recorded, exceeding the prevalence encountered in such other Tropical areas as Costa Rica (85%), Guatemala (84%), Tahiti (70%), and Honduras (81%)." Toxoplasmosis is a sporozoal type of infection, usually derived from raw meat or fecal contamination. The disease is generally mild but, under some circumstances, can become severe and include anemia, fever, rash, and chills.

The mode of transmission for some of these diseases—toxoplasmosis, malaria, salmonella, and histoplasmin—may be explained by the natural endemicity for the region over the past centuries. For others, however, it is difficult to understand the source of the infections, particularly when the record of no outside contact is accepted.

Perhaps the most shocking explanation is presented by Cockburn (1971:59):

> The Xavante Indians of Brazil . . . [though] very isolated . . .
> were found to have measles and other acute community
> infections. A year ago, this was difficult to explain. Now,
> however, hundreds of Brazilian landowners and government
> officials have been accused of carrying out biological warfare
> against the tribes. Those to be tried number 134, and 200
> have been dismissed from government service. The charge
> against them is that they sent gifts of infested clothing and
> persons with smallpox, tuberculosis, influenza and measles
> to the communities, with the intent of spreading the disease.

Although effective immunological mechanisms have evolved in human populations over many millennia of exposure to pathological agents, cultural factors perhaps become most critical in instances where illnesses sweep through nomadic or village-based societies. In fact, the catastrophic impact frequently noted stems primarily from the breakdown of the many vital functions of a culture. This concept was vividly demonstrated to Neel and his associates (Neel 1971:577) when they chanced to enter a village caught in the midst of a measles epidemic:

> Our impression . . . is that . . . the response of the Yanomamo
> to measles is not greatly different from that of Caucasian
> populations. . . . When an entire Indian village goes down
> with this disease, there is a total collapse of daily life. In the
> tropics, febrile individuals dehydrate rather rapidly, especially
> if there is no one to bring them water. . . . Imagine the plight

of the nursing children when not only do they have measles but so do their mothers.

We see, then, in the studies of the Ge-speakers of South America, societies where apparent health and vigor mask a critical battle for survival. Through centuries of selection, cultural adaptation, and interaction, human populations have achieved a working relationship with their environments. But today the Xavante and the Yanomamo are experiencing what has been the lot of much of humanity throughout our history: assault by microbial and social forces external to their environment—forces that exert biological and cultural pressures to which only a few may be able to respond successfully.

CONCLUSION

By using the techniques of medical anthropology, we gain a perspective on the vast human habitat subsumed as the New World quite different from that achieved through more traditional approaches. The record demands that the history of a people must include analyses of the diseases they have had to confront as well as the biological and cultural defenses they were able to mount against diseases new to them.

Had there been no introduction of smallpox or had there been adequate immunological resources to draw upon in its presence, a New World with a history that contrasts sharply with the one we know can be imagined—a land in which the European conquerors might have been the conquered or, perhaps more mercifully, the expelled. The archaelogical record attests that if the native American civilizations had not been struck down prematurely and calamitously by newly introduced diseases, they might have enriched the world with their achievements.

Similarly, were it not for the medical events and history of the African peoples who were brought to the New World in chains, it is unlikely that the institution of slavery would have profited its perpetrators. A United States whose cultures had evolved without the social divisions derived from slavery would have become a far different nation from the one we know.

It is not unreasonable to hope that, with the aid of the tools and knowledge now available through medical and social sciences, threatened populations among the few remaining indigenous peoples of the New World may be spared a repetition of the tragic history that the record reveals for so many of their American ancestors. Clearly, a medical anthropological approach provides an impetus to reexamine and reevaluate much of human history. But the knowledge gained carries with it a legacy of social responsibility, for the informed can help ensure that no people will have to relive the medical and associated social tragedies of the past.

THE SYPHILIS CONTROVERSY

. . . this malady we call
Syphilis, tearing at our city walls
To bring with it such ruin and such a wrack
That e'en the King escaped not its attack.

—Girolamo Fracastoro (1530)

Syphilis, the "great imitator," is a disease of many names and many faces. Few other diseases are more intimately related to the cultures, mores, and environments of their hosts. Like many of its victims, the disease itself has a flamboyant and vigorously debated past. Although it has been known as a disease entity for almost five hundred years, there is no other major disease whose origin is more disputed.

The first historic awareness of syphilis appeared suddenly in Europe at the close of the fifteenth century. In rapid-fire order it erupted wherever the explorers, colonizers, and military of the day set foot. In keeping with human propensities, many regions of the world quickly became "syphilized" more rapidly than they became "civilized."

THE "NEW" DISEASE WITH MANY NAMES

When it burst tumultuously upon the European scene, syphilis was quite different in symptomology, morbidity, and mortality from the disease known throughout the world in recent times. Whereas today, first-stage syphilis is often so mild as to escape the attention of its host,

211

when it surfaced in Europe the initial lesions progressed rapidly to painful, massive ulcerations, and—in the absence of adequate hygiene or antibiotics—often to gaping wounds and even to loss of limbs and grotesque disfigurations (Fig. 6–1). In the first years of the recognition of the "new" disease, some of the Spaniards called it "bubas" from the buboes, or great ulcerations, that appeared on the skin and body openings. As the incidence rose among pregnant women, stillbirths and early infant deaths became tragically commonplace.

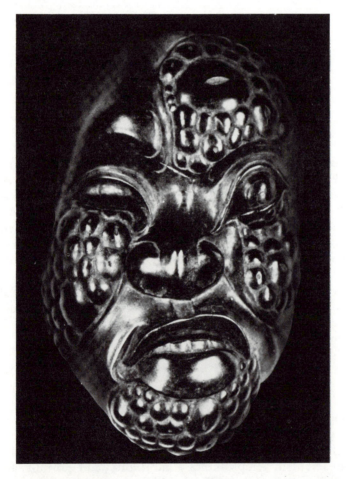

6–1   Mask from Indonesia showing the facial paralysis caused by advanced syphilis. (Courtesy of World Health Organization.)

Spreading like wildfire, the "loathsome disease" soon acquired its many titles: the great poxe, the evil pox, the serpentine disease, lues venera, the French Disease, the Disease of Naples, the Castillian Disease, the Portuguese Disease, the English Pox. Wherever it appeared people tried to place the blame for its existence on someone or someplace else. Francisco López de Villalobos, a famous Spanish physician and scholar of his day, called it the "Pestilence of Egypt," reasoning that one of the Biblical plagues had reappeared to punish the people of Spain for their sins (Dennie 1962). The Turks, perhaps remembering the cross-cultural contact of the Crusades, dubbed it the "Disease of the Christians" (Forer 1962).

By 1530, Girolamo Fracastoro, an Italian physician and poet, had composed a three-part tale in which a shepherd boy, named Syphilis, aroused the wrath of Apollo and was punished by a disease that destroyed him as well as many of the poet's contemporaries. The poem became popular and eventually the name of the disease also, thus ending the name-calling and making syphilis a disease that belonged to all the world.

EARLY SOCIAL REACTIONS TO SYPHILIS

Centuries before the recognition of microscopic agents of disease, causes were sought to every aspect of life. The German nobleman Ulrich von Hutten in 1519 wrote that theologians warned: "God has seminated this malady in anger and in order to punish creatures whose vices have outraged His Majesty" (in Fracastoro 1934:82). In vindictive righteousness, López de Villalobos moralized that victims were suffering from a proper punishment (Dennie 1962:29):

> It seems but just that it should have its beginning
> Only in those parts that do the wicked sinning.

Others looked for explanations in corrupted waters, sea air, impure winds, or infected earth. The astrologically inclined held that the phenomenon responsible was the 1484 conjunction of Mars and Saturn (others said Jupiter and Saturn; some, perhaps more appropriately, claimed Mars and Venus).

Physicians postulated "internal tainted principles," "alterations of the liver," and similar elegantly phrased dysfunctions to veil their ignorance of the pestilence that was sweeping the land. And the spirochete, today called *Treponema pallidum*, continued its own struggle for survival, moving from host to host, usually through the most intimate associations of human life—the genital contact of co-

214

itus, the mother-fetus relationship *in utero*—and, given the lack of hygiene of the day, frequently through less intimate bodily contact as well.

The "law and order" types reacted as might be anticipated. In the late 1490s the city fathers of Paris passed laws that gave all persons with the "Neapolitan Disease" the choice of leaving the city or being hanged. These were followed a year later by edicts permitting the drowning of any infected individual in the Seine River. Similar laws were passed in Aberdeen, Scotland, while nearly every main city of Europe prohibited men with "the evil poxe" from entering barber shops or other public institutions. The hysteria made life particularly harsh for the "light" women of the day. In several cities, infected females suspected of prostitution could be jailed until the symptoms disappeared or until the women died (Dennie 1962).

EARLY ATTEMPTS AT TREATMENT

More pressing than the futile casting about for names and blame were the frantic attempts to treat the "evil poxe" (Fig. 6–2). Von Hutten (in Fracastoro 1934:85) recorded:

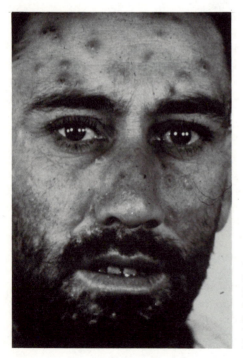

6–2 A case of disseminated syphilitic infection. If this patient is treated with penicillin, his chances for recovery are excellent. Before the days of effective antibiotics the prognosis for such victims was quite poor. (Courtesy of World Health Organization.)

The deplorable results obtained prove the powerlessness of the means that they employed. I remember that it was forbidden me to eat peas because I was told that these grains could enclose little winged insects that cause the infection.

Dennie (1962) notes that some patients who appeared not to be responding to other approaches would be cauterized at the base of the foreskin; others were instructed to wash with lye or with wine in which the poisonous fruit of an American tree had been soaked. He also reports that Ruy Diaz de Isla, who claimed to have treated more than twenty thousand patients in the early years of the sixteenth century, chose to use mercury ointment for thirty days, during which time his patients were not permitted to expose their skin to outside air or to water.

In the 1500s Fracastoro (1934) treated his patients by placing them on a chamber pot, with head and entire body wrapped in a blanket while mercury ore was burned beneath them. Thanks to this drastic procedure, the inhaled mercury frequently caused the patients to lose all their teeth and suffer bone destruction (Fig. 6–3).

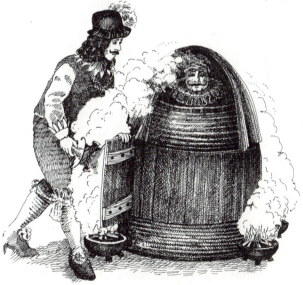

6–3 One method of treating syphilis in sixteenth-century Europe. The patient was enclosed in a chamber and exposed to the fumes of mercury ore that was burned below him. The poisonous fumes often produced favorable interruptions of the spirochete infection, but the side effects, particularly on teeth and bones, made this treatment one of last resort. (Courtesy of National Library, Paris. Adapted from Fracastoro 1934.)

Every traditional treatment and therapeutic concoction gained adherents among the desperate victims and their helpless doctors. As usual, under such conditions, fads and quackery ran rife. Since the disease was no respecter of class or person, patients included kings, popes, and others who wielded great power. Consequently the pressure to find a cure reached extraordinary proportions. Because of the strong belief that the disease was linked with the new discoveries of Columbus, futile expeditions were dispatched to the Americas with orders to find a cure there. For a brief period, great reliance was placed in the efficacy of the bark of the guaiac tree or "holy wood" from the New World.

When the disease entered the second or latent stage—a normal sequence when death does not intervene first—the patient was thought to have recovered and the medications or treatments he had been using would be credited with the "cure." In this way, dozens of useless, frequently painful and destructive treatments earned undeserved reputations for brief periods. Then the frightening affliction would reemerge to destroy or maim the newborn of the syphilitic parents or produce the paralysis, mania, or ruptured blood vessels of the tertiary stage of the disease. Eventually mercury, or "quicksilver," which had been relied on by the ancient Arabs to treat skin eruptions, came to be accepted as the standard remedy and was used in ointments, pills, and plasters, and as a fumigant in sweat chambers. It remained the treatment of choice for several hundred years. As the moralists admonished: "One night with Venus and three years with Mercury."

Since a few individuals were apparently able to effect biological recoveries, it was thought that some cures had occurred. But for the majority of infected people death came quickly, either as a result of generalized infection during the first stage or following the devastating fevers, bone lesions, central nervous system disorders, brain damage, or cardiovascular stigmata of tertiary syphilis.

Not until the discovery of penicillin by Sir Alexander Fleming and Sir Harold Florey in the mid-1900s and its use against syphilis by John Mahoney in the 1940s was a reliable cure available. The use of this extraordinarily effective lowly fungus extract, commonly a contaminant of rotten fruit or stale bread, has probably been one of the most outstanding accomplishments for human health. For the first time it has become possible to think of completely eliminating syphilis from the burden of disease borne by human populations. But, as will be discussed below, although syphilis is now a disease in which a complete cure can be effected, eradication remains a tantalizing dream for much of the world.

SYPHILIS IN THE NEW WORLD

For almost five hundred years, since the first public awareness of syphilis in Europe in 1493, a battle has raged over where this disease originated. As Sigerist (1951) comments, the arguments on each side have been good. The medical historians of the 1500s and 1600s attributed its introduction to the explorations of the New World, claiming that venereal syphilis was unknown in Europe until Columbus's crews returned there (and many historians today concur).

Ruy Díaz de Isla, Fray Bartolomé de Las Casas, Gonzalo Fernández de Ovideo y Valdés, Francisco López de Villalobos, and Fracastoro, all writing in the early 1500s, accepted an American origin unquestioningly. Díaz de Isla, who proposed the name "serpentine disease" ("... for as the serpent is an ugly, fearful and horrid animal so this disease is ugly, fearful and horrid"), wrote:

> It has pleased Divine Justice to give and send down upon us unknown afflictions, never seen nor recognized nor found in medical books, such as this serpentine disease. And this appeared and was seen in Spain in the year of our Lord [1493] in the city of Barcelona: which city was infected and consequently all Europe ...: which disease had its origin and birth ... on the island that today is named Española. ... And this island was discovered and found by the Admiral Xrisptoual Colon [Christopher Columbus].... And as ... the disease is by its very nature contagious it easily attacked [the people] and presently it was seen in the armada itself.... [It is] a grave disease that suppurates and corrupts the flesh: and breaks and rots the bones and disrupts and contracts the nerves. (In Williams et al. 1927:692–693.)

Díaz de Isla claimed to have treated the sailors from Columbus's ships, as well as Vincente Pinzón, master of the *Nina*, for the new disease.

Fray Bartolomé de Las Casas, who spent the greater part of his life after 1503 in the West Indies, wrote that bubas was picked up in Hispaniola when Columbus returned from his first voyage and that it then permeated Seville:

> I was at times diligent in asking the Indians of this Isle if this disease was very ancient here, and they said that it was,

before the Christians had come and that there was no memory of its origin, and of this there can be no doubt. (In Ashburn 1947:181.)

Oviedo reported in 1526 and 1535 that two of the pilots of Columbus's ships informed him that they had seen bubas on the island at the time of the first and third voyages, while two other men who had gone on the second voyage reported the same observations to him (Ashburn 1947). Convinced that the disease originated in the Americas and eager to search for a cure there for his own syphilis infection, Oviedo manipulated an appointment for himself from King Charles V as inspector of all the gold mines of the new lands (Dennie 1962).

Ashburn (1947:182) reports: Columbus's son tells us that on his arrival at Santo Domingo on August 30, 1498, Columbus found "all the families of the island in great tumult and sedition, from which many people were already dead, and there remained only 160 men, full of the French disease."

Parran (1937:33) suggests that Columbus himself contracted the disease. Noting that by the time of his third voyage Columbus began to hear voices and to regard himself as "ambassador of God," he states that Columbus's death in 1506 was precipitated by symptoms typical of tertiary syphilis.

As Ashburn (1947) and others have pointed out, the bubas cited by the witnesses of the fifteenth and sixteenth centuries may not have been related to the inflammatory process that the name implies today. It is possible, but not probable, that a completely different disease, one that no longer exists, was involved. The origin controversy is far from settled.

IDEAL TRANSMISSION CONDITIONS

No one disputes that many cultural and political aspects of life in fifteenth- and sixteenth-century Europe provided ideal conditions for the continual transmission of venereal disease. In Ashburn's (ibid.:183) words:

> The rapidity and extent of the spread of syphilis suggest a state of sexual promiscuity not since equaled. . . . It is possible that in that Rabelaisean period and under such leadership and example as were furnished by Pope Alexander VI, Emperor Charles V, King Henry VIII of England, and Francis, all reputed syphilitics, and by that clergy whose

incontinence and corruption so many medieval writers
scourged and ridiculed, this may have been true.

In the early decades of the outbreak, from 1503 to 1521, three
popes, Alexander VI, Julius II and Leo X, died of the "great pox"
before, as Wright (1971:301) puts it, "the papacy became alive to
the dangers brought to Europe by Columbus." Francis I of France
and Edward VI of England were reported to have contracted the
disease; and Ivan the Terrible of Russia earned his title after his
purported infection progressed to the paranoia of the tertiary stage
(Wright 1971).

Even the humor of the day revealed a distorted attempt to deal
with the mysterious malady that made no distinction between the
purest love and garden-variety lust. During the Restoration, the plots
of many comedies revolved around the predicaments of the victims
of syphilis. In all levels of society, the imprecation "A pox on you!"
became a commonplace and all-too-pertinent epithet.

Parran (1937:41) points to Henry VIII of England as the most
famous example of syphilis acting upon the fate of a whole nation.
He notes that the first four children born to Catherine of Aragon,
Henry's first wife, were all stillborn or died immediately after birth.
Finally came the birth of her one child able to survive, who became
known as "Bloody Mary" and showed many evidences of congenital
infection. Anne Boleyn, Henry's second wife and mother of Eliza-
beth I, had three miscarriages; Jane Seymour, his third wife, bore
only one child, Edward VI, who died at age fifteen; and Henry's last
three wives apparently never conceived. Historians hold that Henry's
drive to sire male heirs, probably frustrated by the syphilis he carried, underlay the struggle between the Crown and the Church that
was to bedevil English politics for years to come.

In addition to the examples set by the religious, political, and
social leaders, objective conditions of the day could not have been
better for ensuring further spread of venereal syphilis. In early 1495,
Charles VIII of France had assembled from many European countries
an army of some fifty thousand mercenaries with an attendant train
of about eight hundred female camp followers, all of whom gathered
outside of Naples for a projected siege. Instead of the anticipated
battle, the Spanish troops sent to aid Alfonso II of Naples fled; the
citizenry of Naples practically welcomed the mercenaries; and the
military and civilian populations were thus thrown together under
conditions of extreme disruption.

Historic accounts indicate that the people conducted themselves as humans will under such circumstances. Pusey (1933:5) notes that it "was more a triumphal march of debauchery than a serious military campaign." In a few months the celebrations came to an end and the mercenaries and prostitutes dispersed, bearing with them spirochetal souvenirs to pass on to the loved ones at home. By the end of 1495, venereal syphilis was reported in France, Germany, and Switzerland; the next year it appeared in Holland and Greece; England and Scotland were struck in 1497, and Hungary and Russia in 1499. During this period the Portuguese were carrying it to Africa and the Orient (Pusey 1933).

The transmission was unfortunately abetted by environmental factors. The year 1495 had been one of extremely poor weather with subsequent ruined crops and hunger, which drove many country people to the congested medieval urban centers in search of work. Poverty and lack of employment produced a population of wandering, unattached males and forced many homeless girls into prostitution—conditions that could only add fuel to the raging syphilitic epidemics.

In short order, as a result of postmedieval Europe's social disruption, wars, crop failures, forced migrations, growing urbanization with attendant culturally accepted licentiousness and prostitution, plus the seemingly eternal human attribute of attraction to new places and new sexual partners, venereal syphilis became a fact of life throughout the entire "civilized" world.

THE "DELICATE" SPIROCHETE

By 1905, Fritz Schaudinn had discovered that venereal syphilis is caused by specific bacteria. These were soon categorized as members of the genus *Treponema*, in the family Treponematacene and the order Spirochaetales. In the same year that Schaudinn announced his findings, August von Wassermann, Albert Neisser and Carl Bruck developed blood tests for the diagnosis of the disease.

The corkscrew-shaped microorganism (Fig. 6–4) was found to be most fastidious in its requirements: precise degrees of moisture and temperature and an apparently exclusive preference for humans and an occasional primate as hosts. This treponeme has been described (Brown 1962:22–23) "as frail as a germ can be and still survive." It is not viable upon exposure to air for more than a few minutes or to temperatures in excess of 104 degrees Fahrenheit and is completely destroyed by penicillin.

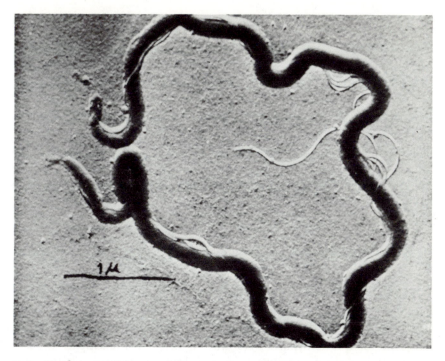

6-4 *Treponema pallidum* by electron microscope. Even at this great magnification, experts are unable to establish major points of differentiation among the various members of the treponeme family that cause diseases such as pinta, yaws, endemic, and veneral syphilis in human hosts. (Courtesy of Center for Disease Control, Atlanta.)

Humans and a few other primates provide ideal hosts for these delicate spriochetes. The basic primate needs for intimate, frequent body contact and the propensity for promiscuous and nonseasonal sexual activities guarantee the continuous recruitment of new hosts. And, prudently, the treponemes persist to the extent that they usually do not destory their hosts quickly.

Over the many centuries of continual exposure and interaction between host and spirochete, a "truce" has been achieved. Through their own evolutionary pressures, the treponemes have selected for the most invasive organisms. Hackett (1963) estimates that a single organism injected properly into the body will produce in thirty-two days about a hundred million progeny—approximately the number required to create a visible skin lesion. Without treatment, the host will live several decades, usually exhibiting only the mildest of symptoms and, incidentally, providing a sanctuary for the parasites. Not until the tertiary stage is reached, and then only in approximately 70 percent of its victims, will the disease destroy the host, through brain, heart, blood vessel, or central nervous system damage.

THE GENUS *TREPONEMA*

Until quite recently syphilis was categorized as a skin disease and studies were reported primarily in dermatology journals. This approach appeared quite reasonable because it was found that all the other members of the treponeme family are adapted to nonvenereal skin transfer. They are responsible for the diseases pinta, yaws, and endemic syphilis. It is the relationship among all these diseases and their city cousin, venereal syphilis, that provides the corpus of arguments against the Americas as the site of the origin of venereal syphilis. Before considering the contending theories, therefore, it is necessary to examine and compare the other members of the clan.

PINTA

Pinta ("spotted") is a mild skin disease caused by *Treponema carateum*, with an incidence restricted to humid, hilly or mountainous areas of Mexico and parts of South America to the Upper Amazon Basin. It is a disease primarily of children and yound adults and is contracted nonvenereally through skin contact. Hackett (1963:15) calls pinta "the ancient endemic treponematosis of the Americas." It was reported between 1505 and 1516 by Oviedo and Cortez as being common among the Carib and Aztec Indians.

The initial and early lesions of pinta are scaly, disseminating plaques that usually appear about the age of four. Later, the patches of the skin become blue. In still later stages of the infection, hues of pink, brown, blue, and black develop; and eventually complete dyspigmentation occurs in the infected areas, producing an individual who appears to possess a multicolored skin (Fig. 6–5). Along with the color changes, the affected skin loses its ability to sweat or to secrete oil. So far as is known, this treponemal infection produces no symptomatology other than these skin changes. Interestingly, pinta patients cannot be infected artificially with yaws, and venereal syphilis is extremely unlikely to afflict them.

In the early 1960s, according to Langagne (1962), an estimated 400,000 people in Mexico were infected with pinta. He notes that, although it is a relatively mild disease, its victims are "imprisoned in cruel psychological barriers," and its eradication would involve "a health campaign with deep psychological, social and economic repercussions" (ibid.: 172, 173).

The attitude of the people toward the "spotted ones" has varied markedly depending upon the particular social conditions of their

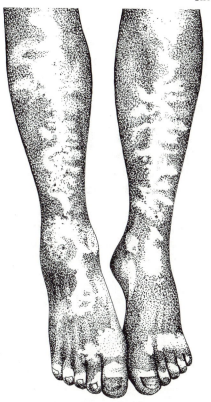

6–5 The multicolored skin of late pinta. The areas of the skin that undergo permanent pigmentation changes also lose their ability to secrete oil or perspiration.

society. Shunned and scorned at times, the "Pintados" in other circumstances have enjoyed high status because of their distinctive appearance. These were the people selected by the powerful Emperor Montezuma to bear his litter as a complement to the displays of precious stones, feathers, and other brilliantly colored objects he preferred for his retinue. Through many of Mexico's wars, the Pintados have formed their own battalions, composing a subgroup within their society as a result of their childhood encounters with the mildest of the treponemal infections, pinta.

YAWS
Yaws ("frambesia" in parts of Africa and "priam" in the West Indies) is also a nonvenereal skin disease. Like pinta, it occurs primarily in

childhood and is spread through skin contact. Unlike pinta, it is widespread, affecting mainly children living unclothed in the humid tropics. The agent responsible for yaws is *Treponema pertenue*, which generally enters a child's uninfected skin, particularly below the knee, through cuts and abrasions as a result of close contact with another child's infected lesions.

According to Hudson (1965), yaws is the commonest of the treponemal syndromes and is found in almost every populated humid tropical region. As Lomholt (1972:668) puts it, "It is a disease of rural areas where living conditions are poor. It is said that yaws begins where highways end." Hackett (1963:27) notes:

> In Africa, yaws has so flourished that some observers have thought that it was the cradle of the disease. The prevalence and severity of yaws in tropical Africa during the first 30 years of this century were probably much greater than anywhere else. More than one observer regarded yaws as a bigger burden to some African populations than all other infections put together . . . affecting most of the population by adult life.

Infectious lesions containing vast numbers of treponemes may remain for several months and recur, either through self-infection or through reinfection from external contacts. Yaws is particularly prevalent in communities where large numbers of children are in frequent contact, personal hygiene opportunities are limited, and humid conditions keep the skin moist. Quite often polygamous families and sedentary village life provide the large numbers of children and the social conditions that court yaws transmission. Observers have also noted that the number of cases tend to increase in rainy seasons.

In contrast with the benignity of pinta, yaws is often both painful and debilitating. Beginning as a localized lesion, commonly on the legs, the infection usually remains latent for a brief period and then erupts as generalized lesions and ulcerations on the face, buttocks, and extremities. Without the magic of penicillin, which produces cures almost overnight, the sores are slow to heal, frequently progressing to destructive lesions of periostitis, particularly of the tibiae (Fig. 6–6) and the nasal area. Occasionally the eyes are severely involved as well. Unlike venereal syphilis, yaws rarely involves the central nervous system or cardiovascular organs.

Frequently, in the late stages, painful eruptions appear on palms and soles, requiring the victims, when walking, to transfer the weight

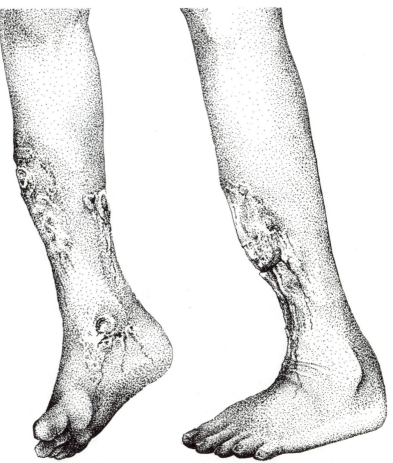

6-6   Yaws, caused by spirochetes, is often both painful and debilitating. Found primarily in humid tropical regions "where the paved roads end," it is frequently transmitted from child to child through contact in play.

of the body to unaffected parts and producing a characteristic "crab walk," hence the name "crab yaws." On the little island of Kar Kar, off the northeast coast of New Guinea, such deformities from yaws were so pronounced that the area was called "the Island of Crooked Men." Among other affected populations, the ulcers were more likely to attack the nose and palate, giving the voice a strange nasal quality. Under these conditions, the common name for the disease was "gangosa," the Spanish word for "nasal voice."

In 1962 an estimated 50 million active cases and 150 million latent cases existed worldwide (Guthe 1962). But through the combined efforts of the World Health Organization and local agencies, yaws has been eradicated in many areas of the world. Venezuela provides a notable example of the possibilities of such campaigns. Unfortunately, many people who in the past would have been yaws victims are now caught up in urbanization or other social turmoil and, lacking yaws' gift of immunological resistance to venereal syphilis, are prime targets for that disease, which is rapidly assuming epidemic proportions and will necessitate additional antitreponemal programs.

Willcox (1974) reports witnessing this change take place in New Guinea, where venereal syphilis had been practically unknown before 1970 but yaws had been prevalent. A mass campaign against yaws was undertaken in 1957. Shortly after yaws eradication was achieved a new highway was begun across the island. Subsequently, venereal syphilis was introduced by infected truck drivers and the passenger-prostitutes who sought clients in the villages along the truck route. Willcox (1974:174) notes:

> The dissemination of the disease amongst the local population is in proportion to the prevailing sexual freedom, the spread being most extensive amongst the promiscuous Chimbu. . . .
> Thus, even now, towards the end of the 20th century, an opportunity still exists of observing the rapid "syphilization" of a susceptible community.

ENDEMIC SYPHILIS

The final member of the unsavory treponemal quartet is endemic syphilis, called "bejel" by the Bedouins, "njovera" in Rhodesia, "dichuchwa" by the Bushmen, "irkintja" by the Australian aborigines, and "franji" in the Middle East. Like the other treponemal diseases, endemic syphilis is intimately related to the environments and social conditions of its hosts. It characteristically attacks poor, rural populations. Gasparini (1962:158) comments, "The isolation and the poor living conditions of some countries where non-venereal syphilis is endemic today contributed to its resistance and survival." Willcox (1960) notes that it may be found anywhere in the world except where yaws is endemic.

Endemic syphilis occurs most commonly in warm, semiarid or arid areas. The causative agent is the same as that of venereal syphilis,

Treponema pallidum. Infection stems from simple contact with infected companions or through contaminated drinking, eating, or play objects (Fig. 6–7). Because this disease occurs in environments where clothing is required, the possibilities of extensive skin-to-skin contact are limited. The bacteria survive by producing lesions about the mouth so that transmission is achieved through kissing, through fondling of children, occasionally through wetnurse practices, and frequently through the common use of cups, toothpicks, pipes, cigarettes, and moist towels.

The infection may begin as a small mucous patch on the buccal mucosa, followed by lesions on the trunk or extremities. Periostitis of the legs is common and in later stages gummatous lesions of the nose and soft palate may appear. Occasionally, no initial lesions can be observed and the disease may lurk in the body with no external manifestations until late stages are approached.

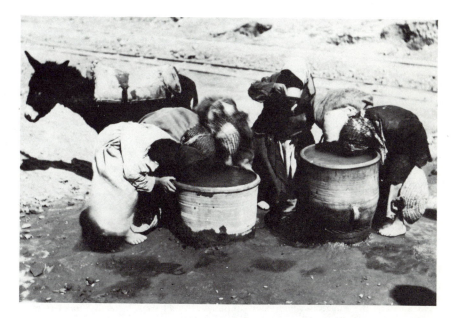

6–7   A quick but dangerous way to quench thirst. One of the possible modes of transmission of endemic syphilis as well as other diseases is shown here as workers in the dry countryside of Kish, Iraq, stop for a drink of water at a watering spot and share the one communal cup—and bacteria. (Courtesy of Field Museum of Natural History, Chicago.)

Hackett (1963) cites evidence that the early, repeated superinfections that occur in childhood in endemic areas result in a few years in the immunological protection of the heart and central nervous system of the victim.

> This is in contrast to adult infection and less frequent superinfection in venereal syphilis. In this way they account for the rarity, mildness . . . or absence of late neurosyphilis and cardiovascular lesions in rural populations in whom endemic syphilis is present. (Ibid.:13.)

This nonvenereal syphilis has been known for several centuries— since the arrival of the Ottoman invaders in parts of Europe. At present it is estimated to affect about a million people over an extremely wide range (Fig. 6–8). It used to be common among the

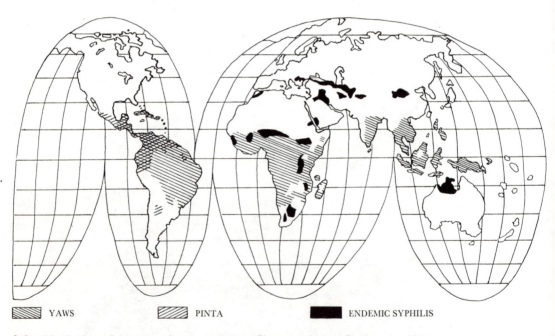

YAWS   PINTA   ENDEMIC SYPHILIS

6–8 Distribution of nonvenereal treponematoses. Pinta remains confined to dry highland areas of the Americas while yaws continues to hold sway in many humid tropical regions. Endemic syphillis has a patchy, widespread distribution particularly among peoples in semiarid, nonindustrialized areas. The continuation of all these debilitating or disfiguring diseases, despite the relatively low cost of antitrepomenal drugs such as penicillin, reflects the inadequate use of social, political, and economic resources. (Adapted from Guthe 1962.)

nomadic peoples of the Central Asian steppes but has not been observed in the Americas. Mass eradication campaigns, involving treatment of whole populations, have been undertaken, with promising results, in Syria, Iraq, Bechuanaland, parts of West Africa, and the Bosnia region of Yugoslavia.

ONE DISEASE OR MANY?

All of the treponemes examined, *T. pallidum, T. pertenue, T. carateum*, are indistinguishable, one from another, whether examined under light microscopy or electron microscopy of the highest magnification, or subjected to elaborate serological testing. A summary of the differences and similarities within the genus, as humans are affected, is shown in Table 6–1.

Table 6-1
Characteristics of the four human treponemal diseases

	Pinta	Yaws	Endemic syphilis	Venereal syphilis
Agent	*T. carateum*	*T. pertenue*	*T. pallidum*	*T. pallidum*
Populations affected	Children, young adults	Children	Children, adults	Adolescents, adults
Geographic regions	Hilly, mountainous, rural	Humid tropics, rural	Warm, arid, rural	Worldwide, primarily urban
Organs affected	Skin	Skin, mucosa, bone	Skin, mucosa, bone	Skin, mucosa, bone, eyes, central nervous system, heart, arteries
Means of transmission	Nonvenereal	Nonvenereal	Nonvenereal	Venereal
Usual site of initial lesion	Any exposed part of the skin	Skin, generally on legs, below the knees	Frequently mouth or mucosa; occasionally unobservable	Genitalia, occasionally other areas of sexual activity
Potentially infectious period	Many years	Three to five years	Three to five years	Three to five years
Response to penicillin	Effective cure	Effective cure	Effective cure	Effective cure
Congenital infections	No	No	No	Yes

Infections with any one of the bacteria will produce a positive blood test. Penicillin has remained unfailingly effective in curing early infections. Nevertheless, as has often been shown, no disease is eliminated from a population by treatment alone. As will be discussed, eradication of syphilis and related treponemal infections is profoundly dependent on the ability to effect changes in the attitudes, behavior, and social conditions that maintain these diseases throughout the world.

According to Hudson (1965), 90 percent of the world's treponemal infections have been acquired nonsexually. The natural history of the treponemes reveals a vicious circle of poverty creating disease and disease creating poverty. In today's world the possession of an effective cure is a powerful start but does not ensure the elimination of these diseases. The social and behavioral sciences can supply many of the required data, particularly by delving into the history of syphilis and various theories about its origin.

ARGUMENTS IN THE ORIGIN DEBATE

It is generally agreed that the original treponemes were probably microorganisms that parasitized decaying organic matter and opportunistically established themselves in human hosts by penetrating traumatized human skin, perhaps hundreds of thousands of years ago (cf. Hudson 1965). Hackett (1963) differs to the extent that he believes the organisms probably went through an animal-host stage before opting for humans.

WHERE AND WITH WHOM?
The debate that began almost five centuries ago, and continues hotly today, centers fundamentally on the question of where and with whom venereal syphilis began. Did it originate in the Americas to be carried to the rest of the world as the sixteenth-century historians unanimously agreed? Or, as others claim, did the transmission move in the opposite direction? Did the disease originate in Europe to be borne by European sailors to the American Indians and later to the rest of the European-explored world? With the increasing information available concerning the worldwide distribution of the various

treponemal diseases, the arguments have become much more complicated than a simplistic origin debate would indicate.

ONE TREPONEMA WITH MANY FACES?

Hudson (1962, 1963, 1965, 1972), a physician and medical historian, argues that the treponematoses constitute a single but extremely flexible disease that manifests itself in various ways depending on the environment and culture of the host. He claims
(1965:890), "Every social group has the kind of treponematosis that
is appropriate to its geographical and climatic home and its stage of
cultural development." Thus, venereal syphilis "probably sprang
from endemic syphilis in many places at many times as a result of
local improvement in levels of hygiene and changes in sexual mores."

Hudson, as well as Willcox (1974), suggests yaws as the original
syndrome, affecting forest hunters and gatherers, beginning in sub-
Saharan Africa in Paleolithic times and continuing in susceptible populations through most of human existence. When infected Neolithic
societies established sedentary village cultures, the propagation of the
infections would have been encouraged by increased numbers of
children and by unhygienic conditions. Yaws would have been maintained in hot and humid environments but endemic syphilis would
haved emerged under cooler, drier climes where less skin was exposed
for direct skin transmission.

Hudson (1965) contends that with the rise of urban centers in
the Fertile Crescent, approximately six thousand years ago, endemic
syphilis changed to venereal syphilis as a result of several factors
operating simultaneously. Urban life engenders more clothing plus a
minimal degree of public and private hygiene, thus reducing the
opportunities for nonvenereal transmission. At the same time, the
atmosphere of urban life tends to promote more opportunities for
varied sexual interaction as well as the establishment of prostitution,
an institution that Hudson claims has never achieved importance in
small village structures.

According to this hypothesis, the spirochetes remained the
same, but the site of entry shifted from skin to buccal mucosa to
genitalia. Further, in ancient and medieval urban centers, the stigmata of primary syphilis would not have been differentiated from
other skin eruptions, all being lumped together under the generic
umbrella of "leprosy," until, at the end of the fifteenth-century, a
separate identity was achieved.

Earlier, the treponemes would have crossed the Bering Strait with the first Americans. As the migrants settled in various regions, symptoms of yaws would have emerged in the humid tropics, pinta in the drier highlands, and venereal syphilis when urban centers arose. Thus, Hudson's "unitarian" theory tends to eliminate the argument of transmission from Europeans to Americans or vice versa; he postulates the presence of syphilis on both continents long before Columbus's men were born.

Hudson's proposals appear to gain support from the studies of Grin (1961), who found, while conducting treponemal surveys in Sudanese villages, that some villages were undergoing a treponemal "transitional stage." For example, among the Dinka tribe in Bor district, yaws was in slow regression while endemic syphilis was on the rise. But, Grin's, view diverges somewhat from Hudson's, for Grin suggests that venereal syphilitic infections have been brought in from the towns and have become endemic, nonvenereal syphilis in the village environments: "In some villages in the Kadugli area of the Nuba Mountains region it was possible to establish how the first sporadic venereal syphilis infections were imported and then spread as non-venereal endemic syphilis on account of the generally low hygiene and living conditions of the population in the rural areas" (ibid.:236).

THE MUTATION THEORY

Hackett (1963) offers a history of the treponemal diseases quite different from Hudson's. He (ibid.:13) believes that "the differences in clinical manifestations of the various treponematoses are probably due to [changes in] the treponeme strains themselves." He thus introduces the concept of mutations to account for the changes in the varying diseases. His reconstruction begins with pinta as the choice candidate for the original human treponemal infection. In support of this hypothesis, Hackett proposes that the longer infectious period characteristic of pinta makes it likely that it was the original treponeme, since a longer infectious period helps ensure continuous transmission in a small population. As further evidence of a more ancient parasitic relationship, he points to pinta's relative mildness and lack of invasion of the deeper body tissues.

According to Hackett, pinta arose from an animal infection some twenty thousand years ago in the Euro-Afro-Asian landmass, and then spread throughout the world, including the Americas when the Bering Strait permitted human passage. It was then cut off when the ice receded and closed the land passage, isolating the American continent. Cockburn (1971:46) also suggests an animal origin, but an earlier one. He cites evidence of infections in various primates as support for a very early origin, "many millions of years, possibly as far back as the Miocene."

As Hackett sees it, around ten thousand years ago the humid tropical conditions in Afro-Asia favored mutants that evolved in the direction of yaws infections. These then spread and flourished throughout the tropical regions of the world except for the American landmass, which by then was completely isolated by the surrounding waters. In the arid, warm regions bordering the tropics, the mutated treponemes of yaws would have been selected for, evolutionary pressures favoring those with the ability to adapt to the different climatic conditions and endemic syphilis would have been added to the treponeme genus (Fig. 6–9). With the rise of urban centers, mutants of

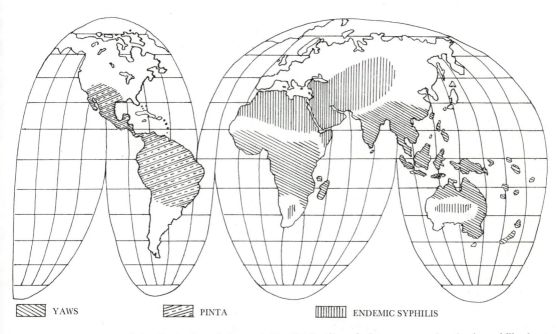

YAWS   PINTA   ENDEMIC SYPHILIS

6–9 Projection of the probable distribution of pinta, yaws, and endemic syphilis about nine thousand years ago, before the advent of widespread agricultural communities and associated cities. The distribution appears to stem primarily from climatic conditions and the relative isolation of particular peoples. (Adapted from Hackett 1963.)

endemic syphilis would have been favored if they possessed the ability to infect clothed hosts genitally. In this manner, venereal syphilis would have appeared about 3000 B.C. in the eastern Mediterranean region and southwest Asia.

Cockburn (1961) also favors a process based on mutations of the treponemes, particularly as their transmission depended on human population size and access to body orifices as influenced by clothing, hygiene, and related cultural factors. Cockburn and Hackett (1963) also argue for the presence of venereal syphilis in pre-Columbian Europe in the guise of "leprosy," but, Hackett raises the possibility that the original mutants may have produced a "mild disease" until, at the end of the fifteenth-century in Europe, more virulent mutations arose. The latter would have been responsible for the grave disease recorded in post-Columbian history. The newly emerged venereal syphilis would then have been carried to the regions of the world where it had formerly been unknown.

The final argument to be considered here supports the pre-Columbian presence of syphilis only in the Americas. This is the position of Williams (1932; Williams et al. 1927), Pusey (1933), Sigerist (1951), Dennie (1962), Kerley and Bass (1967), Morse (1969), and others. In addition to the previously reported accounts, of the historians and physicians of Columbus's day, this position is the only one that can claim support from osteological evidence.

In contrast, Hudson, Hackett, Cockburn, and others derive their hypotheses from a reasoned examination of the treponemal diseases as they are known today. From current knowledge they extrapolate back in time and, further, they argue for a broad interpretation of pre-Columbian references to leprosy as actually including symptoms of syphilis as well as other diseases affecting the skin. Hudson (1962, 1972) also offers evidence of an early presence of venereal syphilis in Europe based on various examples of pre-Columbian literature, which, he argues, refer to symptoms that can be interpreted only as belonging to venereal syphilis.

THE TESTIMONY OF THE BONES

Neither Hudson, Hackett, nor any other supporters of the case for a pre-Columbian presence of syphilis in the Old World have been able to point to any bones of Old World, pre-Columbian populations that reveal evidence of syphilis infections. Indeed, Smith (1930:xxvii) reports that . . . "after examining the remains of something like 30,000 bodies of ancient Egyptians and Nubians representing every period of the history of the last sixty centuries, and from every part of the country, it can be stated quite confidently that no trace whatever even suggesting syphilitic injuries to bones or teeth was revealed in Egypt before modern times."

Similarly, Møller-Christensen (1967), alone and with teams of other experts, examined more than nineteen thousand skulls, skeletons, and mummies from Scotland, England, France, and Denmark and recorded no evidence of syphilis. Williams (1932:974) reports two personal communications from Professors Boldt of Amsterdam and Manouvrier of Paris, who "had studied many thousands of skulls taken from burial places of various periods [in Europe and] had never found a syphilitic skull of pre-Columbian date."

On the other hand, the case for the presence of syphilis in the pre-Columbian New World is strengthened by the accumulation of an impressive body of skeletal material containing indications of syphilitic infections. Goff (1967) provides an osteological summary of the changes that must be present in order to constitute a reasonable case for a diagnosis of syphilitic bone damage. He also stresses the points of differentiation between venereal syphilis, yaws, and other destructive bone pathologies, and adds that the most commonly involved bony areas affected by venereal syphilis are the skull and tibiae. Goff (ibid.:283,286) describes how syphilitic damage was identified:

> An inflammatory process, beginning on the periosteum, was soon separated from the underlying bone, which became necrotic. The skin over these necrotic areas frequently formed ulcers and sloughed away. A sequestrum formed within the necrotic bone and discharged through the broken down areas. Sometimes, however, instead of becoming necrotic, a new growth of spongy bone formed on the surface on the old cortex, appearing rather like a coating of pumice stone when the bone dried.

As Sigerist (1951:55) remarks in regard to a syphilitic skull, "Whoever has seen such a skull will never forget it" (Fig. 6–10).

According to H. U. Williams (1932:781), a physician and professor of pathology: "Most of the specimens of bones supposed to be ancient and syphilitic reported in recent years have been found in America." He hypothesizes that syphilis was introduced by migrants who crossed the Bering Strait from Asia some ten thousand years ago and brought with them a nonpathogenic organism that later acquired pathogenic properties.

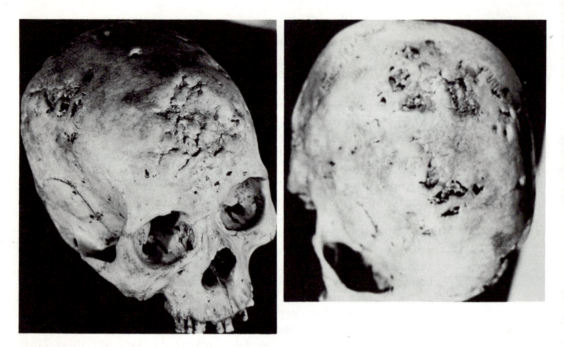

6–10 Front and rear views of the skull of a prehistoric Eskimo showing severe damage from long-standing syphilitic infection. Prehistoric bones with these characteristic stigmata of advanced syphilis are found in many areas of the New World. (Courtesy of San Diego Museum of Man. Photo by Mary Edgecomb.)

Williams personally examined virtually every collection of prehistoric American skeletal remains available in his time and asserted (ibid.:977) that the specimens he diagnosed were syphilitic, "as nearly free from suspicion as any that can be found." Apparently bending over backward to avoid error or prejudice, he discarded every bone that was the least bit questionable. To avoid any possibility of bias, he enlisted the expertise of many eminent medical specialists, including roentgenologists who X-rayed the bones he presented and invariably concurred with him.

Williams reported on skeletal material from the burial mounds of the Ohio, Mississippi, and Tennessee valleys that contained bones strongly suggestive of syphilitic infection. In the Pueblo region of the Southwest, from sites dated A.D. 919, 1073, and 1130 by tree-ring analysis, he records finding "some of the most important bones that in all reasonable probability are syphilitic." Williams points further to pre-Inca bones with clear evidence of syphilitic disease from Peru and Argentina, and concludes: "In contrast with the small number of bones from the eastern hemisphere that are suspected of showing ancient syphilis, the amount of material in America is almost embarrassing." (ibid.).

Stewart (1940:42) complains that Williams's unquestionably syphilitic skulls and long bones are unexplainably sparse, arguing that this is "an attribute not characteristic of this disease." He questions the pre-Columbian origin of some bones but does not contest the diagnosis of syphilis, adding at one point (1940:36): "Although the age of the specimen is in doubt, there seems to be good evidence that syphilis was present, if not common, among the Ohio Hopewellians." More recent authorities have concluded that the Hopewellian cultures emerged in various parts of the eastern United States from 500 B.C. to 100 B.C. and disappeared by A.D. 500 (Smith 1974, Ritzenthaler 1970).

Nevertheless, even the skeptical Stewart (1940:45) concedes that in regard to the Pueblo skeletal material, "where the skeletal remains of the Pueblos can be accurately dated, it is recognized that the custom of deforming the head goes well back into prehistoric times. A few of these old remains show lesions that may be due to syphilis."

Goff (1967) examined a small collection of skeletal material from Santo Domingo that failed to reveal any lesions resembling cranial bone syphilis or yaws, but he notes that other West Indian collections have yielded an occasional specimen that he accepts as characteristic of syphilis. He also examined two skulls with a certain date of A.D. 900–1000 excavated in Guatemala and found these to demonstrate positive characteristics of cranial venereal syphilis. He also notes a collection, first described by Martinez Del Rio (1953), that contains some twenty skulls and nearly a hundred postcranial bones from ancient caves in the Candellaria Mountains of Mexico. From this assemblage, both investigators agree that three of the skulls are definitely marked by syphilitic lesions.

Cole et al. (1955) report studies made on fifty-seven more or less complete skeletons from Kinishba and from Vandal Cave in Arizona. Analyses of forty-five or seventy-five datable specimens of pine and piñon roof beams of Kinishba gave overall dates between A.D. 1233 and 1306 and equally early dates were found at Vandal Cave. Six of the skeletons yielded material suspicious of syphilitic lesions; two were definitely accepted after intensive examination.

Morse (1969:33) presents more recent discoveries from Illinois that "would tend to support the hypothesis that syphilis is of American origin." He adds (ibid.:28): "We now know that almost all collections of Indian skeletons show some examples of generalized osteitis and periostitis which would be difficult to explain unless we would consider treponeme infection." In central Illinois, Morse found the skeletons of two males, aged approximately forty, who had lived between A.D. 1000 and 1200 and both of whom showed evidence of treponemal infections. He cites the work of McGimsey in 1966 who reported similar periosteal reactions in the shafts of the tibiae and femorae in thirty-one out of sixty-seven skeletal remains from Panama dated 4853 B.C. ±100.

Morse reviews four hundred Illinois skeletons dated from 1500 B.C. to A.D. 800. In this collection he found nine cases of multiple periostitis, which involved all tibiae and some crania and was generalized in some specimens. From another, incompletely studied Illinois site, containing hundreds of skeletal remains, he notes two dated approximately A.D. 800. Both were females in their late thirties and manifested severe periostitis of the tibiae and slight involvement of a femur. One exhibited two holes surrounded by erosive pitting in the top of the skull.

Table 6–2 presents a partial summary of undisputed syphilitic skeletal material from pre-Columbian remains discovered in the New World. As new excavations appear and old finds are reexamined, the numbers of syphilis-stigmatized bones from the Americas continue to increase.

THE HUNG JURY

There are, then, at least three fundamental theories, with numerous variations, concerning the origin of human venereal syphilis. Each proposal has attracted a devoted, well-informed following but the very proliferation of theories attests to the lack of agreement. The absence of pre-Columbian, Old World skeletal remains with treponemal stigmata, contrasted with the growing abundance of ancient syphilitic bones from the New World, makes it difficult to refute the argument that the human disease originated in the Americas and was transported to Europe and then to other human habitats by the European colonists and explorers. As Parran (1937:39-40) remarks:

> It would be extremely interesting from the academic point
> of view if here, indeed, were an instance of a major plague
> imposed . . . upon the white civilizations of the day, in

Table 6-2
Pre-Columbian American skeletal remains with undisputed syphilitic lesions

Bones	Number	Source	Age	Investigator or reference
Skulls and femur	3	Pecos Pueblo	"undisputably prehistoric" (Hooton 1930:311)	Williams 1932
Skull, long bones	1	Argentina	"pre-Columbian"	Williams 1932
Skull	1 (elderly person)	Peru	"pre-Inca"	Williams 1932
Tibiae	8	Ohio	Mound Builders	Williams 1932
Skeletons	3	Ohio	Mound Builders	Williams 1932
Various bones	9 (individuals)	Tennessee	Mound Builders	Williams 1932
Femur	1	Toltec	A.D. 1200-1300	Williams 1932
Tibiae and fibulae	6	Jersey Bluff	A.D. 800	Titterington 1935
Skulls	2	Guatemala	Qankyak or Xinabahul phase	Goff 1953
Skulls	2	Arizona	"none later than" A.D. 1300	Cole et al. 1955
Tibiae	2	Arizona	"none later than" A.D. 1300	Cole et al. 1955
Tibiae and femorae	31	Panama	4835 B.C.	McGimsey 1966 (in Morse 1969)
Skulls	3	Mexico, Candellaria caves"	"ancient caves"	Goff 1967; Martinez Del Rio 1953
Variety	2 males, aged 40	Central Illinois	A.D. 1000-1200	Morse 1969
Tibiae and crania	9	Illinois	1500 B.C.- A.D. 800	Morse 1969
Tibiae and right femur	1 female, aged 38	Illinois	A.D. 800	Morse 1969
Skull and left tibia	1 female, aged 36	Illinois	A.D. 800	Morse 1969

contradiction to the usual practice whereby the white man adds his civilized diseases to the other miseries he brings to the aboriginal.

Occasionally, new findings serve to cloud rather than to clarify the issue. Research conducted by investigators (cf. Hume 1962) have used strains of treponemes from human yaws cases that initially produced yaws lesions in experimental animals. After numerous passages of the treponemes through rabbits, however, lesions appeared that were considered typical of venereal syphilis. Although the reverse trend has not been reported, the apparent flexibility of the treponemes must be weighed and further studies conducted before a completely satisfactory origin theory can be appraised.

Further, we cannot summarily dismiss the possibility that by the time human occupancy had occurred, members of the treponeme family were present on all the continents but that the Old World contained forms with which the world is no longer familiar. Finally, in considering the origin of syphilis as well as other human diseases, customs and culture have to be examined as critical determinants of the form taken by the parasite responsible for the disease.

TODAY'S PROBLEM

SOCIAL FACTORS UNDERLYING CONTINUED TRANSMISSION

In today's world, particularly in urbanized and urbanizing areas, the trend has been toward the replacement of all other forms of the treponematoses by the venereally transmitted *Treponema pallidum*. Health agencies confront the dilemma of the continued presence, indeed the frequent proliferation, of a disease for which there exists a cure that is not only completely effective but also painless, cheap, and readily available.

Medical and biological sciences have contributed all that could be desired toward the goal of totally eliminating syphilis. Its persistence, as well as the even greater incidence of the diseases caused by treponemal kin, now becomes a problem requiring contributions by the behavioral sciences. In order finally to eradicate these diseases, it is necessary to learn what factors operate to prohibit or discourage the afflicted from availing themselves of the promise of penicillin.

Leona Baumgartner (1962:27, 29) sums up the problem succinctly:

> Much of the answer seems to lie in human behavior. . . .
> Penicillin was such a magnificent weapon against
> syphilis that near-miraculous powers were attributed to it. . . .
> It was very nearly assumed that the drug would somehow
> seek out the afflicted and inject itself.

For many populations today, the primary obstacle to freedom from syphilis is poverty. This is particularly true of newly urbanized people who, beset with myriad problems of adaptation to an unfamiliar way of life and concomitant breakdown of familiar cultural patterns and mores, frequently do not have access to medical facilities that make possible the diagnosis and treatment of syphilis. Very often these people live in "developing" countries in which limited financial resources are overwhelmed by urgent demands that must be given priority over syphilis eradication.

At this stage in their development, the only realistic approach for these countries is to depend on the services of worldwide agencies such as the World Health Organization of the United Nations. In its comparatively short existence WHO has demonstrated the efficiency and wisdom of the "total approach" in the complete eradication of treponemal disease from many areas of the world.

Eradication of syphilis in richer, industrialized nations such as the United States was optimistically (and prematurely) anticipated in the early decades following the discovery of penicillin. Indeed, after World War II, mass programs of diagnosis and treatment were initiated and the subsequent incidence rates did indicate the predicted decline. Intensive investigations aimed at an effective vaccine appeared promising but, as of 1976, results remained experimental and clinical use far distant (Ross 1976).

Schambert (1962) suggests that the decline of syphilis after the introduction of penicillin was at least partially due to the phenomenon known as "happen-stance" therapy. This was a result of the initial widespread, indiscriminate use of penicillin for almost every ailment in the human disease catalogue, including those of the most trivial nature. Under these circumstances, unknown and undiagnosed cases of syphilis would often be cured inadvertently as an individual sought relief from a completely unrelated disease.

Unfortunately, many government officials confused decline with eradication, so they reduced appropriations drastically and, as results showed, quite prematurely. As put ironically by Brown

(1962:21): "As a disease control program approaches the end-point of eradication, it is the program, not the disease, which is more likely to be eradicated."

In the United States the goal of eradication slipped away as funds to finance research and public health measures were reduced. Moore (1963) reports that in 1962 syphilis continued to kill a minimum of 3,000 persons each year and that many others died from syphilitic disease that was not officially recorded as the cause of death. Some 124,000 cases of syphilis of all stages were reported during that year, but as Moore points out (ibid.:831):

> The actual incidence of syphilis is believed to be between 75,000 and 100,000 cases a year. . . . Because many of these are not found and treated at all, there exists a large reservoir of persons needing treatment, probably close to 1,200,000 [or] 25,000 potential paretics, 6,000 potential syphilitic blind, 23,000 who will develop tabes dorsalis, and 90,000 who will develop cardiovascular syphilis.

Incidences similarly increased around the world, as reported in 76 out of 106 of the countries participating in a WHO study (Guthe 1962).

As the decade of the sixties progressed, public health officials began to report upsurges in syphilis until, at present, many regions are experiencing near-epidemics. DeMuth et al. (1974) estimate that in the United States over one-half million persons have syphilis, with one American contracting a venereal disease every fifteen seconds.

EFFECTS OF CULTURAL ATTITUDES AND PRACTICES
Lacking adequate support, social science research nevertheless attempts to find the answer to the apparent inability of people to avail themselves of the cure at hand. In addition, the reason for the soaring increase is sought in changing patterns of belief and behavior. Lomholt (1972:634) writes:

> The reason for [the marked increase] is not known but it may be concerned with the changed attitude of the modern welfare-society to morals . . . and with increasing tourism and movements of populations. . . . The spread has everywhere taken place mainly among the younger age groups and in men. . . .
>
> In recent years the influence of the use of contraceptive gestogen pills and intra-uterine devices (I.U.D.) on human-

sexual behavior and the widespread use of drugs among young people are, without doubt, factors of importance in the spread of venereal diseases.

The world has moved a long way from the days when drowning was considered an appropriate treatment for the syphilitic. Nevertheless sufficient prejudice against the disease and its victims persists to impede attempts to deal with it rationally. Biegel (1962) points to the rise of Puritanism as largely responsible for Western attitudes toward syphilis and the sexual activity with which it is associated.

He states, (ibid.:400) "The rise of Puritanism . . . made syphilis a whip for sinners in the hand of God" and adds (ibid.:401):

> Three hundred years have passed since syphilis . . . was declared a deserved punishment for immorality, yet the condemnation of both the disease and the diseased is still with us. V.D. to certain groups is not a sickness like any other, but an exposure of evil and lust to which compassion must be denied.

In a revealing illustration of Biegel's thesis, Hodann (1937:80) quotes a public figure, one I. Clephane, who, "far from considering syphilis an evil, regarded it, on the contrary as a blessing. Could the disease be exterminated . . . fornication would ride rampant throughout the land."

It is not just the attitude toward syphilis itself that plays a critical role in eradication efforts but also such attitudes as those toward women, marriage, and extramarital relations. As Baumgartner (1962:32) sums up the situation:

> Neither the [Surgeon General's] Task Force nor anybody else knows precisely why syphilis is on the increase. . . . There is a critical lack of knowledge about the attitudes and habits of people who contract syphilis. . . . So we need enormously expanded research into human behavior, into mores, attitudes, motivations.

In the United States the average number of sexual contacts made by the syphilitic patient during the period in which he or she is most infectious is about five, but studies show that fifty, seventy-five, and even more than a hundred contacts are not uncommon (Moore 1963:832). In numerous areas of the Western world, the activities of female prostitutes have become a far less potent factor than formerly in the transmission of syphilis because of the changing pattern of male homosexuality.

244

Sachs (1962) reports that half of 506 male patients interviewed in the Health Department of Los Angeles, named male sexual contacts exclusively; approximately one-third named heterosexual partners only, while 18 percent named both male and female contacts. Judson (1976) adds that in studies performed in Colorado, nearly 50 percent of all the syphilis cases seen were likely to have resulted from homosexual encounters. Waugh (1972) reports a similar trend reflected in studies conducted in Europe as well as in other areas of the United States.

TECHNOLOGY IS NOT ENOUGH

One of the primary requirements in any less than "total approach" program aimed at eradication is to find and treat all contacts. This becomes an extremely troubled area because the social attitudes of guilt and shame that surround sexual activity couple with the strong cultural proscriptions against "informing" on another person. These two attitudes act to prevent the hidden reservoir of infection from surfacing to accept treatment.

Although physicians are legally and ethically required to report positive cases of syphilis to public health agencies in order that contacts may be found and treated, very often considerations of patients' embarrassment and fear of exposure are given priority over the general public welfare. Moore (1963) estimates that private physicians in the United States report fewer than one-quarter of the cases of syphilis they diagnose. Orgel (1964:482) notes that in a study conducted in Los Angeles, physicians "tended to report those patients whose social, racial, and economic status varied most from that of the doctor and the more the bonds of similarity between the patient and the physician, the less likely he was to report it."

It is apparent that many physicians also share the attitudes and prejudices that confine venereal syphilis or other venereal infections to "lesser groups." Pariser (1964:227) states:

> I know of no disease in which diagnosis is influenced more by non-medical factors than that of syphilis. . . .
> A tie, jacket and a generally well-groomed, clean-cut appearance influence against the diagnosis, as does an air of prosperity, evidence of education, and social or family prominence. Under these circumstances, the patient is often deprived of even an elementary investigation for syphilis.

In like manner, education about venereal disease evokes protest from parents or community leaders fearful of exposing children to information that might be interpreted as an acceptance of sexual activity as a normal part of life. In many urban areas, syphilis among fifteen- to nineteen-year-olds has reached appalling heights (Sachs 1964). Nevertheless, knowledge that could be critical in preventing infection or inducing victims to seek treatment remains shrouded in ignorance, superstition, and secrecy.

It is possible also that a generation that has grown up in an era comparatively free from many of the traditional infectious diseases of the past has lost the fearful respect for disease that characterized much of the behavior of their parents and grandparents. Most likely, one or more of these factors is relevant in every case of syphilis that continues to elude available treatment. The precise proportion contributed by each factor—and others that have not yet surfaced—will become known only through intensive investigations of this crucial aspect of human behavior. Through such knowledge, and with strong financial support from government agencies, syphilis may someday join the other parasites that have ceased to affect human life.

CONCLUSION

The struggle to reduce or eliminate syphilis is greatly hindered by the lack of an effective immunization agent. Consequently, the eradication strategy must differ significantly from that used in the recent almost worldwide eradication of smallpox, for which a completely effective vaccine does exist. Syphilis must be treated, as it were, *ex post facto*. Nevertheless, as stated before, the treatment, usually one or two injections of penicillin, is dependable; side effects are unusual; supplies are readily available; and the cost is minimal.

The barriers to the elimination of syphilis, then, are today not in the realm of the medical and biological sciences; except for producing a reliable immunization technique, little more can be asked of them. The barriers are primarily in the social arena. A puritanical, know-nothing attitude puts blinders on public officials in many parts of the world who fear political reprisals for raising the questions required to effectively screen vulnerable segments of the population.

In areas of the world such as the urbanized United States, where a "new morality" includes a sexual freedom to experiment with multiple partners at an early age, much unnecessary suffering could

246

be avoided by introducing routine testing for syphilis in high school as well as in new-employment examinations. Discreet treatment and contact follow-up for those who have become infected could markedly reduce the number of hidden infections. As a very minimum, straightforward instruction on all aspects of human sexuality, without the current judgmental opprobrium, should be instituted in public schools at an early age (Fig. 6–11).

In many other parts of the world, syphilis is a rapidly growing new problem. Particularly in areas that formerly were "protected" by endemic yaws, former immunities no longer obtain now that yaws has been successfully reduced or eliminated. New opportunities for travel, new partners in the form of tourists or other individuals, augur a new treponemal disease that can be eradicated as was yaws only if social attitudes to the new form do not intervene with sources of treatment.

The studies and contacts of anthropologists whose research takes them to many areas of developing nations could greatly assist health agencies attempting to head off impending new diseases. Knowledge of attitudes and practices of affected or threatened groups within a society could be invaluable in determining the acceptable avenues through which treatment should be introduced.

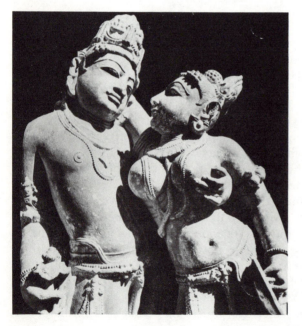

6–11 Ancient Hindu art of India depicting the ecstasy and joy of sexual love. Healthy, informed, and responsible attitudes toward sexual activity, based on mutual respect, could do much to check the rising tide of veneral disease, particularly in urban societies. (Courtesy of World Health Organization.)

7

MALARIA AND THE HUMAN FACTOR

Nature is not a faithful ally of man; she
seems always to be quite as deeply interested
in the success of the parasite and of
the mosquito.

—L. W. Hackett (1937:267)

Malaria has played a major role in much of human history and today is still the greatest single destroyer of human lives. Perhaps equally important is malaria's impact on the lives that it touches but does not entirely destroy. Bates (1965:223) expresses this with a depth of feeling that many malaria victims would echo:

> The force of malaria should not be judged by the number of people that it kills, or by the number of man-days of human energy lost in the course of clinical attacks. It is reflected more staggeringly in the accumulated misery of the populations in which it holds full sway.

WORLDWIDE PREVALENCE

Those populations over whom malaria "holds full sway" were estimated by the World Health Organization in 1952 to constitute more than 350 million persons, or 6.3 percent of the world's population (Livingstone 1971). Despite more than half a century of organized efforts to eradicate malaria, by 1976—because of increased population and other conditions to be considered—343 million people still lived in malarious areas that were not yet protected by specific antimalarial measures (Noguer, Werndorfer, and Kouznetzov 1976). In 1978 some two billion people were reported to reside in malaria-infested regions (Fig. 7–1). The disease strikes 150 million people

247

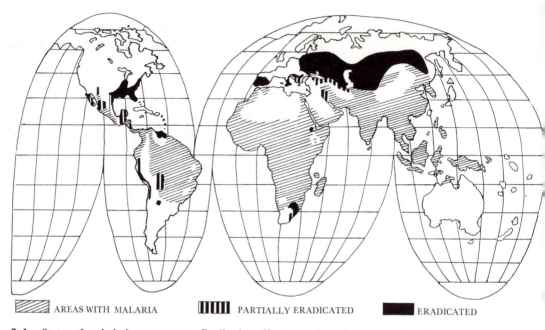

AREAS WITH MALARIA   PARTIALLY ERADICATED   ERADICATED

7–1 Status of malaria in recent years. Eradication efforts as well as changing social and economic conditions have acted to compress the distribution, which was once almost world-wide. But increasing human populations, plus growing insecticide resistance among the anopheles vectors, maintain this disease as the foremost destroyer of human life.

annually. In Africa alone each year a million children die of it and one-quarter of the adult population suffers recurring bouts.

Even these figures may be understatements. Because of its frequently deceptive nature, malaria is often overlooked in morbidity statistics. Thus, Bruce-Chwatt (1954) cautions that the amount of mortality due to malaria is so imperfectly known that even an approximate estimate is likely to be a guess.

It has been calculated that in malarious areas, adults who have survived the disease are incapacitated, on the average, for two months of every year. As if adding insult to injury, the most debilitating illness frequently occurs at harvest times when all hands are needed to sustain a full economy. The severity of malaria's challenge to survival is reflected in the selection for such genetic traits as sickle cell anemia, Mediterranean anemia or thalassemia, probably glucose-6-phosphate dehydrogenase deficiency disease, and perhaps other red blood cell anomalies such as hemoglobin E and C, D in India, K in northern and western Africa, and O in Indonesia. Livingstone (1971:48) points out that "all of the elevated frequencies of abnormal hemoglobins are found in populations that are or have been subjected to endemic malaria." Most of these abnormal hemoglobins kill or chronically disable a proportion of the young people who possess the genes in homozygous condition. Nonetheless, such hemoglobins are maintained in populations by evolutionary processes of natural selection because they enable the heterozygotes to survive in malarious regions (Fig. 7–2).

Even before much of today's knowledge concerning the association between abnormal hemoglobins and malaria was available, Hackett (1937:xi) was moved to write:

> [Malaria] is a tolerant and self-perpetuating parasitism
> which aims to enslave rather than destroy the populations
> which succumb to it. The victims ordinarily come to some
> sort of terms with their inveterate enemy, making an annual
> sacrifice of their youth to obtain for the old a certain
> tolerable freedom from attack.

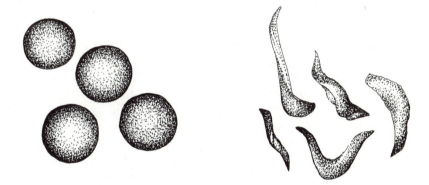

7–2 Red blood cells with two variants of human hemoglobin. *Left*: cells with normal hemoglobin A. A person with this type of hemoglobin will acquire heavy infestations of proliferating protozoa in endemic areas. *Right*: cells with hemoglobin S or sickle cell anemia. An individual who has inherited only this type of hemoglobin will acquire increased resistance to malaria but will suffer the painful disabilities of sickle cell anemia and may die prematurely. A person who has inherited both hemoglobin A and hemoglobin S will be most advantaged in areas where malaria is continuously transmitted. Sickle cell anemia is one of the best-documented variants of human blood known to be selected for in association with a specific disease.

In the same vein, Sambon (1901:349) postulated that the terrible monsters, such as the Minotaur, that figured in many old legends as claiming a yearly tribute of victims were probably symbolic of the prevalence of malaria among ancient populations. To these dismal reflections, U.S. Surgeon-General Hugh Cumming (in Hackett 1937:175) adds, "Malaria has the disastrous effect of permitting human existence while precluding the possibility of human health or happiness."

Nevertheless, Prothero (1965:15) claims that, in spite of the tremendous toll, people do come to accept malaria as a part of life: "In many illiterate communities it is scarcely recognizable as a disease. It is frequently difficult to convince those who are affected by it of the need for eradication measures." This resilience of human beings in the presence of rampant malaria may underlie the dearth of material regarding the disease in anthropological ethnographies.

An illustration of the ability to maintain a high degree of normality under malarious conditions is given by Hackett (1937:229), who describes a Spanish village where one year malaria was so bad that every laborer was stricken. Alternating groups were established based upon the incidence of attacks; each group worked on the days its members had no chills and fever but rested at home on the days when the attacks struck.

MALARIA IN ANIMALS OTHER THAN HUMANS

Malaria is far more common in birds, amphibia, and reptiles than it is in mammals, although bats, squirrels, dormice, buffalo, antelope, and shrews have been found infected in nature. Coatney et al. (1971) claim that every major vertebrate group is susceptible to malaria. But the parasite-host relationship is generally older, hence better adapted, among animals other than man, causing little known harm in wild species.

Occasionally, however, the comfortable relationship fails and the results are disastrous. Fiennes (1965), for example, reports that the entire penguin population of the Antwerp Zoo was wiped out by malaria, though the mosquitoes that transmitted it had fed on local sparrows that apparently were unaffected. Despite occasional reports of this nature, man remains the only animal for whom malaria is a leading cause of death.

THE MECHANISM OF MALARIA TRANSMISSION

Malaria is primarily a disease of red blood cells. It is caused by a protozoa, the smallest of animal organisms, belonging to the genus *Plasmodium* and the class Sporozoa. Four species have been identified as affecting man: vivax, malariae, ovale, and—the most pathological—falciparum (Fig. 7–3). Each species has varying degrees of virulence and is represented by many strains. In highly malarious areas, victims often suffer infestations of several strains and more than one species, each infection impervious to the resistance that develops for the others.

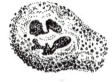

7–3   Human red blood cells showing four different species of malarial protozoa in the schizont stage. From left to right: *Plasmodium vivax, P. ovale, P. malariae*, and *P. falciparum*. Although each form occurs in specific environments, they frequently overlap; thus a person may often host more than one variety of malaria and experience each invasion as a separate illness. (Adapted from Coatney et al. 1971.)

HUMANS, THE INTERMEDIATE HOSTS

For all strains and species the basic cycle is fundamentally the same; variations occur only in time and pathogenicity. As in all cycles, the starting point is arbitrary. (See Fig. 7–4.) One may begin with the probing, infective, female *Anopheles* mosquito, which requires a blood meal for her egg production and selects a human host as the source of this meal. It should be stressed that it is the infective, not merely infected, mosquito that makes the difference in transmission considerations.

Before beginning to withdraw blood from her host, the anopheline makes several probes or injections before settling into one particular site. In her initial probings, she injects "ripened" sporozoites

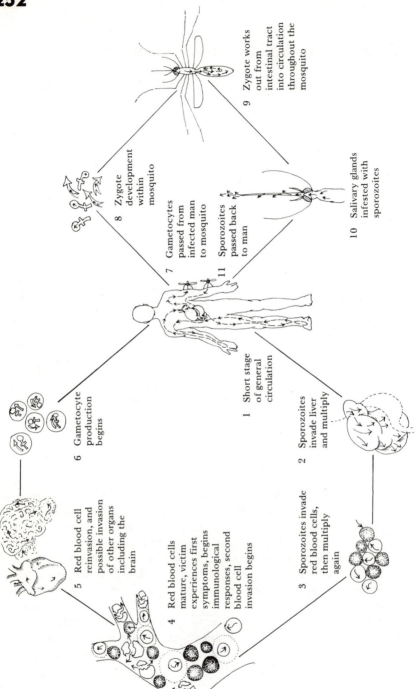

7—4 The cycle required for malaria transmission to continue. The protozoa that cause malaria are able to reproduce sexually only in the body of their determinant host, the female anopheles mosquito. This mosquito, which seeks blood meals in order to produce her eggs, is the only mosquito capable of continuing the cycle. In the human host, transmission occurs only after a long period of multiplication and growth of the parasites in the human liver and then in the red blood cells.

9 Zygote works out from intestinal tract into circulation throughout the mosquito

8 Zygote development within mosquito

7 Gametocytes passed from infected man to mosquito

11 Sporozoites passed back to man

10 Salivary glands infested with sporozoites

1 Short stage of general circulation

2 Sporozoites invade liver and multiply

6 Gametocyte production begins

5 Red blood cell reinvasion, and possible invasion of other organs including the brain

4 Red blood cells mature, victim experiences first symptoms, begins immunological responses, second blood cell invasion begins

3 Sporozoites invade red blood cells, then multiply again

from her salivary glands into the victim's blood stream. The number of sporozoites per injection may be 1,000 or more; the quantity varies from several hundred to 10,000.

Upon entering the human or intermediate host, the sporozoites, now termed "trophozoites," utilize the blood stream for little more than sixty minutes in order to reach the parenchymal cells of the liver and some endothelial cells of the capillary vessels as well as certain elements of the bone marrow. At these sites they begin a series of intense multiplications. This "exoerythrocytic phase," first confirmed as recently as the 1930s, persists for seven to ten days, during which time the host exhibits no clinical symptoms of malaria, nor is he infective to mosquitoes taking blood meals. The parasites apparently utilize the large stores of purines and folic acid in the mammalian liver and other tissues during this period of growth and multiplication.

The products of the multiplication within the liver, or pre-erythrocytic phase, are called "schizonts." At a species-specific time, the schizonts leave the liver and reenter the blood stream. Each schizont finds its own red blood cell, which then becomes the site of a new series of nuclear divisions and manifold multiplications, utilizing the adenine triphosphate, glucose, and oxygen in the hemoglobin of the red cells. The results of the new proliferations are termed "merozoites." For each mosquito-injected sporozoite, as many as 30,000 merozoites (McGregor 1964:88) may be the end products of the exoerythrocytic and erythrocytic phases.

The first clinical manifestations—chills, shakings, and fevers that may reach as high as 107 degrees Fahrenheit (41.7 degrees Celsius)—occur when the red cells rupture and spill the merozoites as well as their toxic products of metabolism into the host's circulation. It is also at this time, and only at this time, that the human immunological resources are stimulated to react against the foreign invastion and that antimalarial drugs become effective (no biological or medicinal mechanism is known that destroys the original sporozoites). In addition, during this phase, the parasite is for the first time demonstrable through laboratory techniques in which the microscopic bodies are seen as pale discs or ring forms.

Some of the merozoites will develop into sexual gametocytes, or crescent forms. These male microgametocytes and female macrogametocytes may reach maturity but they cannot undergo sexual conjugation in the human host. The crescent forms are never found in the blood at the early stages of the infection; rather, they appear seven to ten days after the first clinical attack. If at this point, when the sexual gametocytes are in the peripheral circulation, they fail to be ingested by a susceptible mosquito, they will be phagocytized by fixed reticular cells of the host and no longer constitute a source of new infection to another human. It is only the sexual form of merozoite, the gametocyte, that can infect a mosquito and continue the malaria parasites' life cycle.

MacDonald (1957:6) notes that at first the erythrocytic forms apparently multiply freely but that within a week after the first clinical symptoms appear there is a marked reduction in the rate of multiplication. He postulates that in this way some balance of numbers is achieved even though there is a fairly dense parasitism, approaching 100,000 parasites per cubic millimeter of whole blood.

As Kitchen (1949b:966) describes this "balancing" process:

> It might be said that the course of an uninterrupted infection is characterized by the appearance of one or more waves, each comprising four or five successive generations of trophozoites, which evoke a febrile reaction until the patient develops a degree of tolerance for the parasite and/or its products that terminates his responses, although the parasitemia may continue for a variable period beyond this point.

This scant human immunological response perhaps constitutes the crux of the malaria problem, giving singular vigor to the parasites' perpetuation and making the disease one that presents tremendous obstacles to eradication.

Hackett (1937:250, 251) speculates that if one hundred malaria infections were distributed completely at random among one hundred humans, thirty-seven might escape infection; for another thirty-seven there would probably be one infection; for eighteen, two infections; for six, three infections; and for two, four or more infections. He adds, "The incidence of malaria can go no higher, of course, than 100 percent, but the intensity of infection may still increase almost indefinitely, bringing about what is known as a *hyperendemic* situation." Thus, where the anophelines are abundant and active, and where human social conditions expose people to their stings, until some resistance is achieved through years and years of continuous infection—or death intervenes—human malaria seemingly has no saturation point.

EFFECTS OF MALARIA ON HUMAN HOSTS

In general, severe parasitic infestations cause a rapid loss of red blood cells, with consequent disturbances in the body chemistry. According to Clark and Tomlinson (1949), the destruction may amount to as much as one million cells per cubic millimeter for each paroxysm. Their estimate appears applicable only in cases of overwhelming, fatal infestations. The human body, as a rule, will not survive infection of 20 percent or more of its red blood cells, although, as in all human diseases, occasional unexpected recoveries do occur. Kitchen (1949a), for example, describes the recovery of a six-year-old boy with an infestation of 26 percent of his erythrocytes. For falciparum, a parasite count of 750,000 per cubic millimeter of whole blood is generally accepted as the limit of tolerance.

To clarify the parasite-erythrocyte ratio, it is helpful to use some calculations (in Boyd 1930:20) of Sir Ronald Ross, who proved the mosquito's role in transmitting malaria. According to Ross, when the number of parasites has increased to approximately 50 per cubic millimeter of blood, the patient starts having the first definite symptoms. An average healthy adult male, weighing 142 pounds, may be estimated to possess some 15 trillion red blood cells; thus the above ratio equals about one parasite for every 100,000 erythrocytes, or 150,000,000 parasites in the victim's body. The limit of tolerance (750,000 per cubic millimeter of whole blood) becomes more meaningful when seen in this light.

The extensive red cell destruction severely taxes the body. To the burden of severe anemia is added the equally onerous problem of eliminating the many products of red cell breakdown. The spleen, congested with millions of destroyed red cells, shows the most dramatic reaction as it enlarges to many times its normal size, giving the characteristic "ague cake" or "swollen belly" appearance to so many inhabitants of malarious areas.

Probably no part of the body remains unaffected by the violently disrupted biochemical balance, so that death, when it occurs, may be attributed to any one of a multitude of immediate causes. Although the sequel to most infections, particularly in adults, may be recovery, a long period of debilitation as well as recurrence of symptoms is likely to follow. And, as already noted, one, two, three, or more infections give no adequate protection against additional incursions. Each new inoculation by an infective mosquito assaults the human host with a new disease, with new symptoms and additional burdens on an already overtaxed body.

MOSQUITOES, THE DEFINITIVE HOSTS

Mosquitoes taking blood meals from hosts with gametocytes in their peripheral circulation may at that time acquire plasmodia that can continue the parasitic cycle if the necessary circumstances obtain. Susceptibility of individual anophelines to infection, varies, depending on heredity and probably also on how well the biochemistry of the ingested blood has fulfilled the metabolic and nutritional requirements of the plasmodia. Again it may be stressed that neither the sporozoites, nor the liver forms, nor the primary forms developing in the red cells are able to infest the mosquito; only the sexual forms, the gametocytes, can continue the cycle in the mosquito.

Gametocytes ingested by susceptible mosquitoes undergo a sexual phase. In the anopheline stomach the male exflagellates, or emits germinative threads. These fertilize the female elements, producing zygotes that become capable of independent movement and thus can encyst themselves in the mosquito's stomach wall. A maturation period follows, lasting ten to fourteen days, depending on atmospheric conditions. During this entire phase the mosquito may take numerous blood meals, all accompanied by salivary injections, but she is not infective to humans.

By a special process not completely understood, the encysted elements perforate the insect's gut and, as sporozoites, some reach the mosquito's salivary glands. If the mosquito then inoculates an animal susceptible to malaria, the parasite continues its cycle, going again into the asexual multiplication phase in the vertebrate host and so on ad infinitum.

In view of the extremely complicated and demanding mechanisms required for malaria's transmission, its persistent prevalence on a world scale is a striking illustration of the operation of a "mechanism for generating a high degree of the improbable," or as aptly put by Hackett (1937:68): "The most astonishing thing about malaria, considering the chances against its successful transmission in nature, is the appalling amount of it in the world."

The basis for the above statements becomes patent through a brief recapitulation of some of the factors required for successful transmission: (1) *Anopheles* mosquitoes must prosper in the environment, which means that they must be near an appropriate water source where they can lay their eggs and the larvae can hatch (Fig. 7–5). This requires at least one or two weeks, during which time the water must remain undisturbed and the larvae must not be consumed by any predators. (2) A healthy female adult mosquito must take a

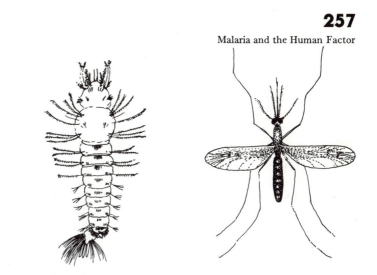

7–5 *Left*: larva of *Anopheles quadrimaculatus* adhering to water surface. *Center*: external anatomy of larva. *Right*: adult stage of mosquito. The larva and the pupa (not shown) require water for their successful development; thus eradication attempts often focus on water supplies, using various substances that interrupt the growth and development of this vector of malaria. In some circumstances it is deemed more effective to spray walls of homes to destroy the adult mosquito. Occasionally mass irradiation of males is attempted when other antimosquito attacks have failed.

blood meal not just from an infected person but from someone in one particular stage of infection—the exact time when gametocytes have appeared in the circulating blood. (3) Gametocytes must be passing through the site from which the mosquito is withdrawing blood. (As cases become more chronic, fewer gametocytes appear and those present seldom tend, for some unknown reason, to be found in the peripheral circulation.) (4) The mosquito must survive in nature long enough for sporozoites to enter her salivary glands. Hackett (1937) suggests that, theoretically, only one in four mosquitoes will live long enough to achieve this condition, requiring as it does at least fourteen days of adulthood. (5) Both the number and the vitality of the sporozoites decrease the longer they have been in the mosquito, and before those in the salivary glands degenerate and die (approximately six or seven weeks), the female anopheline must find another blood meal in a susceptible host. (6) The human host must, of course, survive the length of time required for the gametocytes to be produced and must be in a situation where the mosquito can take a blood meal. Indeed, the degree of improbability of all these events occurring at the proper times is staggering; nevertheless, the fact that they do is testified by the calamitous incidence of malaria among human populations.

IMMUNOLOGICAL STIMULATION TO TRANSMISSION RATES

> A balance must always be struck in nature between a parasite
> and its host. The most successful parasitisms are those
> which do not disturb too profoundly the normal life of the
> host; and malaria is one of the most successful of all
> parasitisms, since through vast lapses of time the attack
> has developed a counter-resistance which can only check but
> not destroy it. (Hackett 1937:170.)

In endemic areas such as are found in most of tropical Africa and much of the Far East, malaria is a year-round menace. Tolerance to the parasites builds up over many years of constant exposure.

Immunity to malaria is not innate; although a newborn may receive a transitory passive immunity from its mother, there exist no inherited exemptions, no racial immunity. When the short-lived passive immunity has gone, the child of an infected mother becomes as susceptible as all other infants to the threat of malaria. In endemic areas, regularly one-third to one-half or more of all infants die of malaria in the first few years of life. Among those who do survive are likely to be those children who have inherited an allele for one of the abnormal hemoglobins. This alters the red cells in such a way as to offer a somewhat less hospitable environment for the parasites and therefore reduces the severity of the infection. But even these children do not escape malaria; they survive as a result of the attenuating effect of their hemoglobin on the malaria they contract.

Russell (1952:38) claims that it takes fifteen to thirty years of continuous exposure to develop sufficient immunity to effect a truce between the parasite and the host. Significantly, resistance is effective only against the clinical manifestations of the infestation, because immunity develops only against the merozoites that are produced after the exo- and erythrocytic cycles are completed. Immunity, therefore, does not preclude active infection, but the height and constancy of the immunity do depend largely on the inoculation rate and the strength of the victim's immunological responses.

One result of continuous immunological challenge is reflected in the results of McGregor's (1964) study of differences among various populations in levels of gamma globulin in the serum. This blood substance is basic to the synthesis of antibody formation. McGregor compared four populations: (1) unprotected Gambians, that is, those receiving no antimalarial medication; (2) protected Gambians; (3) West Africans living in London for several years; and (4) Europeans who had had no malaria exposure. He found a gamma globulin level of 175 milligrams per kilogram for the first group, 100 for the second, 50 for the third, and only 25 for the unexposed Europeans.

Similarly, a World Health Organization study (1963) showed that adult Ghanaians with a high degree of immunity synthesized and catabolized gamma globulin at a daily rate eight times greater than that of nonimmune Europeans. McGregor (1964) and others suggest that prolonged heavy infections perhaps constitute stronger stimuli to immunological response than do transient light infections. Similarly, Boyd (1930) and Hackett (1937) stress that variations in clinical manifestations as well as immunological response depend primarily on an individual's history of exposure to malaria.

Apparently, the human response to various strains and species proceeds at differing rates. Hackett (1937:164) reports that J. G. Thomson "found among the native children of Nyasaland that while the parasites of *P. vivax* and *P. malariae* had practically disappeared from the blood by the age of nine, all the children continued to show ring forms of *P. flaciparum.*" He adds that "no gametocytes of any kind, however, were to be found after that age," thus, incidentally, implicating the young children as the reservoirs of active transmission.

In addition to being the most seriously affected, children apparently are the chief source of gametocyte production in endemic areas. In Hackett's (1937:246) words, "Babies are non-immune immigrants and add dry fuel to the fire of malaria." As early as 1899, Robert Koch noted that in endemic areas malaria is frequently confined almost wholly to the children (Howard et al. 1912:197). Christophers and Bentley (1911:24), reporting on a study conducted among the tea garden labor crews in Duars, India, lamented:

> It is very doubtful if one child in many hundreds will be found whose blood is not more or less thin and watery and whose whole physique is not modified by malaria. . . . In some instances, seen by us, malaria seems responsible for the almost complete absence of children among certain communities, nearly every child dying within a year or two of its birth.

Boyd (1930:115) maintains that "true endemic malaria probably exists only in the tropics." Falciparum, the most virulent species, occurs over most of tropical Africa below 5,000 feet and in many parts of India and the Far East. The malaria situation in other regions of the world differs sharply. As many investigators of malaria have stressed, the human barriers against being completely overwhelmed by malarial onslaughts develop in response to the pressures exerted by the disease, and then only slowly over many years.

Epidemiological evidence suggests further that the pressure must be a continuous, steady type such as is found in endemic regions. Where numbers of anophelines are erratic—decreasing in cold or dry weather, increasing in hot, rainy weather, reacting to modifications in agricultural techniques—transmission becomes sporadic and human immunological systems of defense become disorganized and ineffectual. Populations lacking constant stimulation are unable to sustain strong communal immunological barriers. The result could be this seemingly incongruous situation described by Hackett (1937:216): "A native of Nigeria can remain in relatively good health while he is being infected almost every night, but if the rate of infection were reduced or interrupted for a long period he might not do so well."

Consequently, any changes in transmission balance—for instance, increases in numbers of mosquitoes, deviations in mosquito biting habits such as a switch from cattle to humans, the arrival of new gametocyte reservoirs in the form of human immigrants from malarious areas—may set fulminating epidemics into motion. MacDonald (1957:52) charges that, most commonly, epidemics stemming from the abnormal multiplication of anophelines are properly described as "man-made malaria." To illustrate his point, he writes:

> South East Asia has suffered particularly, and much from the construction engineer whose borrow-pits and obstructions to natural drainage by roads, railways and ill-laid culverts have provided innumerable breeding places for *A. culicifacies* and other carriers. The health of the entire State of Bengal, for instance, deteriorated during the last century largely owing to this cause.

The pattern of malaria found in much of India, particularly the Punjab, and of Ceylon has been historically one of dormancy interrupted by violent upsurges due to intermittent transmission. With no opportunity to acquire steady immunological reserves, populations periodically have been devastated by sweeping epidemics. The record suggests that similar patterns marked much of European and American history when the onset of cold weather regularly interrupted transmission or social factors introduced disruptive population changes.

Malariologists have claimed that the contrasts between these two patterns of transmission—the steady, stable endemicity of the tropics versus the sporadic, fickle upsurges and alternating periods of quiescence found in other parts of the world—are so great as to betoken different diseases. Hackett (1937:266) adds to this concept emphatically: "Everything about malaria is so moulded and altered by local conditions that it becomes a thousand different diseases and epidemiological puzzles."

HISTORICAL BACKGROUND

> For as long as man has had a history, malaria has been at
> work, more effectively than any secret agent, undermining
> whole nations, attacking, killing men, women and children
> by the millions and holding back progress everywhere . . .
> [It is] the greatest single destroyer of human life. . . .
> Malaria-infested societies never prosper and often in his-
> tory they have gone down into decay, victims of the marshes
> and the mosquitoes and their own chronic ill health. (Leff
> 1953:176.)

Although a cursory consideration of this dramatic statement might lead one to dismiss it as so much rhetoric, even a brief review of the historical record tends to lend some credence to it. As Fiennes (1965:53) remarks, "Malaria may perhaps be the oldest disease in history; if not it has been in the past, and still is today, the most important."

PREHISTORIC EVIDENCE OF MALARIA

Emerging humans probably were subjected to malaria, according to Russell (1955:2), who maintains that "when man appeared, mosquitoes were already an ancient form of life with needles sharpened and adapted to the procurement of vertebrate blood." Evidence of fossilized mosquitoes, many trapped intact in amber, is widespread, and evidence of parasitism dates back almost three billion years.

Malaria's ubiquity in the animal kingdom suggests an evolutionary history predating hominids by many millions of years. Coatney et al. (1971) propose a primeval parasite originating in an invertebrate host somewhere in the jungles of Southeast or South Central Asia. They postulate a spread to early tree-dwelling reptiles and, at a much later stage, a proliferation throughout Asia, particularly through the cercopithecoid ancestors of Old World monkeys. It is believed that the parasite was introduced into Africa by early apes and man in relatively recent times, perhaps five hundred thousand to one million years ago. Further, it is generally agreed that the rigorous requirements for continuous transmission make it unlikely that malaria became consequential in human existence until the advent of settled village life in association with agriculture.

THE FAR EAST AND THE MIDDLE EAST

Bruce-Chwatt (1965b) postulates that Mesopotamia was one of the most historically important malarious areas of the ancient world. In evidence he offers Mesopotamia's geographical location plus frequent cuneiform notations of both lethal and intermittent fevers that appear in the eight hundred clay tablets dealing with medicine that were found in the library of Ashurbanipal, a king of Assyria, and date as far back as 2000 B.C. Additional circumstantial evidence, suggesting not only the presence of malaria but also some native suspicion of its carrier, derives from the early depictions of Nergal, the Babylonian god of pestilence, who appears in the form of a double-winged insect. And there is also Russell's (1955:4) suggestion that the Hebrew *gaddahath* in Leviticus XXVI:16 was perhaps malaria, which "doubtless was endemic in Palestine."

Apparently malaria was well known in China long before the Christian era, and, not surprisingly, a demonic origin was advanced. Hoeppli (1959) notes the depictions in Chinese mythology of three demons thought to be responsible for the characteristic headache, chills, and fever of malaria: one demon, equipped with a hammer, knocks on a skull and causes headaches; a second demon, holding a pail of cold water, gives rise to chills; and a third, seen with a stove, produces fever. By the second century a popular treatise on fevers appeared, attributed to a physician named Chang Chi.

One of the earliest recorded unmistakable mentions of malaria is attributed to Susruta, a Brahmin priest and founder of Aryan surgery, who about 500 B.C. gave a clear description of malarial fever, which he thought was caused by mosquitoes. Bruce-Chwatt (1965b:376) records the following incantation that suggests an unhappy familiarity with the symptoms of malaria. It is taken from the Atharva-Veda and is addressed to Takman, a fever demon:

> To the cold Takman, to the shaking one, and to the deliri-
> ously hot, the glowing, do I render homage. To him that
> returns on the morrow, to him that returns for two succes-
> sive days, to the Takman that returns on the third day,
> homage shall be.

After examining the lost cities of Ceylon, including the ancient capital, Anuradhapura, founded in 437 B.C., Nicholls (1921) concluded that the once vigorous populations that left "picturesque ruins comparable to the Egyptian pyramid of Gizeh" were victims of malaria. He traces the introduction of rice cultivation as primarily responsible for providing favorable breeding sites for the mosquito vectors and notes (ibid.:123) that the culture "was not overwhelmed by a single great catastrophe. The energy of the people waned through many years." As he explains it:

> Diseases such as cholera and plague are terrible in their
> visitation; the majority of those who are infected die, a
> few recover and in a few years the effects of the outbreak
> will have disappeared and leave behind no permanent damage
> upon the population. It is different in the case of malaria;
> the children of the fever-stricken areas are in a continual
> state of ill health and those who live grow to an enervated
> manhood. And the decay is persistent and accumulative
> through generations. (Ibid.:124.)

THE MEDITERRANEAN REGION

In the Mediterranean region malaria has figured prominently throughout recorded history and continues to do so today. The Iliad of Homer, dating back about a thousand years before Christ, contains a reference to "autumnal fevers" that are attributed to the stagnant marshes and the destruction of the forests during the Bronze Age.

As Hippocrates observed in the fifth century B.C., swollen spleens were common among the inhabitants of the marshy regions. The four cardinal "humors" of Hippocrates include black bile, thought to originate in the spleen, the Sigerist (1943:150–151) observes:

> It may seem queer that the spleen should have assumed
> the rank of a cardinal organ, since it is rather inconspic-

uous and systematic dissections were not performed in those
days. The explanation may be that these theories were
elaborated in malaria regions. Megalospleny is a symptom
of chronic malaria. . . . Thus the spleen, located in the
left part of the abdominal cavity, seemed to balance the
liver on the right.

Laderman (1975) speculates that the deforestation that made
way for intensification of agriculture and provided wood for the
many ships required for the Persian Wars in the fifth century B.C.
enhanced conditions for the spread of malaria vectors. And the wars
themselves, she proposes, introduced new reservoirs of parasites, as
did the Olympic Games, which by the sixth century B.C. were drawing competitors from possibly infested areas.

The record indicates that malaria was well established, perhaps
endemic, in Greece by 400 B.C., although Jones (1909:30) offers
evidence suggesting that the typical fevers and chills became common
in that region more than a century earlier. He cites the Greek scholar
Athenaeus, who describes the city of Sybaris as lying in a valley that
was torrid around noon but extremely cold during the morning and
night hours. "Hence arose," writes Jones, "the saying that he who
did not wish to die young ought to avoid, in Sybaris, seeing the sun,
either when it rose or when it set." Jones interprets this as a likely
reference to the biting times of the indigenous mosquitoes.

Malaria had much to do with the fall of Greece, according to
Jones (1909:107–108), who claims that largely as a result of malarial
devastations, "under the Roman dominion the general character of
the Greek race was no longer what it had been in the glorious days of
the past." This metamorphosis was, he believes, partially wrought by
the disastrous epidemic that ruined agriculture, flooded the cities
with "sluggish and unenterprising" sick people, decimated the youth,
and effected a "habit of laziness" and "psychical disturbances."

In Italy, as early as the fifth century B.C., Empedocles, a states-
man and philosopher, rescued the Sicilian town of Selinunte from the
"fevers" by draining the swamps, thus converting the stagnant, mosquito-breeding sites into flowing streams. Jaramillo-Arango (1950:4)
records that for his efforts Empedocles received "the same honours
as those bestowed upon a warrior or a poet."

Malaria played a significant role in the history of Rome, particularly in the Campagna, the land surrounding the city. Sigerist
(1943:126) states, "There is no doubt that malaria was the history-
making factor in the Roman Campagna." Russell (1955) suggests

that malaria may also have been a critical factor in the decline of the Etruscans who had inhabited the Campagna before the days of the Republic.

The cult of the Fever Goddess, *Dea Febris,* was extremely old. She was depicted as "a hairless old hag, with prominent belly and swollen veins, . . . half-naked and in the act of drinking" (Sambon 1901:350). Hackett (1937:5) notes that "to Cicero it was already 'the *old* Fever Temple on the Palatine.' " The goddess Febris was still worshipped immediately prior to the advent of Christianity and with its establishment "found expression among the Romans in the veneration of the Virgin Mary under the title of *Madonna della Febbre,* whose painting now hangs in the Sacristy of St. Peter's in Rome" (ibid.:6).

References to malaria-like fevers in Rome around 200 B.C. are found in Plautus, Terence, Cicero, Celsus, and Pliny the Elder (Russell 1952:2). Horace (Ep. I, vii) wrote: "The first figs and the heat bring out the undertaker. . . . Every father and fond mother turns pale with fear for the children, while diligence in the Forum's petty business brings on fevers and unseals wills." In Haggard's (1929:180) view, it was after centuries of malarial debilitation that Rome was pillaged by the barbarian tribes from the forests of Germany: "Malaria and plague were as much its conquerors as were these Goths and Vandals."

The ravages of malaria continued unabated after the advent of Christianity. But the political effects were reversed, perhaps because the indigenous population had acquired some degree of tolerance or perhaps because of an increased (or new) selection for thalassemia, a familial hypochromic anemia that continues to occur frequently among certain Italian populations. Hackett (1937:6) records:

> For centuries malaria was actually the protector of Rome.
> Foreign conquerors found it impossible to take possession of
> the capital of Christendom and make it their residence. The
> invaders were always decimated, but the natives were spared.

In 1167, this concept was put to verse by Godfrey of Viterbo, an eyewitness in Rome to the fevers that destroyed the army of Frederick Barbarossa (Celli, 1933:95):

> When unable to save herself by the sword
> Rome could defend herself by means of the "fever";
> The soldier, of whom but yesterday she was afraid, dies from
>   fever,

Those from whom Rome was unable to defend herself, were
    dispersed by the air
At whose breath the German youth fell;
Thus when Rome is silent, our glory sinks.
Within a short time, vanquished by the Roman disease,
Is vanquished and overcome power and might, the lords of
    the world.

Echoing the old Italian adage *Malaria vien della pentola* ("Malaria depends upon what comes out of the pot"), Bruce-Chwatt (1965a:132) notes that malaria "today still divides the rich world from the poor." Historically, however, malaria was quite democratic in its selection of victims, striking indiscriminately at peasant, poet, pope, or king. It is said that Alexander the Great died of malaria in Babylon (Haggard 1929). And "Plutarch says that Pericles 'seems' to have died of a mild attack of the Plague . . . but the symptoms, as given by Plutarch, are strongly suggestive of malaria" (Jones 1909:36). Dante met his death of fever likely to have been malaria contracted on a journey in Ravenna in 1321 (Celli 1933), and five centuries later malaria claimed the life of Lord Byron in Greece. Henry VII of the House of Luxembourg was struck down in 1313 apparently by malaria "at the very moment he was making preparations to conquer Rome for the second time" (ibid.:83).

Malaria's ability, over the centuries, to vanquish the most highly placed is exemplified in the following report, which is attributed to Tegan, the biographer of Louis le Débonnaire and concerns ninth-century Rome (Celli 1933:73):

Lothar, son of Louis, did not make his appearance at the
Council of Worms because at that time he had a fresh attack
of the fever and was seriously ill. The Emperor's orders
could not be carried out on account of a pestilence which
killed Wala, Abbot of Corby, and kept Lothar in bed for a
very long time. . . . We must in this connection mention,
with great wonder, the widespread and deadly infection
(fever) which seized those who had followed Lothar to Rome;
for within the short period that elapsed between the first
days of September and St. Martin's Day [November 11] there
died the following prelates, the Bishop of Amiens, the
Bishop Elic of Troves, Wala of Corby, Matfrid (Earl of
Orleans), Hugh (of Tours, Lothar's father-in-law), Lambert
(Earl of Nantes), Geoffrey Agimbert, Earl of Pertens and
Burgarit, the former Royal Master of the Hunt. Richard
narrowly escaped death; soon afterwards he also died. These

were the men by whose loss France, as it was said, was
bereft of her nobility and her strength destroyed, for it
was as if her nerves had been cut through and her wisdom had
sunk into the grave with their passing.

By the fourteenth century, foreign popes were no longer
allowed by the Church to reside in Rome. "The letters of Petrarch
make it unmistakably clear that the obstinate refusals of Popes and
cardinals alike to transfer the papal court from Avignon to Rome
were due solely to their fear of the 'Roman fever,' " according to
Warshaw (ibid.:23). When the move eventually was made, their ap-
prehensions were validated. In Rome, in 1590, Sixtus V died of malaria, and a month later, Urban VII, his successor, succumbed from
the same cause. In 1623, eight cardinals and thirty secretaries of the
Vatican died and many more fell ill—all, Hackett (1937) claims, from
malaria.

Warshaw (1949:23) notes that "it was an attack of malaria that
prevented the notorious Cesare Borgia from placing all of Italy under
his power." Anticipating his father's imminent death, Borgia had
fully prepared himself to seize authority but when the critical
moment came, he was down with fever and chills. The list of malaria's victims is interminable; Celli's (1933) fascinating history of the
Roman Campagna includes more than twenty-five pages on some of
the historical figures who were felled by the "Roman fever" in the
late Middle Ages.

ENGLAND

Malaria had a long history in England, lasting well into the middle of
the nineteenth century. It was responsible for the death of James I
and for the severe illness of Charles II. When Sir Walter Raleigh was
condemned to die on the gallows, he reportedly pleaded with his
jailers to arrange his execution for a particular time of day, when he
would be free of the malarial shaking that he thought might be
construed as a sign of fear (Warshaw 1949).

Although the name "malaria" (implying a relationship to the
bad air of the swamps and marshes) was bestowed on the disease
early in the 1700s by a young Italian physician named Tonti, in
England "ague" became the vernacular description for the same disease and its common symptoms. Russell (1955:182) reports that
when Defoe visited the Essex marshes in 1722, he was told that the
local men went to the uplands to obtain their wives but that these
women, having been raised in relatively mosquito-free regions, pos-

sessed no immunological resistance to malaria and often succumbed
to the "ague" soon after going to live in the marshes. Defoe reported
that he frequently met men who had had "five-six-fourteen wives,
nay, and some, more!"

The ardent Protestant Oliver Cromwell "succumbed at White-
hall from a 'bastard tertian ague' in 1658, a bad malaria year" (Ship-
ley 1908:238). Ironically, about three years earlier, aid to malaria
victims had become available in the form of powdered bark from the
South American cinchona tree, a source of the still-useful quinine.
But the popular names of this Peruvian import—"Jesuit's Bark,"
"Cardinal's Powder," and "the Popish powder"—suggest why none of
Cromwell's physicians dared administer the medication to him. As
Warshaw (1949) records, rumors circulated throughout the Protestant world implicating the Jesuits in an international plot: they
were, it was said, using the bark as an insidious poison to destroy all
those who had renounced Catholicism to embrace Protestantism.
Consequently, the zealous Protestants, including Cromwell, were
denied the one possibly effective therapy for their malaria, succumbing, in a sense, as much to the religious hysteria of the day as to the
plasmodia.

A number of illustrious patients, including Charles II, the
Dauphin son of Louis XIV, and the Queen of Spain, were reportedly
cured of malaria by the spectacular English charlatan or physician—
the record is not clear—Robert Talbor, who did use the bark from
the New World but so ingeniously disguised it that the secret of his
remedy was revealed only after his death.

An unexpected dividend of an encounter with malaria crops up
in a statement attributed to the English naturalist Alfred Russel
Wallace. Apparently the key to evolutionary theory, the idea of
natural selection, flashed into his mind while he struggled with an
attack of the fever acquired in his travels (Dobzhansky 1962).

Russell (1955) notes that the chief vector of malaria in the
English marshes was *Anopheles messeae*, a mosquito that has a strong
preference for animals other than man but will accept humans as
hosts when its preferred blood meals are not available. With the
introduction of turnip culture in England in the mid-nineteenth century, enough food became available for cattle so that the former
annual herd slaughter was no longer necessary. Subsequently, as the
cattle population increased, sufficient numbers of mosquitoes turned
from humans to the preferred, and now abundant cattle to effect a
significant reduction in malaria transmission among the English.

Unfortunately, the tolerance formerly possessed by the men of the marshes, as implied by Defoe's anecdote, was no longer maintained at a functioning level once the immunological stimulus of continuous transmission subsided. When these unprotected men were later sent to fight in malarious areas of the world, the upshot was at least 30,000 malaria-downed troops in 1916, 70,000 in 1917 and, as Hackett (1937:21) says, "No one knows what might have happened in 1918 had they not repatriated 25,000 of the worst and most chronic cases." Similarly, during 1942 and the first half of 1943, malaria casualties among the Allied troops exceeded battle casualties in ratios sometimes as high as thirty to one.

EUROPE

Russell (1956) estimates that the maximum worldwide expansion of malaria occurred sometime between 1885, when an epidemic occurred in southern Canada, and 1922–1923, when the disease approached the Arctic Circle in the Soviet Union. Although "malarial fevers were always rampant in Russia" (Garrison, 1929:794), the stresses of war, drought, and famine combined in 1914 to extend the range of malaria to the shores of the Arctic and the Caucasus. By 1923, in the Soviet Union, there were six million reported cases, which Garrison estimates were probably only one-third of the actual number affected, and mortality reached 40 percent in some areas.

Similar epidemics occurred during World War II in many countries of Europe. Leff (1953:230) reports there were 150,000 cases in Belgium in 1946; 14,000 in Poland as compared with the annual average of 250–300 cases in the preceding decade; 470,000 in Italy as compared with 58,000 only six years earlier; and comparable large-scale epidemics in Spain, Portugal, and Greece following the disruption of the long war years.

Even today areas formerly thought to be free of malaria pose new threats. The Adana area of southern Turkey is a case in point. Here crops requiring steady supplies of water—rice, many vegetables, citrus fruits, and cotton—are grown successfully. Between May and September each year, 700,000 seasonal workers migrate to the Adana region to work in the fields. Anderson (1978) reports that by the early 1970s malaria had been virtually eradicated not only in this region but in all of Turkey. But then control measures were relaxed, and by 1974, 2,877 cases of malaria were confirmed in Turkey. The number shot up to 9,828 in 1975, 37,320 in 1976, and 115,350 in

1977—and the bulk of the cases were in the Adana region. Antimalaria agencies are employing all means available to halt the invasion: larvicides are used on pools of dirty water; antilarvae fish are added to mosquito-breeding lakes and ponds; houses are sprayed thoroughly and regularly; radio and television are employed to encourage people to obtain antimalarial medication; and testing is done on a mass scale. Knowledge of the past history of malaria's impact on Europe has prompted many European countries to contribute cash and goods to help Turkey fight this unexpected battle.

THE CONTROVERSY OVER MALARIA IN THE NEW WORLD
By contrast with the Old World, the New World lacks indisputable historical evidence of malaria in pre-Columbian times. There is no controversy regarding the presence in prehistoric times of suitable vectors for transmitting plasmodia; the arguments hinge on when the parasites arrived and with whom.

According to many workers in the study of disease (Boyd 1941; Cockburn 1971; Dunn 1965; Effertz 1909; Johnson 1969; Modell 1968; Thomas, 1956), malaria was completely unknown in the Americas before the arrival of the Spaniards and their African slaves. On the other hand, the Ecuadorian historian Arcos (in Jaramillo-Arango 1950), Hoeppli (1959) and Jaramillo-Arango (1950) assert that malaria existed in America from pre-Columbian times.

Arcos contends there is linguistic proof that malaria was rampant in the armies of Pachacutec in A.D. 1378. Jaramillo-Arango (1950:31) agrees, arguing that since it is definitely known that prehistoric Asian people had malaria, "we see no reason why these primitive discoverers and colonizers of the New Continent should not have brought malaria with them." This position is upheld by Hoeppli (1959).

The advocates of a preconquest origin offer evidence in the form of pictures of mosquitoes on prehistoric pottery from New Mexico. In addition, they point to several Mayan words that they translate as "malaise, headache, chills, and fever." Unfortunately, the linguistic evidence derives from manuscripts translated after the Spanish conquest and most likely bears much European influence. Guerra (1964:43), for example, cautions, "The books of *Chilam Balam* are copies, of copies, of copies of codices."

A third possibility is raised by Bruce-Chwatt (1965b), who introduces the likelihood of a preconquest source of malaria parasites into the New World through an early human population that could have reached the American landmass by crossing the Pacific à la Kon-tiki. This is an even more difficult position to prove or deny since a sea route virtually precludes the possibility of much archeological information. However, one opposing argument is that Hawaii and other Pacific Islands are known to have been free of malaria vectors prehistorically.

The case for a late introduction, either after or very shortly before the conquest, rests upon biological, immunological, and historical grounds. Dunn (1965) offers a strong biological argument. He notes that whereas in Africa and Asia, plasmodia have been found throughout the primate and mammalian world, in the Americas they are found in nature only in human populations and in some cebid monkeys. Therefore, "the vagaries of host and geographical distribution of American primate plasmodia support the conclusion that these parasites have not been established in the New World for a very long period of time" (ibid.:389–390). Dunn notes further that the many genetic red blood cell polymorphisms such as sickle cell anemia, G-6-PD deficiency, and hemoglobin C and E, all found in association with malaria in other parts of the world, apparently do not exist among the New World aborigines.

An earlier advocate of the "late introduction" school was Otto Effertz, who practiced medicine in East Africa and Mexico in the early 1900s. Remarkably ahead of his time in basing his arguments on immunological evidence, Effertz (1909:250) marked the "extreme malignity" of malaria when contracted by natives of America as contrasted with its "extreme benignity" among adults in Africa. He said that in his day, much of coastal tropical America was inhabitable only by "pure Africans because, on account of malaria, Indians cannot live there," whereas in the days of the conquest these areas were the sites of large Indian populations (ibid.:260). There is general agreement today that extreme pathogenicity indicates a newly established parasitic relationship.

Effertz also recorded that his Indian patients absolutely refused to take quinine because, they insisted, it was too strong for their blood. "Quinine is taken out of a tree of American origin. Yet native healers knew nothing of its febrifuge properties," Effertz wrote, commenting that it "is probably the only American remedy which escaped Indian healers" (ibid.). Effertz praised the skill and knowledge of Indian healers when they treated such diseases as syphilis, which he claims had a long American history, and he concluded that his findings strongly suggested that the Indians "could not yet ac-

commodate themselves to the new circumstance of recent malaria"
(ibid.:261).

Several advocates of the post-Columbian origin of malaria in the
New World (cf. Boyd 1941; Bruce-Chwatt 1965b), countering
Arcos's and Hoeppli's position, stress that the requirements for continued malaria transmission make it highly unlikely that the disease
could be maintained by small groups of people moving from Asia to
the North American continent across the cold and arid regions of the
Bering Strait. They add that historical records of the early *conquistadores* give no indication that these Europeans encountered malaria-
like symptoms in their many American expeditions.

IMPLICATIONS OF A RECENT INVESTIGATION

Wood, Harrison, and Weiner (1972) and Wood (1974, 1975) provide
additional inferential evidence supporting the case for malaria's late
introduction to the New World. They found that 3,500 female
Anopheles gambiae tested on human volunteers took preferentially
more blood meals from hosts who possessed blood group O. From
this finding, it follows that, if the same choices are made consistently
in nature, then many persons belonging to this blood group would be
sufficiently disadvantaged that a degree of selection favoring a certain proportion of blood groups A, B, and AB would result. Conversely, in the absence of this selection by malaria, the naturally
occurring selection against blood groups A and B due to mother-child
incompatibility (Cohen 1970; Matsunaga and Hiraizumi 1962) would
result eventually in the virtual elimination of the A and B genes from
the population.

Serological investigations of Asian populations reveal comparatively high and widely dispersed values of groups A and B. The
distribution of the polymorphisms found suggests a long period of
adaptation. It is most unlikely that the Asian immigrants to the
Americas would have failed to possess a certain portion of these
genes. Nevertheless, among the aboriginal populations in the Americas, where there has been no European or African contact, blood
group distributions tend, with only one or two exceptions, to approach 100 percent frequency for blood group O.

The implication of this unique distribution is that no forces
selecting for the presence of blood groups A or B, such as malaria,
existed until relatively recently. As a result, ABO incompatibility
pressures remained unopposed and A and B genes declined to their
present near-zero level. The findings of this investigation may there-

fore add fuel to the argument favoring malaria's comparatively recent arrival in the New World.

In addition, scientific investigations substantiate the common claim that individuals within the same population differ markedly in their relative attractiveness to mosquitoes (Hackett 1937). The dynamics of malarial transmission indicate that the role of the vector, particularly the factors influencing her choice of hosts, is of crucial importance. A new avenue of exploration is opened by the above-noted investigation of the host's blood group as one factor influencing the malaria vector. Sequels to this investigation might focus on why the *Anopheles gambiae* chose as they did, possible relationships of their choice to other blood group systems, the choices of other species of anophelines, and how choices are made by the vectors of many other human diseases.

IMPACT OF MALARIA IN THE UNITED STATES

The malaria-origin controversy continues, but there is no dispute regarding the prominent role malaria assumed after the conquest. One of the reasons the Pilgrims in 1620 went to New England instead of the originally projected Guiana in South America, was according to their leader, William Bradford (in Childs 1940:28), because "such hott countries are subject to greevous diseases and many noysome impediments, which other more temperate places are freer from, and would not so well agree with our English bodys." Unhappily, the Pilgrims did not escape malaria by changing their destination to the Atlantic seaboard; outbreaks were disastrously frequent there.

The Jamestown colonists were recruited primarily from London and its vicinity, which at that time, according to Boyd (1941), had high rates of malaria. Late in April 1607, they arrived at the small, marshy island. By the end of June, an epidemic had progressed to the point where scarcely ten people could either "stand or go." Of the original 105 settlers, fifty were dead by mid-September of that year. The capital of the colony was moved finally from Jamestown to Williamsburg in 1699. To the north, a series of epidemics, very likely malarious, swept through the Massachusetts Bay colony in 1647, 1650, and 1668.

To the south, the volume of African slave trade was rapidly building up by the 1560s. In addition to contributing large reservoirs of plasmodia, the African slaves demonstrated a superior resistance to the infestations of malaria. The latter attribute was recognized as essential to the successful exploitation of agriculture in the coastal regions and became the foundation upon which the West Indian sugar industry developed (Boyd 1941).

Childs (1940:30) maintains that the strength of the Africans' immunological response to malaria "rendered the Europeans incapable of competing with the Africans in outdoor labor in the southern part of the United States"—and thus, he says, was slavery established. The African's mixed blessing of increased tolerance to malarial parasites became particularly crucial when rice culture was introduced into the Carolina low country around 1690. This region became the most intensely malarious along the Atlantic seaboard, and again the African laborer, with his high level of hard-earned immunity, was granted an unsought labor monopoly.

Malaria did not lose much time in joining the pioneers, and, with the implementation of "Manifest Destiny," the plasmodia were borne rapidly across the entire United States. The spread was hastened by the custom of using streams and rivers for main routes wherever possible in crossing the country and by the proclivity of the pioneers to settle on the banks of these water routes. The indigenous *Anopheles quadrimaculatus* were on hand to serve as vectors.

By 1829, ague and fever appeared around Fort Vancouver on the lower Columbia River and, among the Indians, produced epidemics that annihilated entire tribes—or nine-tenths of the aboriginal population, according to Boyd (1941). After the discovery of gold in the West in 1849, the flood of immigrants from all parts of the world provided additional malarial reservoirs—new plasmodia strains as well as malarially virginal human hosts—all of which readily attracted California's indigenous *Anopheles freeborni*.

The Civil War, with its disruption of normal life, food shortages, lack of public hygiene, and displacement of populations, created epidemic conditions in many formerly quiescent areas and, via soldiers returning to the North, introduced malaria to regions where it had earlier been relatively unimportant. In the decades that followed, malaria became a nationwide fact of life.

Recalling impressions of his youth, Dr. V. C. Vaughan (in Warshaw, 1949:29) recorded: "In 1865, every man, woman and child in southern Illinois, at least in my range, shook with ague every other day. . . . The minister made his appointments to preach so as to accommodate his shakes." Warshaw (ibid.:200) says that in the Middle West "in some towns the church bells were rung daily at dusk to remind the inhabitants to take their Dr. Sappington's pills." (The pills were quinine disguised with licorice, myrrh, and oil of sassafras.)

During this period, the new American settlers, suffering from the omnipresent malaria, developed characteristics reminiscent of Jones's description of the Greeks around 400 B.C. These settlers, in sharp contrast to the more familiar Hollywood legends, are described by Warshaw (1949:29) as "Thin, sallow, pale and sickly, their chronic debility ... often reflected by an indolence of speech and movement."

Warshaw (ibid.:29–30) augments his descriptions with a carica-ture drawn by the medical historian Fielding Garrison, who pre-sented the malaria-ridden American of his day in terms one hopes are at least slightly exaggerated:

> He was literally hamstrung by the malaria and so-called typhomalarial fever. . . . All along the watercourses, from the Mississippi to the Potomac, the salient physical type of the caricaturists was pale, gaunt, haggard, attenuated, narrow-chested, spindle-shanked, sharp-featured, lantern jawed, lank-haired, anxious-eyed, with care-furrowed brow of pasty, sallow, bilious or dyspeptic complexion, of serious concen-trated, careworn expression and languid or irritable mien; his womankind, like himself, scrawny, without incentive to dis-play the meager charms concealed by ruffles and pantalettes, and of forbidding aspect, as if about to call the police, or, like the celebrated Miss Baxter who "refused a man before he axed her."

Until the early 1930s, more than 100,000 cases of malaria were reported annually in the United States. By 1942, eradication efforts, improved social and economic conditions, and changes in agricultural techniques had combined to reduce the number of malaria victims to 60,000 annually (Pratt et al. 1963). Finally, by 1947 there was be-gun a United States Malaria Eradication Program, which succeeded in a few years in eliminating malaria in the general population.

MALARIA AND CULTURE—AN INTIMATE RELATIONSHIP

THE LINK BETWEEN TRANSMISSION AND SOCIAL AND CULTURAL PRACTICES
Considering the elaborate requirements for continuous malaria trans-mission, one would be hard put to find a disease more directly de-pendent on social and cultural practices for its persistence among

human populations. And, given the impartiality exhibited by nature, the plasmodia and their winged vectors have been unerringly adept in adjusting to the habits and vagaries of the human hosts. Even the peaks of activity of many of the species of mosquito vectors coincide with the times that gregarious humans are likely to congregate out-of-doors for their various social activities.

Indeed, it might be argued that the mosquitoes themselves, as well as their accompanying protozoa, could probably not have done better if they had been the directors of the human social and cultural practices that would provide the easiest marks for their needs. Amorous liaisons, for example, which most cultures deem best conducted with discretion, almost invariably involve clandestine meetings at times when the mosquitoes are poised for attack and often take place in the bush where no protection from the mosquitoes is feasible, even if one could assume that the couples indeed ever had mosquitoes or malaria on their minds.

Prothero (1965) notes another covert, mosquito-enticing activity in the illegal movement of Sudanese across the dry or shallow river beds into neighboring Ethiopia to buy *arragi*, an alcoholic liquor forbidden in Muslim Sudan. He (ibid.:60) observes, "Those who travel for this purpose do so at times when mosquito activity is at a maximum and there is every likelihood of them being bitten."

Even where eradication measures have been introduced, social practices frequently are found to favor the parasites rather than human health. A prime example is what happened after the colonial division of Somalia created artificial borders and intense political tensions. When eradication procedures were initiated, water tanks where mosquitoes bred were treated with insecticides on one side of the border but, less than a hundred yards away, the mosquitoes were unopposed and could subsequently infect both sides of the border with impunity, irrespective of political affiliation. Prothero (1965:75) warns that such populations "will continue to be ravaged by malaria and other diseases until adequate interterritorial coordination and cooperation are established."

RELATIONSHIP TO AGRICULTURE

Historically, perhaps the most common source of new opportunities for the encroachment of malaria has been the felling of virgin forests to create agricultural land. The conversion frequently disturbs the ecological balance and at the same time provides new sites as well as susceptible human hosts for the opportunistic vectors and their nefarious passengers. As Bleibtreu (1969:290) comments on the sequence of events:

> [Frank] Livingstone has traced the genesis of this complex
> relationship between man, mosquito and protozoan as a sequel
> to the introduction of iron tools for clearing the tropical
> forest, the cultivation of food plants giving high yields of
> calories on tropical soils and the formation of settled
> agricultural communities which provide both an ecological
> setting favorable to the *Anopheles gambiae* and a human
> population higher in density than that of the hunters and
> gatherers who were earlier occupants of the region.

Hackett (1937:90) describes how the pioneering phase of land occupation and development provides social conditions that are frequently linked with intense malaria transmission:

> There are many non-immunes in the labour aggregations,
> while infected immigrants bring new strains of parasites
> and acquire others. There is a shortage of accommodation,
> with overcrowding, which greatly facilitates the spread of
> infection. There is a local increase in mosquito production,
> resulting from a disturbance of the natural balance . . . ,
> leading to a high inoculation-rate. There is increased
> severity of clinical symptoms with an associated increase
> in gametocytes, due to primary attacks, new strains, young
> sporozoites, lowered resistance, and multiple infections . . .
> and finally, there are few or no domestic animals.

At other times, since the advent of agriculture, the shift to different crops, such as rice, with its requirements of extensive irrigation, has fostered additional breeding sites for the anophelines as well as the increased human population densities under conditions described by Bleibtreu and Hackett. Such a situation, and concomitant malaria intensification, occurred in the Carolina lowlands, as mentioned above, and far more recently in California, when vast land holdings and irrigation projects initiated the present "agribusiness" approach to farming. Likewise, severe epidemics began in Holland when land reclamation sufficiently reduced water salinity to invite mass mosquito production.

By no means are all the mosquito proliferations due to large-scale agricultural changes; on the contrary, as Boyd (1930:209) illustrates, the most seemingly insignificant ecological changes can often lead to the development of new mosquito-breeding sites:

Although gambiae occurs in a great variety of types of water, the most striking are the shallow, open, sunlit pools with which every field worker in Africa is familiar. The origin of such pools is legion and may range from barrow-pits, drains, brick pits, ruts, car tracks and hoof prints around ponds and water holes to those resulting from the overflow of rivers, pools left by receding rivers, rain waters. . . . The stamp of human activity is implicit.

Similarly, Sarkad (1975) reports that the water used for settling cement floors in half-constructed multistoried buildings in Calcutta were found to be the source of prodigious mosquito production.

EFFECTS OF HUMAN ACTIVITIES, MIGRATIONS, PILGRIMAGES, AND WARS

Intensified malaria transmission is often the inadvertent by-product of many other human activities and institutions. Prothero (1965), in examining the activities of the market women among the Hausa and Yoruba peoples of West Africa, shows how the market institution itself, by providing meeting places for friends and relatives from the hinterland, serves as a mechanism for increased malaria transmission.

Pottery, frequently introduced in association with agriculture, became a potential lure for mosquitoes because it made possible the storage of large supplies of water. Villagers living a safe distance from mosquito-breeding river banks may unknowingly import mosquito nurseries into their villages through the use of large, clay storage jars that are too cumbersome to clean frequently but will hold sufficient water for the parturient anophelines to deposit their eggs. McClelland (1973:34), reporting on the significance of these jars among the Makonde tribespeople in southeast Tanzania, notes, "Such water storage habits, once necessary for human survival, have become ritual so that the practice persisted even when piped water was available."

Prothero (1965:41) also documents the vast movements of Africans from villages "to large farms, plantations, mines, factories, commercial centers, and ports" for purposes of migratory labor—at least five million people on the move in sub-Saharan Africa each year. Many of these migrants are males in search of a bride price; occasionally, as reported by a group of migrants from West Cameroon, tension from witchcraft threats has provoked an exodus from certain villages. Prothero's study reveals that migrants, particularly farm workers, can expect to be housed in temporary shelters with roofs and walls of straw that quickly become the choice resting places for the *Anopheles gambiae* and prove quite resistant to spraying when eradication with insecticides is attempted.

The migrants are frequently gone from their villages for more than a year, during which time they may introduce gametocytes into virgin territories or, in other instances, may return to formerly uninfected villages with red blood cells that contain parasites acquired while in their labor camps. Even when infected workers travel to infected areas, new strains of plasmodia are exchanged and general conditions tend to encourage the process. In all cases, demographic disturbances inevitably seem to work to the advantage of malarial transmission.

Religious customs that entail pilgrimages and mass convergences in specific places often set the stage for intensified transmission (Fig. 7–6). Prothero (ibid.:33) describes the Islamic requirement for

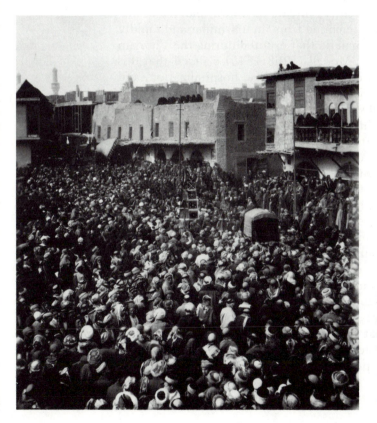

7–6 Pilgrims and funeral procession in Iraq. In such crowded conditions, where sanitation is at risk, new populations, including the infected and the infectious, are in intimate contact and the transmission of malaria as well as other diseases is intensified. (Courtesy of Field Museum of Natural History, Chicago.)

making the *Kaj*, the pilgrimage to Mecca or Medina, at least once in a lifetime. He then shows how this practice, resulting in the massing of hundreds of thousands of infected, along with susceptible, people under conditions of exhaustion, inadequate housing, and haphazard nutrition, virtually ensures widespread transmission.

On a less massive scale, clan and tribal convergences for feasts, funerals, weddings, and other universal human rituals often bring together the same hazardous combinations: unsettled housing, susceptible humans juxtaposed with infected ones, and all accompanied by vectors ready to go into action. Here again, much of the celebrating is frequently accomplished at the end of the day and continues through all or most of the night, giving the mosquitoes once more a distinctly unequal advantage.

War, conquest, and related man-made institutions have, as discussed earlier, substantially heightened rates of malaria through much of human history. Recently, threats of a new man-made malaria situation have emerged, stemming from an unfamiliar and rapidly spreading malignant form of malaria that erupted during the Vietnam War. In the midst of the war, Modell (1968:1346) claimed that this new falciparum strain "caused more disability, hospitalization, and demoralization among American soldiers in Vietnam than enemy fire did." Shortly after Modell's report appeared, there was a marked increase in aerial bombing. In addition to the immediate tragic consequences, these actions created thousands of bomb craters that retained water and thus became ideally suited for lavish mosquito breeding and, no doubt, assured the production of inestimable numbers of vectors to transmit the new falciparum strain. This form of malaria, which, Modell (ibid.) warns, "threatens to envelop the world," is resistant to chloroquine and most other synthetic antimalarial drugs as well as to quinine. But, through military medicine, a one-dose cure has been found in the combination of sulfalene and trimethoprim. These drugs cause a folic acid deficiency, to which protozoa are sensitive. Though successful as a quick treatment, the drug combination is, unfortunately, not feasible as a prophylactic, so the search for a preventive goes on. A sinister note is sounded in reports of experiments that have shown the South American night monkey *Aotus* to be capable of acting as a reservoir for this form of malaria, thus opening the possibility of new pathways of transmission of the disease.

A HANDFUL OF MOSQUITOES—FOURTEEN THOUSAND DEATHS

Although some 150 species of *Anopheles* have been described in the world, only about 10 percent have been implicated as malaria vectors and these have generally been thought to be rather rigidly dependent on the specific environment in which they evolved. But in recent years, as Boyd (1941) notes, the freshwater gambiae has shown itself capable of hitchhiking rides on modern transport and then establishing itself with distressing versatility in the new home. Studies have indicated that the epidemic that struck Brazil in the 1930s was the result of the surreptitious entry of a few infective *Anopheles* on board planes that flew from Africa to Brazil. They soon spread from the city to the hinterland, creating, in Boyd's (ibid.:206) words, "the most dramatic epidemic ever seen in tropical America." By 1938–1939, deaths reached fourteen thousand—a toll resulting from less than a handful of venturesome mosquitoes!

Recognizing the emergency, the Brazilian government, with the aid of private U.S. foundations, launched a massive mosquito extermination program, costing two million dollars, over an area of fifty thousand square miles. Twenty Brazilian doctors, five sanitary inspectors, and some two thousand men plus mobile laboratories were employed (Shannon 1942). Apparently, enough gambiae were destroyed to halt the epidemic and, in addition, a valuable lesson was learned. Today, every plane arriving in Brazil from Africa is thoroughly sprayed and examined.

HUMAN PRACTICES THAT REDUCE MALARIA TRANSMISSION

On a more optimistic note, occasionally human activities have acted to divert the hungry mosquitoes, sometimes protecting one segment of the population while exposing others, but sometimes shunting the mosquitoes to nonhuman hosts. In villages where subsistence depends largely on fishing, the men who are away at sea through most of the anophelines' biting times have fewer infections than the women and children left at home with the mosquitoes (Boyd 1930). Conversely, in societies such as those in the Islamic world and many parts of India where the women are cloistered and swathed in heavy clothing, a considerably lower parasite rate occurs among the females than among the males (Russell 1952).

Boyd (1930) and others have found that most anophelines, if given a choice, prefer large livestock over humans for their hosts.

Consequently, in many formerly endemic regions, where changes in agricultural practices have led to animal husbandry, especially dairying, and special enclosures have been constructed for the animals, the blood-sucking vectors have been diverted to their preferred bovines and human malaria rates have dropped dramatically. Similarly, in Romania, Noguer (1976) reports that the indigenous carrier *A. maculipennis* switched completely from human hosts to domesticated animals as a result of recent improvements in the people's habitations.

Boyd (1930:103) notes that in some instances the establishment of agriculture has served to reduce mosquito infestations. Specifically, he points to a zone of the coastal plain in Malaya where the vector *A. umbrosus* breeds only in undrained jungle pools. Here the people living in the virgin jungle are often heavily infested with malaria parasites but become practically free of the disease when the jungle is cleared and the land drained.

Occasionally, certain cultural practices have evolved in response to the assaults of the mosquitoes and, in the process, have reduced or eliminated malaria rates. Howard, Dyar, and Knab (1912) report that in many areas of the world, during the heavy biting seasons inhabitants of sporadic malarious regions established temporary living quarters in nearby hills where the mosquitoes would not follow. A similar tack was followed by the shepherds of the Roman Campagna who customarily constructed scaffoldings several meters above the ground so that they could spend their nights relatively secure from heavy mosquito attacks. And, Laderman (1975) notes that in northern Vietnam, the hill people build their houses on stilts so that they live much of the time about eight to ten feet above the ground, with their domesticated animals directly below. The anophelines specific for that area seldom fly to the heights of the living quarters and also prefer to obtain most of their blood meals from the more conveniently situated animals.

For some areas of the Americas as well as in Mauritius and Ceylon, Boyd (1941) cites reductions in mosquito numbers and malaria rates due to the practice of washing clothes in streams where mosquitoes would ordinarily breed. The washers use strongly alkaline soaps that change the pH of the water to such an extent that the mosquito larvae are destroyed.

Even where no relationship between mosquitoes and malaria is recognized, most people will readily acknowledge that life is more comfortable without their nettlesome presence. Consequently, many attempts are made to persuade the mosquitoes to go elsewhere. Shipley (1908) catalogues some of the many folk remedies employed to discourage the mosquitoes. Pyrethrum, derived from chrysanthemums, has a long history of use as an insecticide. When blown into corners of a shelter as a powder or burned as "pastilles," it is believed to "stupefy the mosquito." Eucalyptus has been employed for a similar effect: When a few twigs or leaves are placed around the sleeping area a good night's sleep is, reportedly, assured. Other substances used as repellants include castor oil, lavender (chewed and then rubbed over the body), the familiar cooking herb basil (burnt or sprinkled as a powder), tar (used in ointments), and fish grease. In short, as Warshaw (1949) observes, nearly everything that smells has been used at some time somewhere in the world to ward off the voracious intruders, and not infrequently the odors have proved less offensive to mosquitoes than to humans.

MALARIA ERADICATION AND SOCIAL PROBLEMS

Leff (1953) stresses the direct dependence of diseases such as malaria on social conditions. He argues, and is substantiated by even the most cursory historical review, that though malaria is now largely confined to tropical regions and therefore often classified with such truly tropical diseases as yaws, yellow fever, and sleeping sickness, it was not long ago that malaria was common in all countries of the temperate zone before social conditions improved and it is still prevalent in countries like Greece, Spain, and Italy where poor social conditions are general.

In support of this position, it has often been noted that malaria as well as diseases like plague, typhus, and leprosy once occurred in widespread areas throughout the world and declined in importance in countries where social conditions and sanitation improved, long before there was accurate medical knowledge concerning their cause or treatment. Bates (1965:307) augments Leff's argument, adding that in any attempts at eradication of mosquitoes and malaria, "the crying need seems to be for concentration on strategic operations in what might be called the social field."

The economics of malaria today remains a fundamental stumbling block to eradication. Malaria affects primarily the poorest parts of the world. Therefore, as Peters (1975) explains, few of the profit-oriented pharmaceutical companies today are prepared to invest in the search for compounds such as antimalarials. Ironically, such progress as has taken place in this direction derives from the pressures of military demands such as the recent Vietnam involvement, which stimulated the development of a promising human malaria vaccine (Silverman 1977).

On the other hand, as Hackett (1937:319-320) cautions:

> Ignorance, poverty and disease constitute a vicious triangle of
> human social inadequacy. An attack on any one of them
> helps to dissipate the other two. But the causes of malaria, at
> least, are in the main independent of the ignorance and pov-
> erty of its victims and can be separately handled. It is easier
> to believe that release from the burden of malaria will help to
> bring prosperity and knowledge than that a higher standard
> of living and education must precede the eradication of
> malaria.

Although the technological means—insecticides, drainage of swamps, deterrent drugs, and other approaches—are available and sufficiently advanced to achieve almost complete eradication of malaria from human populations, again and again agencies attempting this task confront cultural and social forces that have to be recognized and adapted to before eradication measures can proceed (Fig. 7–7). It has been the frustrating experience in many eradication programs, perhaps predictable through the application of anthropological techniques and knowledge, that methods efficacious for one society, or several, were found to be unworkable for others.

An example of this problem was demonstrated in the utilization of the Pinotti method (Prothero 1965), combining common salt with an antimalarial drug, which was first applied on a large scale in the Amazon valley of South America. The procedure achieved a limited, but steady, degree of success there because the product was acceptable to the people and its distribution was in the hands of a small number of agents. Giglioli (1968:113) states that the "entirely primitive" Wai-Wai Indians from the depths of the Brazilian virgin forest "take to the use of the [chloroquinized] salt with great readiness as soon as it is made available." He adds that "at the present stage of malariological knowledge and antimalarial technique, it appears likely that treatment and prevention may be extended more easily to the primitive and semi-primitive Indian through the established channels of intertribal barter trade, in a bag of salt, than through a spray gun or a bottle of tablets."

The Pinotti technique was also attempted in Tanzania and in northern Ghana. The immediate results were spectacular: the parasite rate fell in two months from 80 percent to 5 percent. Nevertheless,

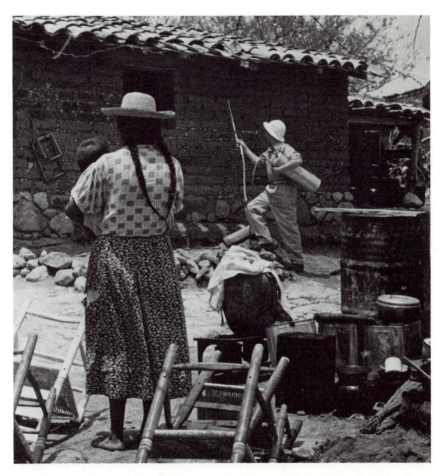

7–7   An antimalarial technician sprays a temporarily vacated home in a rural area of Mexico. In some parts of the world the cycle of malaria transmission has been disrupted by destroying the adult mosquitoes that frequently rest on walls during the day. (Courtesy of World Health Organization.)

the operation failed. The results could not be sustained because the people were accustomed to pillars of hard, grey, crude salt, obtained from many local sources in the Sahara, and soon they surreptitiously began to obtain this familiar, unmedicated salt. This example shows, once again, that innovative technical advances can succeed only when they are adaptable to a people's customs, or when adequate anthropological research prepares the way for innovation.

Even the character and world views of a people, as molded by their traditions and way of life, require the understanding and flexibility of workers in eradication programs. When Sir Ronald Ross (who in 1902 received the Nobel prize in physiology and medicine largely for proving that mosquitoes transmit malaria) proposed the organization of antimosquito brigades in London early in this century, an unprecedented storm of protest flooded the local press. Some argued that mosquitoes could not be destroyed since they spring "naturally" from grass and trees; others more vociferously maintained that mosquito control was basically immoral and contrary to the will of God since these insects were created to punish man for his many sins. Many years were to pass before the program became a reality.

Howard, Dyar, and Knab (1912:16) found that, in South America, those who lived around the Rio de la Magdalena regarded the swarms of mosquitoes as a nuisance but believed that they were good for human health: "These animals, say the inhabitants, bleed us slightly and in an excessively warm country, they preserve us from ... inflammatory maladies." Clearly these people were not likely to cooperate in a program to remove the mosquitoes.

Prothero (1965:36) cites the many nomadic peoples of Africa whose harsh and often cruel way of life has made them independent, conservative, suspicious of outsiders—"resentful of control and direction"; consequently, they often constitute major stumbling blocks in eradication programs for which they have not been adequately prepared. Similarly, the many people who are frequently cited as not recognizing malaria as an important factor in their lives, which are overburdened by more dramatic tropical diseases, have not been convinced that the same chills and fevers that discomfort them for a few days account, in large part, for the appallingly high numbers of infant deaths among them. Mothers, particularly, can become valuable allies in eradication programs when they become convinced that the lives of their children might be spared as a direct result.

CONCLUSION

As a disease that selects young children for its principal victims, malaria has been a significant agent of natural selection, molding exposed populations into forms able to withstand its onslaughts, demolishing those unable to rise to the challenge. A disease primarily of the red blood cells, malaria has probably been the chief selecting agent in the perpetuation of various hemoglobin anomalies that confer some degree of tolerance to the threatened human victims.

As the discussions of mechanisms of transmission and immunity have indicated, malaria is essentially a quantitative disease, achieving a steady rate of transmission and a counterbalancing degree of resistance in those tropical areas where endemicity exists. But even to a person already infected with one or more malaria infestations, new infections bring serious consequences. Inoculation with different species or different strains means new disease, giving rise to fresh cycles of symptoms, postponing recovery, and putting additional burdens on an already overtaxed body.

Under these conditions, an equilibrium, or perhaps more accurately, a precarious truce, is approached between the human host and the plasmodium. Unfortunately, this *entente* becomes operative for the human host only after he has built up stores of immunological reserves sufficient to disarm the invading parasites. The opposing forces are engaged, as McGregor (1964:91) writes, "not on the beaches but subsequently when the plasmodium has been permitted, by cryptic amplification in the cells of the liver, greatly to increase its numerical strength."

Young babies are lost if they receive levels of parasitemia larger than the natural resources of the body can handle. If the numbers of red cells destroyed are so overwhelming that the spleen and other organs cannot cope with the breakdown products and the bone marrow is unable to replace erythrocytes in numbers sufficient to maintain homeostatic mechanisms, a Pyrrhic victory is achieved by the parasites and the child succumbs. Considering that a full-term newborn is likely to possess only about 300 cubic centimeters of blood, the numbers of parasites required to destroy the critical 20 percent of the red blood cells appears precariously low.

At the same time, in the face of continuous threat, no individual living in a malarious area is likely to survive into adulthood unless he has acquired the degree of immunological stimulation required to provoke effective antibody production. Apparently, for malaria, not only is the acquisition of immunological tolerance painfully slow, but it demands continuous challenge in order to be maintained at a functioning level.

Thus the optimal condition for survival in a malarious region before eradication programs were introduced was the possession of any attributes that would reduce, but not prohibit, sporozoite inoculation by the anopheline vectors and grant limited success to those that did get injected. The processes of human evolution have responded to the "no-win" malaria strategy by selecting for the various hemoglobin dyscrasias and, possibly, by the selection for certain human blood groups that are less appealing to some mosquitoes. One is compelled to join with Ashburn (1947:100) in his exclamation:

> It seems a strange thing that such a power on the earth,
> such a great tyrant and oppressor of mankind, should depend
> for its very existence on stagnant pools and should need
> as its agent a fragile and stealthy insect. Yet it is so.

The impressive mechanisms evolved by malaria in its struggle for existence have provoked not only corresponding human social adaptations but also difficult decisions on the part of the international health agencies who have elected to engage it in battle. Stressing the ethnological and sociological implications of malaria control in underdeveloped areas, Bruce-Chwatt (1954:170) raises "haunting questions" confronting eradication agencies such as the World Health Organization: How safe it is to introduce eradication proceedings into holoendemic or hyperendemic areas where populations have made their peace with the disease, acquiring a high degree of tolerance to the parasites at the cost of the sacrificial tribute paid with the lives of the children? "What would happen," asks Bruce-Chwatt, "if the control over a large area broke down because of a financial slump, difficulty in obtaining supplies of insecticide, or political unrest?" Every malariologist knows the answer: epidemics would flare up, destroying not only the children but much of the rest of the then unprotected population as well. And every student of human affairs knows with equally distressing certainty that any of the deterrents to continued success outlined by Bruce-Chwatt are fully within the realm of possibility.

Nevertheless, knowing that the problems of eradication involve complexities that defy theoretical resolution, and perhaps calling on a strength of faith derived from the successes of other programs, WHO, in 1955 initiated a worldwide campaign to eradicate malaria. In so doing, it launched what has been called the greatest venture in public health the world has ever known. The initial attack involved spraying infested areas with suitable insecticides, followed by assaults on the parasites in the victims' blood streams with antimalarial drugs.

These initial skirmishes were succeeded by continuous surveillance for the appearance of new cases and resistant mosquitoes.

The contribution of WHO was to help plan the national campaigns, provide expert advice, stimulate research, and run pilot programs. At the height of the campaign, over 190,000 persons were directly involved—doctors, engineers, entomologists, microscopists, spraymen, and supervisors—covering eighty-five countries inhabited by 740 million people (World Health Organization 1963). The results were immensely rewarding; by 1970, a life free from malaria was granted to over 134 million persons. Yet, despite this success story, by 1978, two billion people lived in malaria-infested areas.

Obviously, the last malaria battle has yet to be fought. Nature, as always the impartial ally of all life, permits both the mosquitoes and malaria to fight for their survival. Drug-resistant anophelines have evolved as well as resistant strains of plasmodia. The human hosts have been beset with political, economic, and social problems that have made them recalcitrant to eradication measures. Nevertheless, the good fight has begun; the odds look better for the much beleaguered humans than for their persistent enemies. This is a "war" in which all humans are allies. And as the proper technologies and the social sciences join forces, eventually malaria will fade like so many other once-insurmountable diseases and become a part of an unlamented past.

THE TRADITIONAL HEALER: HOLISTIC HEALING IN RESPONSE TO STRESSES OF DISEASE

It is an insult to the medicine man to call him the ancestor of the modern physician. He is that, to be sure, but he is much more, namely the ancestor of most of our professions.

—Henry Sigerist (1951:161)

The antiquity of disease is established beyond dispute. From the evidence already reviewed in the bones of ancient peoples, we also know that life expectancy for all peoples known before the most recent times was half or less of that of modern, industrialized *Homo sapiens*. It is reasonable to postulate a parallel, ancient emergence of healers, the unique individuals to whom their compatriots turned for assistance and direction when serious illness or dysfunction disrupted the ordinary course of life. When such stresses occurred, the primary requisite for social survival was the continuation of the social organization with disruption kept to a minimum: water had to be drawn, children tended, and enemies kept at bay. Extended interruption of the ordinary activities could spell chaos and even extinction. Consequently, the functions of the healers who emerged in the presence or threat of illness encompassed far more than the treatment of disease.

Distinctions between physician, counselor, religious adviser, judge, and entertainer are relatively recent cultural innovations. For most of human existence, the members of small bands or tribal units probably subsumed all these roles in the person of the curer. This consolidation persists today for many people still living in social structures that closely parallel those of all human ancestry.

Few concrete data are available on the extent of illness experienced by preliterate peoples. Most commonly, the anthropologists in the field encounter the functioning members of the group; only rarely do they chance upon widespread medical situations such as the smallpox outbreak dramatically recounted by Bowen (1964) or the whooping cough epidemic recorded by Colson (1976). Indeed, even if a medical history, as conceived by modern medical science, were available for any of the societies with which we are concerned, it would be only partially illuminating because sickness is perceived with little predictability from culture to culture.

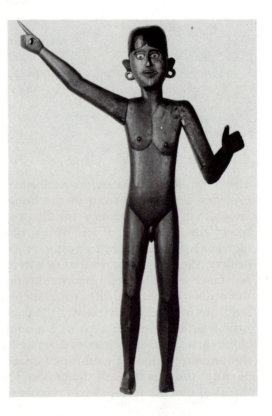

8–1 This anthropomorphic figure from the Nicobar Islands symbolizes the dread and fear of disease found among all peoples. The menacing posture is meant to ward off diseases. (Courtesy of Wellcome Museum of Medical Science, London.)

To be sure, there are some societies that can be cited as possessing so many conditions adverse to good health that they are probably able to function as social entities only through the employment of rigorous cultural mechanisms specifically evolved to deal with disease. The Cēwa of Rhodesia, for example, as described by Marwick (1967:104), live in an environment in which malaria, bilharzia, and severe intestinal disorders are endemic. In addition to these stresses—or perhaps directly derived from them—are poor hygienic conditions and a diet deficient in protein and vitamins. Consequently, for every thousand infants born, more than 250 die before being weaned—an infant mortality rate among the highest in the world. The appalling number of misfortunes in need of explanation and concern in a society in these straits makes the role of healer one of paramount importance for the society's survival (Figs. 8–1 and 8–2).

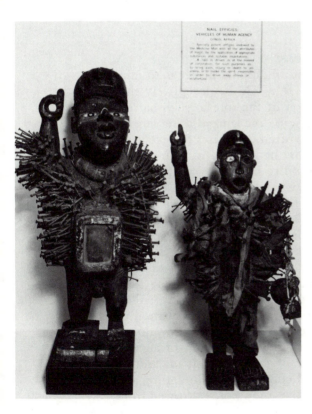

8–2 These nail effigies from Congo were used by traditional curers for more than one magical purpose. The nails were driven into the figure as magic spells were evoked to bring pain, injury, or death to the enemy being conjured. In other instances, the same approach could be used against the spirit of a disease in order to cure the patient. (Courtesy of Wellcome Museum of Medical Science, London.)

Within other societies where the evidence is less direct, it can be reasonably conjectured, from the intense preoccupation with disease made manifest in rituals and religion, that illness constitutes a major concern, playing a role at least equal to, if not greater than, the important one assigned to it by modern, industrialized societies. Further, what statistic could add to the picture of pathos, philosophical resignation, and uncounted "medical events" experienced by someone like the mother in Uganda whose child had just died and who replied to Bowen's (1964:125) offer of consolation: "She has just died. Children often die. It is their nature." What untold tragedies underlie the Nigerian Ogori and Yoruba peoples' belief in a class of spirit children, the *abiku*, "who never stay long in this world, but die and return again and again to plague their mothers" (Gillies 1976:367). Wherever human societies have had to confront conditions of this nature, there have been intense pressures within the group for individuals to emerge who could proffer leadership and succor and elicit an acceptable behavioral response from the afflicted population.

"THE ANCESTOR OF MOST OF OUR PROFESSIONS"

On the surface, the primary task of the traditional healer is to minister to the ills of his or her society. It would be deceptively simplistic, however, to restrict a description of the role to such narrow confines. The traditional healer can also be recognized as serving his people in the role of judge; indeed, he often comprises the exclusive judicial system. Equally important for the survival of human cultures, the effective healer is often found to be a consistent and primary force that welds and maintains what Eliade (1964) calls the "psychic unity" of the culture. And as the local resident "academic," the traditional healer is viewed by his society as the seer who provides explanations in historical contexts that give life a sense of continuity and depth (Fig. 8–3).

In addition, in preliterate societies, it is often the shaman, diviner, or singer who is the chief purveyor of the mythology and folk belief, as well as of the songs, dances, and art forms, of their culture. Not only is the curer's role crucial in the perpetuation of the society's mythology, but frequently the spiritual adventures derived from that role compose the substance of much of ancient mythology: "Probably a large number of epic 'subjects' or motifs, as well as many characters, images and clichés of epic literature, are, finally, of ecstatic origin, in the sense that they were borrowed from

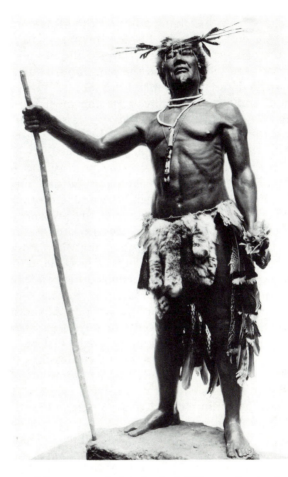

8–3   A Pomo medicine man conjuring the dead. This reproduction in authentic attire demonstrates the dignity and majesty of the traditional North American native healers. (Courtesy of Field Museum of Natural History, Chicago.)

the narratives of the shamans describing their journeys and adventures in the superhuman worlds" (ibid.:510).

THE HEALER AS JUDGE
Given that formally ordained judicial systems were unknown in societies whose state of organization precluded the luxury of nonsubsistence-producing roles, it is not surprising that the judicial function would be subsumed as a vital part of the office of curer. Whereas the

modern judicial system has many adjuncts of enforcement, the curer has one supreme sentence under his administration: it is within the province of his office to discover if any of the morals or mores of his society have been violated; and the sanction for such violations is sickness. As spelled out by Sigerist (1951:157): "Disease thus is a social sanction, and in many tribes it is the most important social sanction they know". Further, if the infraction is sufficiently serious, as testified by the gravity of the illness, then, in a sense, the curer is in the position of pronouncing a death sentence. As Nurge (1958: 1165) has expressed it, "one way to stay healthy and to insure the well-being of one's family is to obey the cultural mores, as they relate to interaction with both the supernatural and other humans."

It may be more precise to state that the presence or threat of disease, particularly as administered by the supernatural world, is the true judiciary, but it must be stressed that the mediator, the one interpreter with whom human exchange is possible, is the curer, the specially endowed person who has achieved his office as a result of direct interactions with these threatening forces. Moreover, as a result of his unique position, as pointed out by Ackerknecht (1971: 168), "the medical practitioner holds the keys to social control. . . . Medical diagnosis becomes thus a kind of 'social justice.' "

Reliance is often placed on extracted confessions from patients because such confessions not only reduce some of the fear and anxiety related to being sick, but also serve to restate the particular norms that have been abused and thereby strengthen the consensus regarding the importance of the rules that have been violated. Among Arctic peoples, for example, important healing sessions frequently involved the participants' disclosures to the shaman of taboos violated: a miscarriage improperly handled or kept secret, a forbidden food eaten, or perhaps an infraction of the rules for proper behavior during menstruation.

The very recitation of an emotionally charged confession acknowledged the antisocial nature of the infractions; the presence of the illness verified the punishment meted out by the gods or spirits, and, as a result, all could witness the precarious position of the shaman who thus had to "plea bargain" with the vindictive spiritual prosecutors. Concomitantly, every participant received an unmistakable message: these are our rules; these are our desirable norms of behavior; witness the troubles that descend upon us when they are violated! The law-enforcement power of such a judge, one who is able to pronounce sentences—bone-wracking fevers, hunger, painful abscesses, or any of the innumerable dyscrasias inherent in human existence—onto the society's lawbreakers, makes the power of the modern, industrialized society's judge, which is generally limited to the imposition of varying periods of incarceration, appear minuscule indeed by comparison.

Again and again, this function of the traditional healer has been impressed on the ethnographer. Turner (1964:262) writes of a Zambian healer, "It seems that the Ndembu 'doctor' sees his task less as curing an individual patient than as remedying the ills of a corporate group." Boyer (1964:397), in a study of Apache curers of North America, defines the shaman as "an individual who is considered to possess supernatural powers which support and are supported by the common values of his culture." Park (1967:234), says of diviner-healers, "In a controlled way [they] intervene in and affect the social process with rather definite and socially useful results. . . . Divination has as its regular consequence the elimination of an important source of disorder in social relationships." Likewise, Lambo (1964:446), in his study of the Yoruba of Nigeria, stresses: "Since disease is viewed as one of the most important social sanctions, 'peaceful living with neighbors, abstentions from adultery, keeping the laws of gods and men, are essential in order to protect oneself and one's family from disease.' "

Leighton et al. (1963:52) make a statement that, though it refers specifically to the Yoruba, could be universally echoed: "More than money, than education, than the city lights, than prestige, more than almost anything, the Yoruba people, like most other people, want to be free of illness and pain." Neither the shaman nor any of today's university-trained scientists can grant the Yoruba dream. But whereas the honest, scientifically oriented physician can seldom answer the cry "Why me?" to his patient's satisfaction, the shaman is not bound by such constraints. Indeed, the essence of his service is to provide the answer precisely to that crucial query. From his intimate knowledge of his patient's entire world, based on his daily interactions with the patient and, for probably a longer period, with the patient's family, the curer is mostly likely to focus on infractions of the social and cultural norms, infractions that his patient readily recognizes.

RESTORER OF "PSYCHIC UNITY"

The need for the healer to assume the role of peacemaker becomes self-evident when one considers the tension-producing elements of much of band, clan, or tribal living. Life in these societies permits little, if any, privacy; individualism is held in low esteem and is rigidly restricted; the "luxury" of social conflict is not affordable. Because of the necessarily close interactions and mutual dependency, internecine conflict could doom the entire village or group. Thus the need for a "psychic unity" becomes crucial and may be justifiably considered a survival mechanism. Much of the healing performed by the traditional curer was, and is, in the realm of forestalling social conflict and reducing social tensions, with the healer as mediator between the victim and his group. As stressed by Eliade (1964:237), the traditional healers see their mission as one "to ensure that the spiritual equilibrium of the entire society is maintained" (Fig. 8–4).

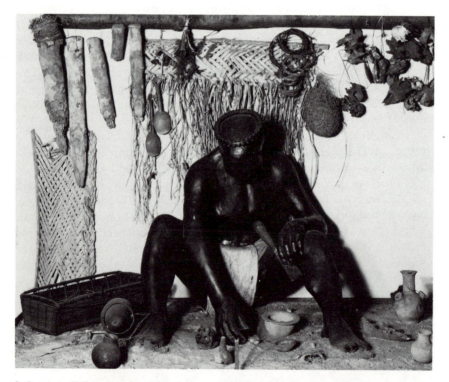

8–4 A medicine man of a medical secret society (Idiong) from Ibidio in southern Nigeria, with all the traditional equipment required in his art. A major part of the healing performed by the traditional curer was, and is, tied to forestalling potential social conflict. (Courtesy of Wellcome Museum of Medical Science, London.)

It is to them that the people come for reaffirmation of the values of the indigenous culture in times of crisis. Describing the *margidbu*, the healers of the native Australians, Berndt (1964:278) reiterates this function:

> In all cases the emphasis is on providing reassurance, on restoring confidence and on doing so in a familiar and therefore comforting way. . . . What they lack in medical skill they make up, to some extent, in knowledge both of the local situation and of traditionally effective means of dealing with crises.

Similarly, Gillies (1976:372) finds among the Ogori of Nigeria that the approach of the healer is to provide "social therapy. . . . A disease is dealt with essentially by righting the patient's life situation, his relationship with the people with whom he is most intimately concerned." The fundamental strategy that emerges in this approach is to present the illness of the individual as the vital concern of the collective body.

This concept is made explicit by Turner (1964:262) in his study of a Ndembu healer of Zambia:

> The sickness of the patient is mainly a sign that "something is rotten" in the corporate body. The patient will not get better until all the tensions and aggressions in the group's interrelationships have been brought to light and exposed to ritual treatment. . . . The raw energies of conflict are thus domesticated in the service of the traditional social order.

He relates how the Ndembu healer summons the kin of the sick person to an improvised shrine where they are induced to confess any grudges or hard feelings they may harbor against the patient. Similarly, the patient is also persuaded to ventilate any hostility he has been incubating. Following this "bush group therapy," which may also be accompanied by dramatic bloodletting, purification, tooth extractions, prayers to the ancestors, and the extraction of some object ostensibly from the patient's body, a restored and rejuvenated social group frequently emerges:

> Men and women who had been on cool terms with one another until recently, shook hands warmly and beamed with happiness. Kachimba even smiled at Makayi, who smiled back. Several hours later a mood of quiet satisfaction still seemed to emanate from the villagers. (Ibid.: 261.)

The same theme is illustrated by Jaspan (1976) in his discussion of the Rajang of Indonesia. The Rajang are acutely aware of the social support required by the sick person and probably contribute, on a different level, to the social unity by investing the time and assistance that the healer and society demand from the group associated with the patient. Jaspan records that kinsmen and friends expect and are expected to be in constant attendance. All night and all day there is always a small crowd beside the sick mat; at no time is the patient left alone to "brood in isolation."

The Navaho curing ceremonies, in particular, have impressed investigators as contributing to a sense of social solidarity. Fox (1964:175) singles out the "nine night sings," which involve "complex rituals and the assembly of thousands of Navaho" and strike him as having a "Durkheimian grandeur." Kaplan and Johnson (1964:228) find that through the active, often intense, participation of so many members of the patient's society the requisite "psychic unity" is achieved, along with

> reaffirmation of the solidarity of the community and indeed
> of the whole pantheon of Navaho deities with the patient.
> The ceremony surrounds him with concern and goodwill and
> serves as a kind of reintegration of the social group, with the
> sick person not only a solid part of it but at its very center.

Even when the cure is not complete, often the support expressed by the group for the sufferer can serve to ease the distress and to cement social bonds that have been strained by the illness (Fig. 8–5).

Far removed in both miles and culture, the !Kung of Africa's Kalahari Desert are, nonetheless, close to their Navaho and Indonesian contemporaries in the shared needs for support and relief in times of pain. Katz (1976:83) reports that one mode of healing requires the healer to wrap his body around the patient. He rubs his own sweat onto the sufferer in the belief that healing properties are contained in the sweat. Then he draws the patient's sickness into his own body, shakes it from his fingers out into space, "his body shuddering with pain." Katz (ibid.: 83, 85) describes, from his own observation, the "psychic unity" achieved through this healing ritual:

> Healing for the !Kung is much more than curing physical
> or psychological ailments, although it includes that. Healing
> nurtures each person's emotional and spiritual growth as well.
> The dance heals the whole person. . . . All receive the protec-
> tion of healing.

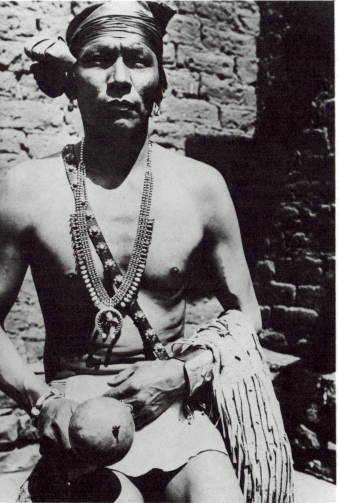

8–5 A Navaho medicine man. Investigators have been particularly impressed by the sense of social solidarity elicited by Navaho curing ceremonies. (Courtesy of Wellcome Museum of Medical Science, London.)

THE HEALER AS ENTERTAINER AND CULTURE HERO

An often overlooked but nonetheless important function of the traditional healer's role is one that stems from the nature of life in a small village or within an isolated hunting and gathering band. The members of such a group have usually been in close association since birth. The daily acquisition and preparation of food occupy the greater part of every day. Except for the events characterized as *rites de passage* or the comparatively rare hunt of a large animal, there are few dramatic interludes to entertain, stimulate, relieve the monotony, or contribute some "spice" to life.

In such a setting, the healer and his dramatic rituals become, if not the only, then certainly the best, "show in town" (Fig. 8–6). Geddes (1969:xv) underscores this aspect of traditional healing in his discussion of the curing rituals of the Land Dyak of Indonesia:

> The ceremonies for the actually sick, together with the larger festivals to keep sickness away from the village, provided the highlights of the peoples' lives. Much of their drama, dancing, singing and feasting depended upon them."

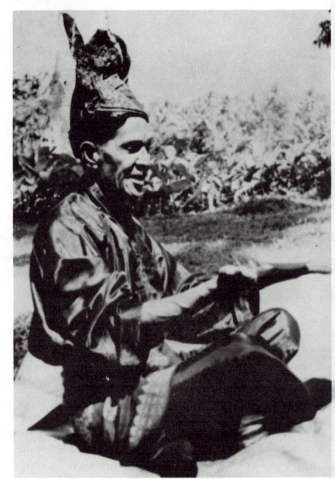

8–6 A Malaysian *bomoh*, in elaborate costume and posturing dramatically, prepares an herbal offering to ward off evil spirits. (Courtesy of World Health Organization. Photo by J. Dauth.)

A vital component of the healing rite is the need to hold and incorporate the attention of the audience. Indeed, as Balikci (1967: 209) points out, "All shamanistic practices [involve] the presence of an audience." To the extent that the curer must continually validate his "call," he must perform in a manner that convinces his clientele that they have chosen well, that he does indeed have powers that transcend those of ordinary mortals, and that, therefore, he is deserving of their support and confidence. The most cursory examination of a shamanic or divining ritual reveals performances that, to achieve these goals, are suffused with all the trappings of true entertainment: drama, pathos, suspense, human interest, music, fantastic costumery, magic, and audience involvement.

Kaplan and Johnson (1964:223) note that the Navaho culture included more than fifty major ceremonials associated with curing. The greatest of the traditional medicine men or "singers" were expected to maintain or restore the desired harmonious balance of nature through the performance of rituals that could require the combined efforts of most of the community and might consume up to nine days and nights. Kluckhohn and Leighton (1962:309) compare the singer's task to that of memorizing a Wagnerian opera, "including orchestral score, every vocal part, all details of the settings, stage business and each requirement of costume."

An intrinsic element of the traditional curing ceremony is the creation of a highly charged, emotional setting, in many ways a communal acting out of the forces of life against the unremitting dark threats that encroach from both sides of the grave. Human vulnerability is surmounted as the assemblage, united in purpose, supports and is supported by their own culture's hero who is willing to brave all on their behalf. As Eliade (1964:182) puts it, in the case of the shaman:

> Through his own ecstatic experience he knows the roads of the extraterrestrial regions. . . . The danger of losing his way in these forbidden regions is still great; but sanctified by his initiation and furnished with his guardian spirits, the shaman is the only human being able to challenge the danger and venture into a mystical geography.

The mood and setting of the ceremonies described by awed ethnographers give some insights into the impact that the curing rituals would have on an even less sophisticated audience. Turner (1964:259), in his description of a Zambian ceremonial, tells of "the intense excitement whipped up by the drums; the patient's trembling; mass participation in the sad-sweet or rousing hunters' cult songs, which are sung to 'please ihamba,' followed by the spate of confessions and the airing of grievances, the reverent or hortatory prayers."

Unquestionably, however, the consummate artists were the Siberian and Alaskan shamans. Relying primarily on hypnosis, ventriloquism, and unequaled feats of legerdemain, they put on performances that probably remain unexcelled in any theater. Witness the shamans' competition among the Netsilik Eskimo as described by Balikci (1967:204):

> A shaman asked . . . , "Do you think I can pass through this tea cup?" Following a negative answer the shaman first pushed his head through the cup, then his whole body, and finally disappeared underground with a rumbling noise. He came back the same way.

This was followed by strange and terrible manipulations of his body that included removing his own leg, piercing himself with spears, growing a full beard in an instant, traveling to the fearsome underworld, then to the moon, and returning from each wondrous trip with vivid descriptions of the bizarre monsters encountered for the now breathless audience.

An equally memorable performance by an Eskimo shaman is described by Eliade (1964:294). Conducted by the shaman because his people were oppressed by unusually poor hunting conditions, the séance began with the shaman journeying to the bottom of the sea. There he encountered Takánakapsâluk, the Mother of the Sea Beasts. She had no fingers, was dirty and slovenly, and her hair hung down over her face—all because the humans had violated sacred rules.

Bravely, the shaman approached her, took her by the shoulders, and gently combed her hair. As he thus soothed her, he pleaded for more seals for his people. But she listed the transgressions of the people—the secret miscarriages and the broken food taboos—that prevented the return of the animals. Then the shaman returned to the anxious group and demanded expiation. His performance was climaxed by a surge of emotional confessions after which all felt comforted and assured that a change in fortune was imminent.

It is worth straining the imagination to try to feel the intensity of emotions that would pervade the entire Pueblo of the Cochiti of New Mexico when a full-scale curing ceremony, involving several curers, was being staged. Fox's vivid description (1964:185–186) permits us to participate, albeit vicariously, in the melodrama.

The stage is set as the medicine men prepare through four nights, chanting in the society house, smoking the magical tobacco, neither eating nor sleeping, but continually building an atmosphere of impending drama. The curers move to the house of the patient, where they manipulate ritualized paraphernalia, invoke the spirits, smoke and chant some more, and add to the tension for four more nights.

> By the fourth night of this ceremony (the eighth in total), the tension is almost unbearable. The witches are gathering to thwart the efforts of the doctors. The doctors maintain that they can only do their best and that the issue is still very much in doubt. Then a final supreme effort must be made. The monotonous rise and fall of the chant, the near-darkness with the flickering fire, the hideous make-up, the cries in the night and rapping at the door and windows, the elaborate precautions—all these elements build up until the doctors, worked into a controlled frenzy, dash from house to house to do battle. Patients describe how they have been nearly mad with fear by this time. . . . Then comes the terrible battle in the darkness. The doctors claim that, although of course they do a lot of the "business" themselves, it is the witches who get "inside them" and make them do it. . . . Finally, exhausted, they return. Those in the house by now are at screaming point. . . . The doctors reappear . . . in the semi-darkness, huddled together fighting with something in their midst that screams horribly. It is the witch who stole the heart [of the patient]. . . . Then, by the firelight, the war chief shoots it, and it disappears. The effect on the patient can be imagined. The incredible relief and tears of joy and gratitude leave him "feeling like all the badness has gone out." The "heart" is returned to the patient. . . . Life returns to normal; the universe is on an even keel again.

These would be hard acts to follow. The most memorable performances would undoubtedly be recounted and reviewed for years to come and eventually might be incorporated into the legendary heritage of the society involved and, perhaps, enrich the imaginations of many beyond the original borders.

TREATMENT BY TRADITIONAL HEALERS

A HOLISTIC APPROACH

The repertoire of the preindustrialized healer was as extensive as human imagination and ingenuity permit. Treatments varied from a few minutes of massage to nine days and nights of incredibly elaborate ritual. Possessing neither antibiotics nor a germ theory nor the thorough understanding of human physiology necessary for predictable surgery, the so-called primitive curer, nevertheless, offered a holistic approach to curing that at least partially compensated for these deficiencies by dealing with the whole person and, particularly, by integrating the individual and the culture for their mutual benefit. As aptly put by Lewis (1976:86) in his study of the Gnau-speakers of New Guinea:

> The traditional sense, the art of healing, implies that medicine is concerned with sick people or patients, with conditions of man; while the modern sense, study and control of disease, implies rather study of a thing, disease.

Perhaps the most significant contribution offered by a study of healing techniques practiced by preliterate societies stems from the totality of their approach to medical and related social problems. Traditional medicine deals with the presenting disease, to be sure, but only as one aspect of the patient, who is also a member of a particular kin group, which in turn is a component of a specific society, and so on. There is no possibility of separating the whole person from his illness, and no attempt is made to do so. Thus the modern tendency to view the sick person as a case of hepatitis or a malfunctioning liver is not encountered in holistic, traditional medicine. Further, as Ackerknecht (1971:25) stresses:

> That old dichotomy between mental and bodily disease, which we seem largely unable to overcome even with psychosomatic medicine, just does not exist among primitives, either in pathology or in therapy. The whole individual is sick, and the whole individual is treated.

Specific syndromes are recognized and frequently dealt with, but are not separated from the total dis-ease of the patient, his family, and his society. The individual's distress is not viewed as his problem alone; every illness touches in important ways the lives of everyone around the sick person.

BIOLOGICAL BASES FOR SUCCESSES

The admirable holistic approach notwithstanding, the prestigious position of the traditional healer derives ultimately from his rate of success in solving the problems presented by his clientele. Fortunately, in this regard, all curers have a staunch ally. Given the millions of years of evolutionary selection for effective immunological response to disease, the normal adult's body is capable of surmounting all but one of the innumerable medical events of a lifetime. Whatever treatment is prescribed, eventual recovery of some sort can be reasonably predicted for the vast majority of diseases experienced past childhood. Only one illness or injury eventually terminates every human life. Before this final event takes place, however, more or less infirmity can be expected throughout the individual's lifetime. This fact of life—and death—is as true for the person living in the most technologically advanced, medically sophisticated society as for the most "primitive" hunter and gatherer living at any time.

An essential function of the healer, then, is to provide support, ease symptoms, and offer reassurance that the particular syndrome being presented is not going to be the final one, or, when there is no escape from the inevitable, to make the going as comfortable as possible. These services are encompassed in the total treatment given by the traditional healer and by the society he embraces—a type of comprehensive care seldom matched by modern medicine.

CONTRIBUTIONS FROM TRADITIONAL HEALING

In his consideration of traditional healing, Landy (1977:418) cautions, "It is an error to downplay the actual medical aspects of the role." In their use of scientifically verifiable ingredients, traditional curers have made noteworthy contributions to the worldwide medical pharmacopoeia. Many important drugs, still in wide use, were derived from the medical kits of "bush healers" and indigenous herbalists. Among these, to name just a few, are digitalis for heart disease, morphine for pain, rauwolfia derivatives for mental illness and hypertension, chaulmoogra oil for leprosy, and quinine for fevers. Bryant (1966) notes also "the curiously correct insight of the Zulu doctors" who utilized powders made from the slag of the iron smelting for the treatment of conditions possibly associated with anemias resulting from iron deficiency.

The frequent accompaniments of treatment sessions—massage, sweat baths, rest, and social concern—remain valuable adjuncts to the most modern course of therapy for a broad spectrum of illnesses (Fig. 8–7). Some instances of sound immunological awareness occasionally appear. For example, among the Ogori of Nigeria, as reported by Gillies (1976:372), a version of vaccination was practiced

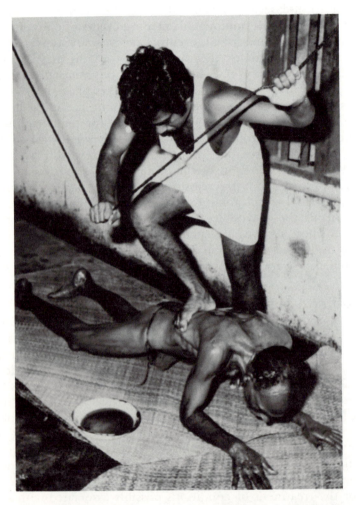

8–7 A healer giving "Thirummal" treatment to a patient in southern India. The patient's body is covered with medicated oil and massaged delicately by hand or foot. This is one of the accepted techniques of Ayurveda, the "science of life." (Courtesy of World Health Organization. Photo by P.N.V. Kurup.)

as an indigenous method of attenuating smallpox epidemics. When word was received of a smallpox outbreak in a neighboring village, a young girl was selected by the diviner to be sent to the stricken village, where she was inoculated with lymph taken from a pustule of the victim. Gillies explains that the passage through the body of a young virgin was believed to "soften" the disease. On the girl's return to her home village, all the young children were similarly vaccinated from her lymph.

FOLK DECISION-MAKING IN TREATMENT OF ILLNESS

All cultures studied appear to differentiate between serious dysfunctions and those that are minor, transient, or "natural" and likely to respond to home treatment. The full magical treatment, with its accompanying appeals to the spiritual world, is not accorded all medical problems. Common ailments of childhood and conditions that are endemic or regularly prevalent in the area are explained as "natural" and generally treated with home care or herbal medications prepared by the mother. Gillies (1976) reports that among the Ogori, curers are not called upon to intervene in cases of malaria, hepatitis, sunstroke, or yellow fever, all unfortunately common events in their lives. Similar categorization of diseases that "just happen," and therefore require no special spiritual intervention, is noted by Ngubane (1976) among the Zulu peoples. The common cold, seasonal diarrhea, measles, malaria, or smallpox may be thus classified and are considered appropriately treated in the home by the mother, the universal first line of defense, or, in acculturating areas, the victim may seek the assistance of Western medical personnel.

Similarly, Erasmus (1952) finds that the Indians of Quito, Ecuador, consider infected wounds, measles, "anger sickness," and skin infections susceptible to home care. The gravity of a disease, as measured by modern medical standards, is not necessarily a reliable determinant of whether a healer's intervention is needed. Malaria, for example, perhaps because of its widespread endemicity as well as its typical pattern of periodic remission of symptoms, is frequently deemed "natural." Thus, among the Sarawak of Borneo, Geddes (1969) finds that most symptoms of malaria are attributed to an overindulgence in sugar cane. Likewise, Edgerton (1977:122), in a study of the Hehe of Tanzania, observes that when they fall ill—"as they often do"—they assign three primary categories of causation, each of which requires different types of treatment: "natural" causes (worry, impure water, or faulty inheritance), witchcraft, and retribution for the violation of Hehe norms.

Beyond the occasionally predictable, mundane conditions that most societies consider responsive to home remedies, there are the myriad other illnesses, special problems, and conditions of nature for which the services of the indigenous specialist are required. Counterparts of the many ills to which the human body is subject are found among all people, with variations dependent primarily on environmental conditions. But the problems considered appropriate for the ministrations of the traditional healer span an even broader spectrum of human concerns. They extend far beyond the realm of ailments generally encountered by a modern practicing physician. Thus, the native curer may be called upon to provide love potions, to induce weather alterations, to appease the restless dead, and occasionally to project an illness onto an implacable enemy. These are indeed leaders with formidable responsibilities!

CATEGORIES OF HEALERS

Just as the pantheon of ailments that afflict humans can be categorized broadly into divisions of bioculturally defined causes, so the associated roles of healers lend themselves to convenient ordering when viewed in panhuman perspective. The curers being considered here are indigenous to the cultures in which they practice. They are granted their society's license to practice through a series of rigidly prescribed, culturally specific experiences. In the majority of cases they have inherited or achieved special relationships with members of their society's spiritual world.

Kiev (1964) notes how the configurations of healers vary according to the economic base of the society. Thus, he finds healing in food-gathering societies dominated by magic and almost exclusively in the hands of individuals who have had special experiences with social forces. On the other hand, specialization appears in agricultural societies, accompanied by increased competition for the roles associated with healing. For example, among the hunting and gathering Australian Murngin, the Cheyenne, the Shoshone, the

Eskimo, and the Andaman Islanders, there is one basic type of healer. Inevitably, this is someone whose powers are believed to be supernaturally bestowed. Conversely, among the Chiga of Uganda, the Mano of Liberia, and many other agricultural societies, diviners, herbalists, midwives, and medical guild members compete for the patronage of the biologically as well as the culturally defined sick members of the group.

THE SHAMAN

The best studied of the indigenous healers is the shaman, a name, according to Eliade (1964:4), derived through Russian from the Tungusic *šaman*, and whose prototype is the Siberian healer-mystic. The title and position are conferred upon a man or woman who, with great effort and danger, acts on behalf of his or her clients—at times for the collective society—to intervene with the supernatural forces responsible for the medical or social emergency facing them.

Frequently, the shaman possesses "familiars," or spiritual assistants, who act on his command. These assistants, acquired as part of an initiation process, are viewed by his society as the ultimate determinant of the shaman's power. Among the Tzeltal Indians, for example, according to Nash (1967:127), the curer's strength derives from an animal counterpart, a *nawales*, into whose form the emerging curer can transform himself, wander about at night, and thus learn from the other nawales. Similarly, the shamans of the Arctic regions and of some of the Indians of North America acquire *tunraqs*, or spiritual aides (cf. Balikci 1967), that also protect and guide them throughout their careers.

In a moving biography of the last shaman of the Washo Indians of the western United States, Handelman (1977:427) reports that the shaman, Henry Rupert, as a young boy dreamed repeatedly of a bear that eventually became one of his "familiars." When in his dreams the bear would vanish, Rupert would follow him to the moon. At other times, when awake, he experienced dizziness, fainting, nosebleeds, and various animal-oriented hallucinations. Interpreting these experiences as a summons to help his people when they were ill, he finally hired an older shaman to teach him his culture's healing arts. During a long and successful career he acquired additional spirit helpers to augment his earlier acquired animal familar.

SPECIAL SHAMANIC CHARACTERISTICS

Eliade (1964:5–6) stresses the special characteristics of the shaman as distinct from other healers:

> Every medicine man is a healer, but the shaman employs a method that is his and his alone. . . . [He] specializes in a trance during which his soul is believed to leave his body and ascend to the sky or descend to the underworld. . . .
> . . . The shaman controls his "spirits," in the sense that he, a human being, is able to communicate with the dead, "demons," and "nature spirits," without thereby becoming their instrument.

Thus, the traditional shaman, by being willing to "die" and journey to a fearful place, is truly heroic and often represents the sole intermediary between the threatening, malevolent spirit world and frail, earthbound humans.

Shamans have been the focal point of many anthropological and psychological studies (cf. Eliade 1964; Kiev 1964; Levi-Strauss 1967) for at least two reasons. First, their own societies assign a most important role to them; second, they often attract the attention of the investigator because of their intriguing configuration of personality traits. A picture has emerged of an exotic being, portrayed sometimes as a charismatic neurotic or hysteric, sometimes as a deceptive charlatan. Except in rare cases, these assessments result from attempts to fit the shamanic personality into a role amenable to the cultural concepts of the investigator. Such attempts inevitably encounter severe difficulties, primarily because the true shaman comprises a totality so unfamilar as to be alien to modern, sophisticated concepts of human personality.

Shamans may indeed embody many of the suggested unflattering attributes, but these are often combined with an unswerving dedication to the welfare of their people. Further, shamans demonstrate an unremitting acceptance of supernatural causation of disease and disaster, coupled with a hard-headed practicality and pragmatism. Perhaps the most important characteristic to add to all these seemingly contradictory facets is that the shamans are the embodiment of the common values of their own cultures.

The controversy around the personality of the traditional shamans tends to boil down to two main positions. Sigerist (1951: 176), for example, accepts the psychotic designation and writes in his discussion of the *inyanga* of the Bantu of Africa:

> Mental illness is the starting point and becoming an inyanga or a shaman is the cure. By accepting the career with all its burdens and dangers, the patient makes an adjustment and becomes a useful member of society, while if he refused it he would remain unadapted, psychotic, a burden to society.

On the other hand, Nadel (1946:36) concludes from a study of shamanism among Sudanese tribes:

> No shaman is, in everyday life, an "abnormal" individual, a neurotic, or a paranoiac; if he were, he would be classed as a lunatic, not respected as a priest. Nor finally can shamanism be correlated with incipient or latent abnormality; I recorded no case of a shaman whose professional hysteria deteriorated into serious mental disorders.

Since mental illness has yet to be defined in terms universally and, particularly, cross culturally acceptable to all, it may be argued that it is quite inappropriate to impose such designations across the vast cultural barriers involved in considerations of societies dependent on the services of shamans.

RECEIVING THE "CALL"
Preceding the acceptance of the shaman's role, there is a culturally prescribed path or initiation period that must be experienced by the selected candidate. Often the emerging curer arrives at his or her position partly through inheritance from a parent or grandparent, as is the rule among the Shona of Rhodesia (Gelfand 1964) and the Mgnang of Borneo (Schmidt 1964). Occasionally, as, for example, among the Blackfoot Indians and Seal Eskimos, a promising youth from outside the family is taken on as an apprentice.

In some societies the emerging shaman learns of his life's mission through a "call." Among the Australian aborigines, where, according to Berndt (1964:268), the shaman is named a *margidbu* from the word meaning "to know," the call is not sought; rather, it is thrust upon the chosen one by the spirit or ghost of a dead relative whose unexpected appearance shocks the person into insensibility, during which time the spirit's power is blown into various body orifices. From that time on, the chosen one is endowed with special powers and is able to help his people, who turn to him when crises arise.

Occasionally, the shamanic role is pressed upon a member of the society who has overcome serious illness. The rationale behind such a selection rests upon the assumption that someone who has survived such a life-threatening experience must have special knowledge or unusual powers. As Sigerist (1951:158) eloquently states it:

> In a number of tribes, and particularly among American Indians, it is believed that a man who was seriously sick and recovered will never again be the same as he was before his illness. The fact that he was in close touch with the transcendental world gives him a special position once and for all, and the fact that he was attacked by evil forces but did not succumb to them shows that he has some power over them. As a result, former patients would enroll in medicine societies.

Less frequently, the status of mystical curer is achieved as a result of outstanding prowess in some aspect of life that is highly valued by the society. Evans-Pritchard (1967) cites the Moro of the Sudan who arrive at the role after gaining great reknown as hunters. It should be noted, however, that the hunter's exceptional success is rarely attributed to his skill alone; rather, intervention by the gods or ancestral spirits is taken to be its ultimate source. Therefore, it would follow that the extraordinary hunter must have achieved some unusual power over the spirits and this faculty could serve the community to good advantage if he were directed into the role of healer.

Sigerist (1951) reports that a series of out-of-the-ordinary experiences sometimes marks the individual as having been singled out by the spirits for special notice. He cites the Apache woman curer who was first struck by lightning and survived and later was attacked by a mountain lion but escaped and recovered. Her seemingly miraculous survival was interpreted as a sign of special powers and led to her career of healer.

In sum, validation of the choice of candidate invariably involves a supernatural, mystical experience, generally of an auditory and/or visual nature, frequently followed by the loss of consciousness and, as reported by a Hehe curer to Edgerton (1977), a time of terror. The loss of consciousness, frequently accompanied by a sense of disembodiment, is interpreted by some scholars as a metaphysical death and resurrection, or as Eliade (1964) sees it, as symbolic of a passage into another sphere, the world of the dead, "where everything is known."

SOCIAL INTERACTIONS OF THE SHAMANIC ROLE

Whatever the means of deriving the call, as Mischel (1959:414) points out, "the bush healer is seen as a wise, holy person who basically derives his power from supernatural sources. . . . Such an individual cannot be challenged or criticized since he is only an agent for supernatural gods." Sigerist (1951:169), writing of the Indian medicine man, comments that this healer's social position has always been a very high one: "He is respected because he is learned and skilful, by far the best-informed man of the group." Similarly, Eliade (1964) stresses that recognition of the shaman is bestowed by the whole community. Indeed through many accounts, it is apparent that the role of shaman is not deliberately, or at least not consciously, sought by the individual; it is much more likely to be derived from a confluence of community needs and the presence of a person fit for the role as determined by cultural norms. In fact, Willard Z. Park (in Eliade 1964:109) suggests that usually a candidate is reluctant to become a shaman: he "assumes his powers and follows the spirit's bidding only when he is told by other shamans that otherwise death will result."

Although highly esteemed by their society, the shamans in their close association with powerful, frightening supernatural forces confront less benevolent social attitudes as well. They are regarded with a mixture of fear and awe that separates them from other members of the community; as a result they are likely to lead lives quite apart and lonely. An additional isolating attribute of the shamanic curer is found among the Koreans and the Sea Dyak of Borneo as well as the Chukchee, Kamchadal, and Koryak of Siberia and others for whom the assumption of the curer's role entails the adoption of female attire. This transvestism does not invariably imply a complete reversion to a female role. Eliade (1964) suggests that more likely the transformation reflects an acknowledgment of strong magical powers associated primarily with women or female functions.

Occasionally the hazardous forces held in tenuous control by the shaman may be deemed by his compatriots to be abused or beyond his regulation. In such cases, members of his society may feel compelled to destroy him and his threatening power. Christensen and

Marti (1972) report the machete slaying as recently as 1966 of a village curer and most of his family in San Pablito, Mexico, because he was judged to have used his powers for evil purposes. Similarly, according to Nash (1967), between 1957 and 1967 at least ten Indian village curers in Tzeltal were killed because of charges of witchcraft.

CURING TECHNIQUES OF THE TRADITIONAL SHAMAN

The techniques employed by shamanic healers encompass remarkably similar patterns throughout the world. As outlined by Eliade (1964) and others, curing sessions routinely begin with ritual cleansing and preparation of the site selected for the rites—as Frank (1973) points out, a symbolic separation from the ordinary course of events. Elaborate, ritually prescribed costumes are worn by the shaman and his assistants. There follows the induction of a trance state, sometimes through the effects of chants, dance, and tobacco or hemp smoke or other traditional hallucinogenic agents. Historically, hemp smoke was reportedly used by the curers of the ancient Thracians, Scythians, and Iranians (Eliade 1674); the hallucinogenic mushroom *Agaricus muscaius* was traditionally employed throughout Central Asia and parts of the Americas; while, according to Dobkin de Rios (1973), the bark of an indigenous vine, *Ayahuasca*, is used today in the Amazon. Perhaps just as frequently, the shamans were able to achieve the trance state through their own ability and predisposition.

Evocation of the associated spirits is performed during the trance, and in this way the cause of the problem is traditionally determined. Often the immediate difficulty is found to be either a lost or a stolen soul, or the problem may be diagnosed as the result of the intrusion of some harmful substance into the victim's body. The diagnosis is followed by attempts to recapture the soul stuff through further trance states during which time the shaman's soul journeys to a spiritual world below or above the earth where the shaman must wheedle, cajole, or force the spirits to relinquish their prize. The successful shaman returns to the assembled group dramatically flourishing a material object that contains the lost soul, or if the diagnosis was an intruded substance, he removes it from the patient's body in an equally dramatic manner. The session, which may last a few hours to several days, frequently ends with the shaman eliciting from the patient and his kin confessions of taboo violations, after which the shaman transmits directions from the gods regarding behavior modification or the need for sacrifices to be performed. It is a remarkable commentary on human similarities, or perhaps an indication of the ancient roots of the role of shaman, that this total configuration, with, of course, culturally specific variations, is found around the world—from Nepal to central Australia to the Near East and throughout the Americas and Siberia.

It is frequently noted that the shamanic performance often demands extremes of mental and physical fortitude from the healer. For example, the traditional Washo curing ceremony, as described by Handelman (1977), requires the shaman to work continuously for three consecutive nights from dusk to midnight and on the fourth night until dawn. Likewise, the Cochiti curing ceremony, as described by Fox (1964), requires the shaman to spend four nights in preparation, neither eating nor sleeping during the initial stage, but inhaling vast amounts of tobacco smoke to facilitate his entry into the requisite "altered" state.

Katz's (1976) rendition of the !Kung healing rituals that center on the healer's attainment of the trance state, called "!kia," reveals the stress created in the minds and bodies of the healers (Fig. 8–8).

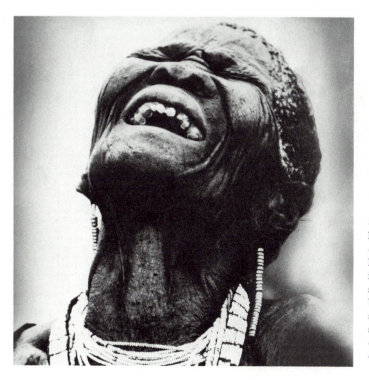

8-8   A !Kung healer of the Kalahari Desert in a state of transcendence, or "!kia." In this trance she lays on hands, draws her patient's illness into her own body, and then shakes it away with her hand as her body shudders with pain. Here the sacrifice and suffering of the shaman on behalf of her people is dramatically portrayed. (Courtesy of Richard Katz. From Katz 1976.)

He explains that some of the actual pain experienced derives from the conviction that healing requires dying and being reborn. Katz, a psychologist, insists that this is not an allegorical rite of passage, but a "terror-filled experience of death and rebirth" that remains deeply embedded in the healer throughout the years of practice. The empathetic and, at the same time, shattering impact of the state is unforgettably revealed in Katz's quotation (ibid.: 85) from Dem, one of the !Kung's most powerful healers:

> In !kia your heart stops, you're dead, your thoughts are nothing, you breathe with difficulty. You see ghosts killing people, you smell burning, rotten flesh. Then you heal, you pull the sickness out. Then you live.

Treatment that aims at expulsion or removal of the disease agent attempts to extract or expel an objectified disease substance that is understood to contain the essence of the illness. Although the most frequent type of expulsion involves the shaman's sucking the substance out of the patient's body (Fig. 8–9), occasionally, as among

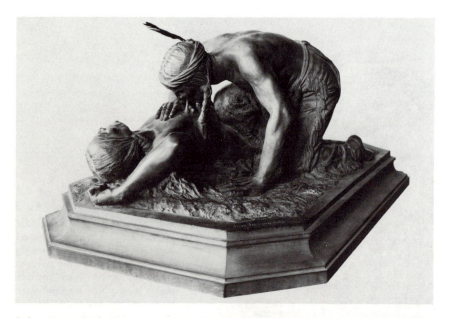

8–9 Removal of disease by sucking through a bone tube, as practiced by the Ojibwa Indians of North America. This approach to treatment is found among traditional healers in many parts of the world and typifies the apparent hazards willingly faced by the shaman. (Courtesy of Wellcome Museum of Medical Science, London. From a sculptured group by J. Jackson.)

the Carib-speakers of Guyana, a ritual blowing on the offending part of the body is practiced. In the Iroquois catalog of medical problems, as described by Wallace (1967), a common source of illness, attributed to malevolent witches, was the magical projection of harmful substances into the victim's body. The healer's task was to locate the intruded object and then, through skillful legerdemain, produce it—a ball of hair, splinters of bone, blood clots, or even bear teeth.

The extraction process has been dramatically described by Lévi-Strauss (1967:31) in his account of a Kwakiutl curer from the Vancouver region of Canada:

> Above all, he learned the *ars magna* of one of the shamanistic schools of the Northwest Coast: The shaman hides a little tuft of down in a corner of his mouth, and he throws it up, covered with blood, at a proper moment—after having bitten his tongue or made his gums bleed—and solemnly presents it to his patient and the onlookers as the pathological foreign body extracted as a result of his sucking and manipulations.

Psychiatrist Frank (1973:63) cautions the skeptical observer:

> Legerdemain . . . is not regarded as trickery, even when the audience knows how it is done. They seem to give emotional assent to the proposition that the bloody bit of cotton is the patient's illness and has been extracted from his body, while at another level they know perfectly well that it is only a piece of cotton. Perhaps their state of mind is analogous to that of the partakers of communion, for whom in one sense the bread and wine are the body and blood of Christ while in another they are just bread and wine.

Often the demands of the healing rituals have required gross bodily insult to the curer. The Maori healer, according to Eliade (1964), was required to plunge his head into water in order to discern the road by which the evil spirit had approached from the underworld. The Fiji shamans, some Polynesian curers, and certain practitioners in southern India gained their audience's confidence by their ability to challenge the offending spirits by walking on burning coals or white-hot stones. Eliade (1964:442) tells of Lolo curers of southern Yunnan who were expected to walk over a number of white-hot plowshares or, in times of epidemics, to build a double ladder of thirty-six knives and climb to the top and then down again on the other side with feet bared. In Eliade's (ibid.:372) view: "The genuineness of such feats is beyond doubt; a number of competent observers have described the 'miracle' after taking all possible mea-

sures to ensure objectivity." Among some of the Indian tribes of
Alaska, Sigerist (1951) reports, the shaman was expected to intervene physically and exorcise the spirit causing the sickness by throw-
ing himself on the patient and wrestling with his body. The shamans
of Samoa and the Nicobar Islands similarly lured the ghostly substance out of the patient's body and then attacked it with a spear.

Though some demands are less vigorous, they nonetheless reveal
the exceptional abilities and the various talents expected of the traditional healers. Among the North American Indian healers who
employ sand painting (Fig. 8–10) in their curing rituals, extraordi-

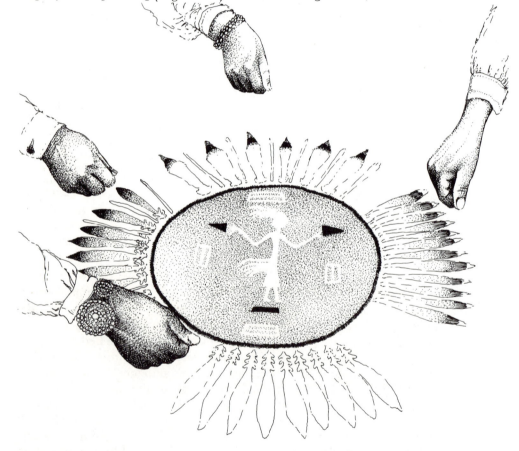

8–10 Sand painting used by several North American Indian healers. Extraordinary artistic
skills are demonstrated in this approach to healing, in which the patient is expected to receive strength and curative power from the ritualized painting. (Adapted from Billard 1974.)

nary artistic skills have been reported. Music also often figured as an important part of the curing ceremonies. Frequently, these required staggering feats of memory among preliterate people who were required to perform, with no allowance for error, songs, chants, and dances that could last for several days before completion. Henry Rupert, the Washo shaman described by Handelman (1977), is an expert hypnotist and uses this skill to hold his patients' attention during the curing sessions. Ventriloquism is another frequently encountered artifice used by shamans in scattered areas throughout the world. The shamans of Siberia and other Arctic regions have earned particular renown for their ability to project their voices as they communicate with the spirit world.

Remarkable surgical procedures are also included among the accomplishments of the shaman of the northern latitudes. Murphy (1964:72) reports that surgical amputations, trepanning, lancing, and bloodletting were practiced regularly by the shamans of the Bering Strait region. She suggests that the ability to employ such procedures successfully in the absence of effective anesthesia or asepsis was, at least partially, a result of the extensive experience gained from the regular dismemberment of animals after the hunt.

More subtle but nevertheless revealing of impressive perception is the ability to extract hidden or subliminal information from the patient as well as from the community around him. This expertise underlies many of the successes accorded the traditional shaman even as it marks the gifted diagnostician in any of today's advanced medical centers. But the medicine man in the traditional society would be at an advantage in this sphere because of his intimate knowledge of his patients and their kin as well as of any existing social tensions that contributed to the medical problem.

NONSHAMANIC TRADITIONAL CURERS

While the traditional shaman was, and probably is, the most representative embodiment of the beliefs, fears, and hopes of traditional peoples throughout the world, in many societies various aspects of the shaman's techniques have been adapted as specialities of different practitioners. Thus we find diviners, singers, magicians, herbalists, spiritualists, and medicine societies at work, particularly in sedentary, agriculturally oriented societies. Although these specialists may be viewed as less dependent on the ecstatic and heroic procedures, they are also generally somewhat more restricted in the categories of problems that they are deemed capable of resolving. In all cases, however, they emerge to fill the otherwise unmet needs of their people, whose illnesses and social problems are so diverse as to seem beyond the power of one individual to resolve.

SPIRITUALISTS

The spiritualist incorporates the shamanic ability to communicate with the dead and to transmit their messages to the anxious living. Called by Rogler and Hollingshead (1961) the "folk psychiatrists," the spiritualists are quite distinct from nontraditional healers in that they use their special faculties, "mystical antennas," to achieve communication and they act to relieve frightening symptomatology by displacing causes onto acceptable bases. But they differ from shamans not only because they lack ecstatic experience, but, more important, because as healers they are viewed as effective for problems affecting individuals rather than as guardians of the well-being of the total society.

In cultures where prestige is accrued from the possession of psychic facilities, as is true, for example, for many areas of Latin America, the spiritualist removes the stigma of illness, particularly those forms categorized as "mental" in modern parlance. As portrayed by Rogler and Hollingshead (1961:19), the aim of reintegration of the troubled individual emerges clearly:

> Does the individual report hallucinations? This clearly indicates to the believer in spiritualism that he is being visited by spirits who manifest themselves visibly and audibly. Does he have delusions? He is told that evil spirits are deceiving him about himself as well as others. His thoughts are being distorted by interfering bad spirits. Is his talk incoherent, rambling and cryptic? This indicates that he is undergoing a test, an experiment engineered by the spirits to see if he is of the right moral fiber.

Since disturbed individuals are prevalent in modern, industrialized societies as well, this particular type of traditional healer readily makes the transition to cultures in which the mystical extremes of the shamanic healer would be less acceptable. A good example is furnished by spiritualist groups in Wales, as described by Skultans

(1976). Here, a patient suffering from a condition such as backache, migraine, or abdominal pain, all of which are often associated with social stress, joins a spiritualist's group. The healer, who is considered to be "sensitive," will claim to experience the pain felt by the patient. This happening, which the healers call "taking on conditions," serves to demonstrate to the patient an empathy that was absent elsewhere in his life situation.

DIVINERS

The diviner, an important figure throughout ancient mythology as well as in many cultures today, is less likely to communicate directly with the spiritual world than the shamans and spiritualists do. Instead, the diviner interprets symptoms, prognosticates, and prescribes courses of action through mechanical, magical manipulations. Allen (1976:528) describes Bàunne, a Nepalese diviner, "who casts handfuls of rice onto a brass plate and pairs off the grains to obtain a yes-no answer to his questions." The answer is determined by whether the number of grains turn out to be odd or even.

Several forms of divination were studied by Beattie (1967) in Uganda. Each was seen as a means of auguring the outcome of a specific illness and varied in relation to the gravity of the problem and the amount of money the patient was able or willing to invest in the rite. One technique involved testing the choice of paths taken by some beetles supplied by the patient. The patient was instructed to place some of his saliva on one branch of a forked stick broken from a special plant. The stick was then inserted in the ground and the beetles placed on the stem. If the beetles moved toward the branch containing the patient's saliva, the prognosis was good. If they moved toward the other, unfavorable side, usually more tests would be attempted. Although only one of two possible answers theoretically is possible under most conditions of divination, the client has the option of holding out for a favorable answer. So the chief purpose of the divination process might be to provide reassurance during a time of anxiety, particularly since close examination indicates that by and large most of the outcomes are subject to a good deal of manipulation by the diviner.

A somewhat more generalized form of divination, haruspication, involves examination of the entrails of animals sacrificed for the purpose. In recent times chickens have become the animal of choice; in more prosperous times oxen were preferred. Again, the patient uses his saliva; this time it is placed on the chicken's beak. The diviner presents a dyadic query to the doomed animal, then carefully cuts the bird open.

At this point, it is believed that the diviner himself is in danger, for if he disrupts certain organs while operating, his own life is threatened. Any culturally defined abnormality of the chicken's insides augurs a poor prognosis. But here again, an initial unfavorable result is not bound to be accepted; in fact, the process may be repeated several times over a period of weeks in the hope of influencing fate. It is worth noting that, since few illnesses remain unresolved for much longer than a few weeks, fate and the prognostication are quite likely to coincide.

The *nganga*, diviners of Rhodesia, use sets of wooden "bones" as the props for their magical determinations (Fig. 8–11). As described by Gelfand (1964), each piece of wood has special markings on it. The nganga interprets the results of the throws to determine

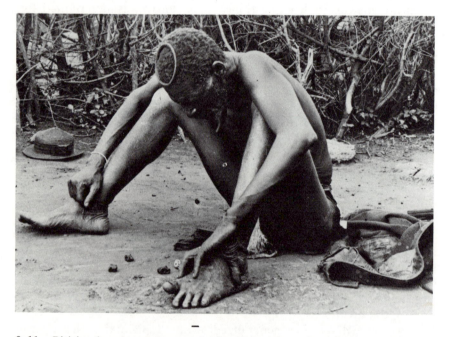

8–11   Divining the source and prognosis of an illness is part of the repertoire of many traditional healers. Here a Rhodesian diviner studies the message in the wooden "bones" he has thrown. The throws of the specially marked pieces are given a discriminating interpretation by the wise diviner.

the cause of the problem presented and the subsequent action for the patient and his kin to follow.

A somewhat different form of divination is practiced by the *janka*, diviners who are part of the Hindu untouchable caste of weavers and village servants in central India. Fuchs (1964) describes the diagnostic procedure in which the janka feels the pulse of the patient with his left hand while pulling at the patient's fingers with his right hand. With each digital manipulation, he mutters the name of a god or spirit. Each crack of the patient's joints is significant and is counted by the janka, who thus determines which spiritual agent is responsible for the problem. Then the curer conducts the appropriate prayers and exhortations to the gods at a religious shrine.

Fuchs (ibid.:125) explains that the somewhat belligerent tone that crops up in the following recitation is meant to impress the urgency of the case upon the offending god:

> Allah! Bismillah! Raheman! Rahim!
> Kali! Mahakali! Brahma's sister-in-law! . . .
> With folded hands I pray: Save!
> But if you don't cure the patient, I shall dishonor your
>   mother!

The punch line, according to Fuchs (ibid.:138), literally translates as "I shall pierce the private part of your mother!" and is believed to "shock the deity into granting the favor."

HERBALISTS

All environments provide some substances deemed useful by the inhabitants for medical treatment. Probably every type of healer at some time has recourse to herbal medicine, and it is particularly associated with the "home curer," most often the mother, as an initial response to an indisposition.

Most accounts (cf. Sigerist 1951) tend to associate the herbal curer with the somewhat mundane, minor illnesses, generally those considered by their culture to be nonsupernatural. Herbs and medications derived from plants and animals are, as a rule, considered "natural" medicines, potent in themselves and effective primarily on diseases with a culturally defined "natural" etiology.

The herbalist is probably the most pragmatic of the traditional healers. Using what resembles the "scientific approach," he or she frequently relies on the knowledge gained during a lengthy training from an experienced practitioner. And nature provides a plentiful storehouse of effective substances for the innovative herbalist to draw upon. Majno (1975:64) states that a review of 2,222 plants revealed some antibiotic activity in 1,362, evolved and selected by the plants for their own protection as resistance to bacterial decay. Through trial and error over thousands of years, herbalists have recognized the beneficial properties of many of these plants and incorporated them into their lore. Five centuries ago, as Ortiz de Montellano (1975:216) notes,

> much empirical research was done by the Aztec doctors and their predecessors. The botanical gardens which so astonished the Spanish conquerors had been established as early as 1467 by Motecuhzoma I. These gardens were maintained primarily to provide the medical profession with raw materials for medicinal formulas and for experimentation.

He notes particularly the use of the plant *Carica papaya*, whose active substance is papase, an enzyme that can remove clotted blood, pus, and dead tissue from surface wounds and ulcers.

Although Ackerknecht (1971) suggests that among traditional herbalists it is stated that the "spirit of the herb fights against disease spirit," studies have nevertheless indicated that 25 to 50 percent of their pharmocopoeia is objectively active. For instance, after examining many of the calculated 700 medicinal plants utilized by the Zulu and Natal healers of southeastern Africa, Bryant (1966) claimed to have found valuable pharmacological properties in at least 240.

Buckley (1976), in an examination of Yoruba herbal medicine, notes that the herbalist is often a distinctive type of person: "sceptical, inventive and individualistic." Buckley also reports that he found little agreement among the native herbalists regarding the nature of the diseases they treated nor consensus on effective cures.

THE "HOT" AND THE "COLD"

Among the herbalists and the common folk in many parts of the world, many diseases and their appropriate treatments are divided into "hot" and "cold" categories. Some medications are so designated because of their intrinsic qualities. Thus, Colson (1976) finds that among the Akawaio Indians of South America, pepper and ginger are considered hot substances and therefore used for treating sicknesses characterized as "cold." These illnesses generally tend to be those accompanied by chills, diarrhea, and extremes of lassitude. River-bank clay and morning dew, as might be expected, are deemed

"cold" and are therefore considered effective for restoring a healthful balance in patients afflicted with "hot" diseases. On the other
hand, there is no obvious reason why some substances are designated
intrinsically sweet or bitter or hot or cold. Salt, for example, is
considered a sweet medicine and appropriate to use only when such a
quality is desirable. Plants and medicinal herbs may also have hot or
cold qualities bestowed upon them by external means. Thus, boiling
a root adds heat to it, while exposing it to the cold night air imparts
coldness.

The concept of restoring balance and harmony to the sick, out-
of-balance patient is generally thought to be derived from the ancient
Hippocratic proposition of the four humors. But Colson believes that
the Akawaio she studied developed the practice quite independent of
European influence. In any case, it is a rationale that underlies much
of the treatment used by healers, particularly herbalists, throughout
the world and, in the process, demonstrates quite admirably a type
of traditional, pragmatic reasoning. Colson (1976:492) describes this
process as practiced by the Akawaio:

> When a condition of cold, weakness and lassitude is diag-
> nosed, hot bitter, energy-giving remedies are sought to restore
> a proper vitality and to force out the sickness. When a burn-
> ing heat, fever and restless discomfort predominate, sweet, cool
> and soothing remedies are applied as the complementary
> opposite.

INDIANS OF NORTH AMERICA, THE SUPERSPECIALISTS

Perhaps in conjunction with the elaborate development of the native
American cultures, and possibly also in reaction to the sudden, severe
burden of devastating disease in the wake of European contact, medical concerns reached an unusual degree of specialization in many
North American Indian societies. Ackerknecht (1971), writing of the
Navaho, cites the reported one-quarter to one-third of their productive time spent in religious ceremonials, most of which are concerned
with disease. He found a similar cultural concentration on disease
treatment and prevention among the Cuna, Chiricahua, Apache,
Cherokee, and Pima Indians. In her study of the Ojibwa Indians,
Landes (1971:178) comments, "The concern with sickness appears
obsessive to an outsider. Every Ojibwa is ridden with anxiety about
his health."

Many tribes had sufficient numbers of curers and specialists to warrant the formation of medicine societies that were dedicated to one particular medical problem. The Omaha, for example, had a Buffalo Society whose members specialized in surgical procedures. The Seneca Indians of the northeastern United States had a group that dealt only with the treatment of wounds. Individual curers also reached a high degree of specialization. The Havasupai of the Grand Canyon region, for example, had a medicine man whose chief concern was weather control, another who was dedicated to particular disease treatment, and others who were responsible only for the treatment of wounds, fractures, and snakebites. Similarly, the Blackfoot tribes were able to call upon specific healers for almost every contingency, and the Chemchuevi had snakebite curers, medicine men who treated only injuries related to falls, and others who were summoned only when horse-related accidents occurred.

CULTURALLY DEFINED CONDITIONS, TREATABLE ONLY BY TRADITIONAL HEALERS

"Soul loss" and "evil eye" constitute distress entities in many areas throughout the world. The patients experiencing these problems probably have many of the symptoms that the modern clinician would recognize and treat as tuberculosis, malnutrition, acute anxiety, or similar conditions that may appear to the victim as vague, generalized, overall distress. But in many societies the same symptoms form a recognizable configuration attributable to supernatural causation and deemed treatable only by their traditional healers.

When the diagnosis indicates the cause of an illness to be loss of soul substance either by spiritual theft, fright, trauma, or any number of possibly offending agencies, the job of the healer is to recapture the missing, vital substance, either by cajoling or by forcing the malevolent spiritual thief to return it. Since this may involve direct trafficking within the world of the spirits, it is considered a trip only the most powerful and courageous curer would dare undertake. The most renowned shamans in this regard are those of the northern latitudes, but soul loss is considered the cause of many problems in other parts of the world as well. Therefore, shamanic-type healers deemed capable of recapturing souls are found in many areas.

The *brujo* or *bruja* curers of Latin America tend to specialize in ailments with a supernatural etiology. The most common problems they encounter, as studied by Christensen and Marti (1972), are "evil eye," loss of heart, and *susto*—loss of soul through sudden fright. Most often soul loss is diagnosed when the victim loses consciousness or suffers a chronic, emaciating disease. For all these conditions, the curer must intervene with the offending spirits on behalf of the patient.

"Evil eye" is basically considered a loss of health caused by the malevolence or envy of an enemy or someone who transgresses the bounds of appropriate behavior. It is treated by traditional curers in such widely diverse societies as the Luo of Kenya, the Yemenites of the Near East, many peasant societies of Europe, and groups throughout Latin America. According to Madsen (1964:426), *mal ojo*, or evil eye in Mexico is thought to be caused by certain persons who are born with "strong vision." When such individuals enviously admire or strongly desire some attribute of another person, harmful emanations leave their body and enter the envied person, who may then suffer symptoms similar to soul loss.

Children, the treasured possessions of their families—and the most threatened by disease—are frequently the victims of *mal ojo* in Mexican cultures. The cure primarily involves social readjustments: the parents of the child diagnosed as suffering from *mal ojo* are directed to consider who may be the one who recently admired the child. The designated person is asked to touch the child on the head, thus neutralizing the foreign force and restoring the lost essence, and, incidentally, mending the disrupted social fences. Should a suitable candidate not be available, the curer can reassure the anxious parent by purging the malicious force out of the child's body by brushing it with certain herbal substances as well as a raw egg in the shell.

Among the Luo of Kenya, a simple disorder such as a digestive problem after excessive indulgence might be attributed to an evil eye spell cast by a particular person, presumably someone less fortunate or filled with envy, whom the patient guiltily recalls having stared at him while he was gorging himself. According to Whisson (1964:288), a combination of extraction and soul recapture might be involved in the treatment. The healer could make several cuts on the body and suck over them with a horn. He could then produce some half-digested food from his own mouth and claim that he had thus removed the chief source of the patient's discomfort, leaving the body receptive to the return of any lost elements. Similar minor social dysfunctions are seen by Middleton (1967:60) as underlying *ole,* or evil eye, among the Lugbara on the Nile-Congo divide. The *oleu,* or evil-eye man, could be someone with unusual facial features such as squinting eyes or someone who has displeased his neighbors or kinfolk because of his "greedy, grumpy" disposition.

Although fear of evil eye is widespread, the "condition" is not a weighty problem in traditional medicine because it lends itself readily to preventive measures. The help of the *mori,* the Yemenite healer, for example, is frequently sought to obtain amulets to be worn by a susceptible adult, but more often by a child, to ward off evil eye. Among the Indians of Ecuador, Erasmus (1952) notes that red ribbons offer the same protection to children. The prevalence of similar charms in many areas of the world suggests a carry-over of the same magical thinking. Thus religious symbols—a cross, star, or saint's image—are used by millions of people who may make no association with the custom's probable origin.

Additional conditions deemed suitable only for treatment by the culture's traditional healer involve problems of sexual dysfunction as well as sterility. In a study of some thirty-three practitioners in a suburb of Zambia, Frankenberg and Leeson (1976) found that 70 percent claimed they specialized in the treatment of barrenness, a condition, they all agreed that Western medicine was unable to treat. Similarly, Last (1976:129), in an investigation of the Hausa of the West African savannah, found that, "loss or lack of children is the commonest cause for seeking treatment by spiritual possession . . . of getting oneself in harmony with the disease spirits."

In a recent study conducted by the present author in Western Samoa, many informants singled out particular types of skin disturbances, called *ila* and *mumu,* as conditions they would have treated by the *fofo,* the traditional healer. These often involved birthmarks that most Western-trained personnel do not consider treatable. To the Samoans, such mysterious stigmata may suggest that some kind of magic or unexplainable force is at work that only the fofo is capable of manipulating.

TREATMENT WITHHELD, DELAYED, OR BORROWED
Further evidence of the innovativeness and pragmatism required for the role of a culturally acceptable traditional healer is found in the many varieties of problems they are expected to deal with. The experienced curer learns all too soon that no matter what course of action is pursued, a certain number of his clients will manifestly be suffering from their final illness; a cure rate of 100 percent is neither achieved nor expected. In these cases, his role of maintaining the integrity of the culture becomes most important. Boyer (1964:403) illustrates how this is handled:

> The Apache shaman was a shrewd and wary person who recognized and as a rule refused to accept responsibility for the cure of serious organic disturbance. Sometimes he resorted to legerdemain to demonstrate that his treatment would be ineffective.

Boyer shows that in cases where the shaman was convinced of failure from the outset, he was prepared to claim that he had been given faulty information, or that his spiritual guide had informed him that the patient's transgression had been too serious for the healer to be effective. Similarly, Sigerist (1951) notes that among the Nias of Indonesia, in some cases of soul loss, presumably when the prognosis was poor, the spirits were deemed to have devoured the soul and therefore no hope was extended to the patient or his family.

A further "out" is possible in that treatment frequently involves the imposition of various taboos or actions upon the relatives of the patient. Violations of these instructions are considered reasonable cause for the failure of a given treatment. Similarly, Allen (1976) found that among the Nepalese, the curer would explain that an outcome was unsatisfactory because only one of several afflicting factors had been recognized.

On the other hand, it is occasionally reported that a curer, recognizing the likelihood of remission of symptoms in some conditions, may accept responsibility for treating certain patients in spite of a recognized poor prognosis. Thus, Appel (1977), in an examination of native healers of Nicaragua, reports that chronic diseases such as particular malignancies, as well as problems such as headache, vomiting, edema, and some convulsions, may have a persistent history of recurrence but are nevertheless considered to be within the province of the *sukya*, or shamanistic healer. It is probably significant that such a healer does not give an instant diagnosis. Instead, the patient, after his initial session with the curer (who, if sufficiently experienced, is likely to recognize a chronic condition), must wait for the curer to receive word from his spiritual advisers in his dreams. Since this delay could conceivably take long enough for the signs of an approaching remission to appear, a temporarily successful cure can be initiated.

The recurring description of traditional healers as innovative, pragmatic individuals is often borne out in examinations of the many instances where their societies are in the process of acculturation. Although it can be, and often is, argued that the traditional healers usually constitute the most ardently conservative members of their cultures, they frequently have not been averse to borrowing useful adjuncts to their practices from the intruding medical system and then intertwining them with their own traditional practices.

Frankenberg and Leeson (1976:254) report a technique once common in medieval Europe and now discovered by them in a suburb of Lusaka, Zambia. In his treatment of a particular medical problem, a Muslim healer would find what he determined was the appropriate passage in his holy book. Using special "therapeutic" ink, he would copy the passage onto the bottom of a plate, add a little water to dissolve the ink, and have the patient swallow the prescription. And then there was the healer who used the traditional scarification, tattooing, and rubbing of herbs into wounds, but, as a result of his contact with Western practitioners and their heavy reliance on medications administered via hypodermics, began to refer to his own traditional treatments as "African injections."

CONCLUSION

The important roles played by the traditional healers in some cultures has, in a few instances, begun to be acknowledged by official government bodies. Thus Meagher (1977) notes that Navaho medicine men's fees have been accepted in recent years by the U.S. Internal Revenue Service as legitimate medical expenses, deductible on Navaho Indians' income tax statements. Further, the international convention of the United Mine Workers of America in 1976 voted to approve a one-year trial program to cover Navaho members' payments to their medicine men. Many enticements are offered to the members to utilize modern medical services but the lure of the traditional healer persists. One of the Navaho questioned is reported by Meagher to have stated, "When medical doctors can provide no remedy, Navajos always go to a medicine man." Another added, "When a patient goes to him, he is reformed in good ways."

In many cases of contact, the combination of traditional medicine and Western practices may benefit the patient. Thus, Frankenberg and Leeson (1976:250) record the incorporation of powdered milk into the pharmacopoeia of one of the Zambian healers. For babies with symptoms of kwashiorkor or marasmus, he would direct the mother to dissolve his traditional herbs in the reconstituted powdered milk, thus, as the investigators comment, "giving the child the best of both worlds." This ability and willingness of traditional healers to innovate as well as to adapt has, unfortunately, been largely ignored in many situations where modern medicine is being introduced into a transitional society. The transition could be made infinitely more smooth and less painful by involving the cooperation of the traditional healers in whom the confidence of the people resides.

It would be futile and misleading to attempt to compare the effectiveness of traditional healing with that of modern medical science in the cases of frank pathology. No social benefits, no psychological spin-offs, none of the acknowledged advantages in the approach of the traditional healer measure up to the immunization techniques that have virtually eradicated smallpox, poliomyelitis, tetanus, diphtheria, and other dread diseases. Few informed people would be willing to trade the efficacy of one or two injections of penicillin in the treatment of such formerly devastating diseases as syphilis, yaws, and gonorrhea for even the all-encompassing ministrations of the traditional curer. Likewise, in light of today's operable conditions, the assurance of recovery and the promise of an extension of life make the advances of modern surgery tower over such techniques as sand painting, spiritual trips to the underworld, and object extraction by sucking, all of which now appear virtually irrelevant.

At the same time, there remains much that modern medicine can absorb from traditional healers. The holistic approach to the troubled victim of some malfunction in his or her life, the involvement of family and friends, the sense of social solidarity and support, the expected and delivered explanations for the troubles at hand—all are vital adjuncts to any medical system. As members of the order Primates, we have a heritage millions of years old that renders us in constant need of the reassurance derived from physical as well as social "stroking."

It can be argued that the exemplary record of the traditional healers in maintaining comforting cultural mechanisms in the presence of illness derives from their lack of the technological know-how that would make such an approach unnecessary. Be that as it may, the record also shows that these healers are vitally concerned with the welfare of their people, and respond effectively to conditions that would otherwise tend toward the disruption, occasionally even the extinction, of the culture afflicted.

Technological solutions to many formerly unremitting medical problems are at hand. Today, when penicillin, protein, and vaccines can be manufactured for pennies, no child should die from diseases, especially deficiency-related diseases, that can be relatively easily prevented or cured. To the extent that the quality of life is marred for so many of the world's people, the remedies are to be sought in expanded knowledge of human interactions. Profound socioeconomic adjustments could solve or ameliorate the overwhelming majority of distribution problems that cause the benefits of modern medical advances to be withheld from appalling numbers of the world's medically burdened populations. An appreciation of the impressive personal efforts by the outstanding leaders we subsume as traditional healers, coupled with knowledge of the tremendous obstacles to survival that have been overcome through the biological mechanisms of evolutionary selection, should contribute to an attitude of optimism, indeed confidence, that the remaining tasks, the social readjustments that lie ahead, should not be insurmountable.

GLOSSARY

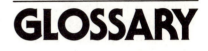

abortifacients   Substances or objects used to cause abortion.

abscess   Inflamed area of tissue, which fills with pus.

achlorhydria   Failure of the stomach to secrete hydrochloric acid.

allele   A variant form of gene for a particular trait, such as eye color.

*arbovirus   A group of viruses that are transmitted to man by arthropods, especially mosquitoes and ticks. Short for "arthropod-borne virus."

*arteriosclerosis   Thickening and loss of elasticity of the coats of arteries, with inflammatory changes; popularly called hardening of the arteries.

artifact   An object made by humans.

bilharzia   Disease caused by a blood fluke transmitted by snails. Also called schistosomiasis.

*bilirubin   An orange bile pigment produced by the breakdown of hemoglobin and excreted by the liver cells.

B.P.   "Before present."

buccal   Of the mouth cavity, especially the cheeks.

C-types   Coxsackievirus, which produces a polio-like disease in humans.

*Definition taken from Benjamin F. Miller and Claire Brackman Keane, *Encyclopedia and Dictionary of Medicine and Nursing* (Philadelphia: W. B. Saunders Co., 1972).

callus   A hard substance that reunites sections of broken bone.

cation   A positive ion.

cerocopithecoid   Referring to the Old World monkeys such as baboons, patas monkeys, and rhesus monkeys.

Chagas' disease   A chronic infection with *Trypanosoma,* involving chills, fever, pains in the extremities, and extreme fatigue; localized in South America but related to African sleeping sickness.

cholesterol   A sterol that is found in animal tissues and may be deposited in the walls of arteries, contributing to arteriosclerosis.

coprolite   Fossilized excrement.

cytology   Science concerned with the structure and functioning of cells.

dermatology   The branch of medicine dealing with skin disorders.

dolmens   Prehistoric monuments of two or more upright stones supporting a capstone. Found especially in Britain and France and thought to be "tombs" constructed by Neolithic peoples.

dyscrasias   abnormalities of the body.

electrolyte   A substance, such as sodium, that will conduct electricity when dissolved in water.

encephalomyelitis   Inflammation of the brain.

encyst   To become enclosed in a capsule within body tissue.

endemic   Constantly present within a particular area or group of organisms.

endometrial   Of the inner lining of the uterus.

*endothelial cells   Cells that line the inside of blood and lymph vessels, the heart, and other closed cavities of the body.

Eocene   Geological epoch lasting 54 to 36 million years B.P.; characterized by the rise of mammals.

*epidemic   Suddenly occurring in a great number of cases at the same time.

erythrocytes   Small, disc-like blood cells that contain hemoglobin and carry oxygen. Also known as red blood cells.

exostosis   An abnormal bony growth.

febrifuge   Any substance that reduces fever.

febrile   Feverish.

femur   The bone of the upper leg. Also called thighbone.

gamete   Mature egg or sperm.

gametocytes   Sex cells from which gametes derive.

gamma globulin   That portion of blood serum that contains the most antibodies.

genus   A category of Linnaean classification comprising related species.

gummatous Describing the soft tumors that arise in the last stage of syphilis.

hemochromatosis Abnormal iron metabolism that results in deposition of iron in tissues, carbohydrate intolerance, and eventual cirrhosis of the liver.

heterozygous Having two different alleles (q.v.) at the same locus on a pair of chromosomes, such as the locus that controls blood groups.

holoendemic Affecting all the residents of a particular region.

hominid The category of primates including modern humans and their fossil ancestors and collaterals but excluding fossil and living apes.

homozygous Having the same two alleles (q.v.) at the same locus on a pair of chromosomes.

host The organism in which a parasite lives.

humerus The bone of the upper arm.

hypochromic microcytic anemia Chronic iron-deficiency anemia, marked by small, pale red blood cells.

ketosis Excessive secretion of ketones by the body due to impaired metabolism.

kilocalorie 1,000 calories.

latency The state in which a disease seems inactive.

macrogametocytes Female gametes of the malarial parasite.

Marburg disease Severe, often fatal, viral disease that impairs the functioning of the liver and kidneys, and causes skin lesions and conjunctivitis.

matrilineality The reckoning of descent through the mother's family.

matrix Nonliving matter in which living cells are embedded.

megalospleny Enlargement of the spleen.

melanin Brown pigment found in the skin and in the iris of the eye.

metaphyseal Referring to the wide part of the shaft of a bone.

metate Stone basin or slab on which foods are ground.

microgametocytes Male gamete of the malarial parasite.

mucosa Mucous membrane, such as the lining of the nose or throat.

necrosis Decay of living tissue.

Neolithic The stage of cultural evolution during which humans domesticated plants and animals. Food production was attained in the Middle East approximately 10,000 years ago and more recently in other areas.

neonate Newly born child.

Oligocene Geological epoch lasting 36 to 23 million years B.P.

osteitis (osteitis deformans)   A disease in the course of which bones lose calcium and soften, then recalcify, becoming thickened and deformed.

osteomyelitis   Infection of the inner marrow cavity of bone.

osteoperiostitis   Inflammation of a bone and its periosteum.

otitis media   Inflammation of the middle ear.

Paget's disease   Another name for osteitis deformans (q.v.).

parasitism   Condition in which one organism lives on another, usually damaging the host.

parenchyma cells   The functioning tissues of organs, as opposed to structural or connective tissues.

paretic   Progressively losing mental and physical power as brain cells degenerate.

parietal bones   Two squarish bones that form the upper sides and the roof of the neurocranium (braincase).

parturient   About to give birth.

pathogenicity   Ability of an organism to produce disease.

perineum   The region between the anus and vagina or anus and scrotum.

periosteum   A fibrous membrane covering all bones except at the articular surfaces.

periostitis   Infection of the outer bone layer.

petrous (petrosal) bones   Two irregularly shaped bones that form the lower sides of the cranium and enclose the inner structures of the ear.

phagocytize   To destroy by means of the white blood cells.

phalanges   Bones of the fingers and toes.

pharmacopoeia   Collection of drugs.

phylum   A category of Linnaean classification ranking below the Kingdom (Animal, Plant, Protist) level: for instance, the Chordates.

plaque   A deposit of fatty material in a blood vessel wall.

Pleistocene   The "Ice Age," a geological epoch lasting roughly 1.8 million to 10,000 years B.P.

polygamy   A marriage system that permits a man two or more wives or a woman two or more husbands.

psychosomatic   Referring to disease that originates in or is aggravated by mental stress.

purine   A colorless, crystalline compound that is the basis of the uric acid group of compounds.

pyorrhea   Inflammation of the gums, leading to loss of teeth.

relapsing fever   A serious but rarely fatal disease marked by periods of normal temperature alternating with periods of fever.

reticular cells   Those cells that form the connective tissue, or the framework, of organs.

sacrum   The large bone, made of five fused spinal bones, located at the lower back between the pelvic bones.

sagittal suture   The suture running from front to back atop the cranium, between the parietal bones.

Salmonella   Genus of bacteria that includes those causing typhoid fever and gastroenteritis.

scarification   Creating designs on the skin by making small incisions or punctures.

sequestrum   A piece of dead bone detached from healthy bone.

species (animal)   The most exclusive category of Linnaean classification: a population or group of populations, of actually or potentially interbreeding animals, reproductively isolated from other populations or groups.

subperiosteal   Beneath the periosteum.

superinfection   Sudden growth of bacteria in a previously infected wound or already diseased tissue.

tapa   A cloth made by pounding the treated inner bark of a paper mulberry tree.

tibia   The inner and larger of two bones of the lower leg. Also called shin or shinbone.

ulna   The longer and more slender of the two bones of the forearm; located on the little-finger side.

zygote   The cell formed by the fusion of two gametes (mature egg and sperm); the fertilized egg.

BIBLIOGRAPHY

Entries preceded by an asterisk are references not cited in the text.

Abel, O.
1924   Neuere Studien über Krankheiten fossiler Wirbeltiere. *Verhandlungen der Zoolog-ische Botanische Gesellschaft, Wien* 73:104.

Ackerknecht, Erwin H.
1971   *Medicine and Ethnology: Selected Essays.* Edited by H. H. Walser and H. M. Koelbing. Baltimore: Johns Hopkins Press.

Albert, Ethel M.
1971   Women of Burundi: A Study of Social Values. In Denise Paulme, ed., *Women of Tropical Africa,* pp. 179-215. Berkeley: University of California Press.

Alfin-Slater, Roslyn B., and Jelliffe, Derrick B.
1977   One Difference between Men and Women Is Their Nutrient Requirements. *Los Angeles Times,* January 30.

Allen, N.J.
1976   Approaches to Illness in the Nepalese Hills (East Nepal). In J. B Loudon, ed., *Social Anthropology and Medicine,* pp. 500-522. New York: Academic Press.

Anderson, Alastair
1978   Bridgehead in Europe. *World Health,* July, pp. 16-19.

Anonymous
1974   The World Food Crisis. *Time,* November 11, pp. 66-68ff.

Appel, Ted C.
1977   The Curandero and the Sukya; Native Healers in Nicaragua. *Medical Anthropology Newsletter* 8(2):16-19.

Armstrong, M. L., Connoe, W. E., and Warner, E. D.
  1967   Xanthomatosis in Rhesus Monkeys Fed a Hypercholesterolemic Diet. *Archives of Pathology* 84:227-337.

Ashburn, Percy M.
  1947   *The Ranks of Death: A Medical History of the Conquest of America.* Edited by Frank D. Ashburn. New York: Coward-McCann.

*Ashmead, Albert S.
  1895   Autochthonous Syphilis in Bolivia and Peru. *Journal of Cutaneous Disease, Including Syphilis and Venereal Disease* 13:415-417.

Augusta, Joseph
  1960   *Prehistoric Animals.* London: Paul Hamlyn.

Bailey, K. V.
  1975   Malnutrition in the African Region. *WHO Chronicle* 29:354-464.

Balikci, Asen
  1967   Shamanistic Behavior among the Netsilik Eskimos. In John Middleton, ed., *Magic, Witchcraft and Curing*, pp. 191-209. Garden City, N.Y.: Natural History Press.

Bates, Marston
  1965   *The Natural History of Mosquitoes.* Reprint ed. New York: Harper and Row (Harper Torch Book).

Baumgartner, Leona
  1964   Syphilis Eradication—A Plan for Action Now. In World Forum on Syphilis and Other Treponematoses, *Proceedings . . .* , pp. 26-32. Public Health Service Publication no. 997. Atlanta: U.S. Department of Health, Education, and Welfare,Public Health Service.

Beattie, John
  1967   Divination in Bunyoro, Uganda. In John Middleton, ed., *Magic, Witchcraft and Curing,* pp. 211-231. Garden City, N.Y.: Natural History Press.

Behar
  1968   Food and Nutrition of the Maya before the Conquest and at the Present Time. In Pan American Health Organization, Advisory Committee on Medical Research, *Biomedical Challenges Presented by the American Indian.* WHO Scientific Publication no. 165. Washington, D.C.

Benedict, Ruth
  1934   *Patterns of Culture.* Boston: Houghton Mifflin Co.

*Bennett, Charles F., Jr.
  1962   The Buyano Cuna Indians, Panama: An Ecological Study of Livelihood and Diet. *Annals of the Association of American Geographers* 52(1):32-50.

Berg, Alan D., with Muscat, Robert J.
  1973   *The Nutrition Factor: Its Role in National Development.* Washington, D.C.: Brookings Institution.

Berkow, Robert, ed., and Talbott, Hohn H., consulting ed.
  1974   *Merck Manual of Diagnosis and Therapy.* 13th ed. Rahway, N.J.: Merck and Co.

Berndt, Catherine H.
  1964   The Role of Native Doctors in Aboriginal Australia. In Ari Kiev, ed., *Magic, Faith and Healing: Studies in Primitive Psychiatry Today,* pp. 264-282. New York: Free Press of Glencoe; London: Collier-Macmillan.

*Bhatt, P. N.; Goverdhan, M. K.; Shaffer, F. F.; Brandt, C. D.; and Fox, J. P.
    1966   Viral Infections of Monkeys in Their Natural Habitats in Southern India. *American Journal of Tropical Medicine and Hygiene* 15:551-560.

Biegel, Hugo G.
    1964   Changes in the Social Climate toward Veneral Disease in the Last Quarter Century. In World Forum on Syphilis and Other Treponematoses, *Proceedings . . .* , pp. 399-406. Public Health Service Publication no. 997. Atlanta: U.S. Department of Health, Education, and Welfare, Public Health Service.

Billard, Jules B., ed.
    1974   *The World of the American Indian.* Washington, D.C.: National Geographic Society.

*Bleibtreu, Herman, ed.
    1969   *Evolutionary Anthropology.* Boston: Allyn and Bacon.

Bleibtreu, John N.
    1968   *The Parable of the Beast.* London: Cox and Wyman.

Boas, Franz
    1928   *Materials for the Study of Inheritance in Man.* New York: Columbia University Press.
  *1930   *The Religion of the Kwakiutl Indians,* pt. 2: *Translations.* New York: Columbia University Press.

Bock, Philip K.
    1967   Love, Magic, Menstrual Taboos and the Facts of Geography. *American Anthropologist* 69:213-217.

Bowen, Elenore Smith
    1964   *Return to Laughter.* Garden City, N.Y.: Doubleday and Co.

Boyd, Mark F.
    1930   *An Introduction to Malariology.* Cambridge, Mass.: Harvard University Press.
    1941   An Historical Sketch of the Prevalence of Malaria in North America. *American Journal of Tropical Medicine* 21:223-244.
  *1949   Epidemiology of Malaria: Factors Related to the Intermediate Host. In Mark F. Boyd, ed., *Malariology,* I,551-607. Philadelphia: W. B. Saunders Co.

Boyer, L. Bryce
    1964   Folk Psychiatry of the Apaches of the Mescalero Indian Reservation. In Ari Kiev., ed., *Magic, Faith and Healing: Studies in Primitive Psychiatry Today,* pp. 384-419. New York: Free Press of Glencoe; London: Collier-Macmillan.

Bradford, William
    1908   *History of Plymouth Plantation.* Edited by William T. Davis. New York: Charles Scriber's Sons.

Brown, Judith K.
    1963   A Cross-Cultural Study of Female Initiation Rites. *American Anthropologist* 65:837-853.

Brown, William J.
    1964   The First Step toward Eradication. In World Forum on Syphilis and Other Treponematoses, *Proceedings . . .* , pp. 21-25. Public Health Service Publication no. 997. Atlanta: U.S. Department of Health, Education, and Welfare, Public Health Service.

Bruce-Chwatt, Leonard J.
  1954   Problems of Malaria Control in Tropical Africa. *British Medical Journal,* January, pp. 169-174.
  1965a   Malaria Research for Malaria Eradication. *Transactions of the Royal Society of Tropical Medicine and Hygiene* 59:105-137.
  1965b   Paleogenesis and Paleo-epidemiology of Primate Malaria. *Bulletin of the World Health Organization* 32:363-387.
 *1971   Malaria: The Persistent Threat. *The Practitioner* 207:143-146.

Bryant, A. T.
  1966   *Zulu Medicine and Medicine Men.* Capetown: C. Struick.

Buckley, Anthony D.
  1976   The Secret: An Idea in Yoruba Medicinal Thought. In J. B. Loudon, ed., *Social Anthropology and Medicine*, pp. 396-421. New York: Academic Press.

Buettner-Janusch, J., ed.
  1964   *Evolutionary and Genetic Biology of Primates.* 2 vols. New York: Academic Press.

Bullough, Vern, and Voght, Martha
  1973   Women, Menstruation and Nineteenth-Century Medicine. *Bulletin of the History of Medicine* 47:66-82.

Carter, Henry Rose
  1931   *Yellow Fever: An Epidemiological and Historical Study of Its Place of Origin.* Edited by Laura Armistead Carter and Wade Hampton Frost. Baltimore: Williams and Wilkins Co.

Castro, Josúe de
  1952   *The Geography of Hunger.* Boston: Little, Brown and Co.

Celli, Angelo
  1933   *The History of Malaria in the Roman Campagna.* London: John Bale, Sons and Danielsson.

Chagnon, Napoleon
  1968   *Yanomamö: The Fierce People.* New York: Holt, Rinehart and Winston.
  _____; Neel, J. V.; Weitkamp, L; Gershowitz, H.: and Ayres, M.
  1975   The Influence of Cultural Factors on the Demography and Pattern of Gene Flow from the Makiritare to the Yanomamo Indians. In F. S. Hulse, ed., *Men and Nature,* pp. 287-300. New York: Random House, 1975.

Chawla, K. K.; Murthy, C.D.S.; Chakravarti, R. N.; and Chhuttani, P. N.
  1967   Arteriosclerosis and Thrombosis in Wild Rhesus Monkeys. *American Heart Journal* 73:85-91.

Childs, St. Julien Ravenel
  1940   *Malaria and Colonization in the Carolina Low Country, 1526-1696.* Baltimore: Johns Hopkins University Press.

Christensen, Bodil, and Marti, Samuel
  1972   *Witchcraft and Pre-Columbian Paper.* 2nd ed. Mexico City: Ediciones Euro-americanas.

Christophers, S. R., and Bentley, C. A.
  1911   *Malaria in the Duars.* Simla, India: Government Monotype Press.

Clark, Herbert C., Dunn, Lawrence H., and Benavides, Joaquin.
  1931   Experimental Transmission to Man of a Relapsing Fever Spirochete in a Wild

Monkey of Panama—*Leontocebus Geoffroyi* (Pucheran). *American Journal of Tropical Medicine* 11:243-257.

————, and Tomlinson, Wray J.
1949   The Pathologic Anatomy of Malaria. In Mark F. Boyd, ed., *Malariology,* II, 874-903. Philadelphia: W. B. Saunders Co.

Clark, Matt, with Hager, Mary, and Shapiro, Dan.
Blight of the Tropics. *Newsweek,* June 26, pp. 83-84.

Clarkson, Thomas
1808   The History of the Rise, Progress and Accomplishment of the Abolition of the Slave Trade. In John Langdon-Davies, ed., *The Slave Trade and Its Abolition—A Collection of Contemporary Documents.* New York: Viking Press, 1965.

Clement, A. J.
1956   Caries in the South African Ape-Man: Some Examples of Undoubted Authenticity Believed to Be 800,000 Years Old. *British Dental Journal* 101:4-7.

Coatney, G. Robert; Collins, William; McWilson, Warren; and Contacos, Peter G.
1971   *The Primate Malarias.* Bethesda, Md.: U.S. National Institute of Allergy and Infectious Diseases.

Cockburn, T. Aidan
1961   The Origin of the Treponematoses. *Bulletin of the World Health Organization* 24:221-228.
*1967   *Infectious Diseases: Their Evolution and Eradication.* Springfield, Ill.: Charles C. Thomas.
1971   Infectious Diseases in Ancient Populations. *Current Anthropology* 12(1):45-62.

Cockerell, T. D. A.
1918   New Species of North American Fossil Beetles, Cockroaches and Tsetse Flies. *Proceedings, U.S. National Museum, Washington* 54:301-311.

*Coe, William R.
1957   Environmental Limitation on Maya Culture: A Reexamination. American Anthropologist 59:328-335.

Cohen, Bernice H.
1970   ABO and Rh Incompatibility: I. Fetal and Neonatal Mortality with ABO Incompatibility and Rh Incompatibility; Some New Interpretations. *American Journal of Human Genetics* 22:412-440.

Cole, Harold N.; Harkin, James C.; Kraus, Bertram S., and Moritz, Alan R.
1955   Pre-Columbian Osseous Syphilis. *Archives of Dermatology* 71:231-238.

Colson, Audrey B.
1976   Binary Opposition and the Treatment of Sickness among the Akawaio. In J. B. Loudon, ed., *Social Anthropology and Medicine,* pp. 422-499. New York: Academic Press.

Coult, Allan D.
1963   Unconscious Inference and Cultural Origins. *American Anthropologist* 65:32-35.

Courville, Cyril B.
*1948   Cranial Injuries among the Indians of North America. *Bulletin of the Los Angeles Neurological Society* 13(2):181-219.
————, and Abbott, K.H.
1942   Cranial Injuries of the Pre-Columbian Incas. *Bulletin of the Los Angeles Neurological Society* 7(3):107-130.

*Crosby, Alfred W., Jr.
  1972   *The Columbian Exchange: Biological and Cultural Consequences of 1492.* West-
         port, Conn.: Greenwood Publishing Co.

Cruickshank, E. K.
  1967   Nutrition in Pregnancy and Lactation. In J. B. Lawson and D. B. Stewart, eds.,
         Obstetrics and Gynaecology in the Tropics and Developing Countries, pp. 11-28.
         London: Edward Arnold.

Culbert, T. Patrick
  1973   *The Classic Maya Collapse.* Albuquerque: University of New Mexico Press.

Curtin, Philip D.
  1968   Epidemiology and the Slave Trade. *Political Science Quarterly* 83(2):190-216.

Davis, Kingsley
  1975   Population Policy: Will Current Programs Succeed? In Priscilla Reining and Irene
         Tinker, eds., *Population: Dynamics, Ethics and Policy,* pp. 27-36. Washington,
         D.C.: American Association for the Advancement of Science.

Day, H. H.; Leakey, R. E. E.; Walker, A. C.; and Wood, B. A.
  1975   New Hominids from East Rudolf, Kenya. *American Journal of Physical Anthro-
         pology* 42:461-475.

De Muth, J. E., Arndt, J. R., and Weinswig, M. H.
  1974   Attempt to Initiate Community Action Programmes in Venereal Disease Educa-
         tion in the United States of America. *British Journal of Venereal Diseases*
         50:151-154.

Dennie, Charles C.
  1962   *A History of Syphilis.* Springfield, Ill.: Charles C. Thomas.

Devereux, George
  1955   *A Study of Abortion in Primitive Societies.* New York: Julian Press. (Reprint ed.,
         New York: International Universities Press, 1976.)

Dingle, John H.
  1973   The Ills of Man. *Scientific American* 229(3):76-84.

Dobkin de Rios, Marlene
  1973   Curing with Ayahuasca in an Urban Slum. In M. J. Harner, ed., *Hallucinogens and
         Shamanism,* pp. 67-85. New York: Oxford University Press.
  1978   An Anthropologist Looks at the Origin of the Sexual Division of Labor in Soci-
         ety. In *Women's Studies: An Interdisciplinary Approach.* In press.

Dobyns, Henry F.
  1963   An Outline of Andean Epidemic History to 1720. *Bulletin of the History of
         Medicine* 37:493-515.

Dobzhansky, Theodosius
  1962   *Mankind Evolving.* New Haven: Yale University Press.

Du Bois, W. E. Burghardt
  1947   *The World and Africa.* New York: Viking Press.

Dubos, René
  1968   *Man, Medicine, and Environment.* New York: Frederick A. Praeger.

Dumond, Don E.
  1975   The Limitation of Human Population: A Natural History. In Priscilla Reining and

Irene Tinker, eds., *Population: Dynamics, Ethics and Policy,* pp. 83-90. Washington, D.C.: American Association for the Advancement of Science.

Dunn, Frederick L.
1965 On the Antiquity of Malaria in the Western Hemisphere. *Human Biology* 37:385-393.
1968 Epidemiological Factors: Health and Disease in Hunter-Gatherers. In R. B. Lee and I. DeVore, eds., *Man the Hunter*, pp. 221-228. Chicago: Aldine Publishing Co.

Dupire, Marguerite
1971 The Position of Women in a Pastoral Society (The Fulani WoDaaBe, Nomads of the Niger). In Denise Paulme, ed., *Women of Tropical Africa*, pp. 47-92. Berkeley: University of California Press.

Edgerton, Robert B.
1977 A Traditional African Psychiatrist. In *Readings in Anthropology 77/78,* pp. 121-136. Guilford, Conn.: Dushkin Publishing Group.

Effertz, Otto
1909 Malaria in Tropical America and among Indians. *Janus, Revue Internationale* 14:246-261.

*Ehrenriech, Barbara, and English, Deirdre
1973 *Witches, Midwives and Nurses: A History of Women Healers.* New York: Feminist Press.

Ehrhardt, Anke A.
1975 Prenatal Hormones and Human Behavior: Implications for the Status of Women. In Dana Raphael, ed., *Being Female: Reproduction, Power and Changes,* pp. 19-24. Paris: Mouton Press.

Eliade, Mircea
1976 *Shamanism: Archaic Techniques of Ecstasy.* Translated by Willard R. Trask. Bollingen Series 76. Princeton: Princeton University Press. (Paperback ed., 1972.)

Engel, George L.
1977 The Need for a New Medical Model: A Challenge for Biomedicine. *Science* 196:129-136.

Engels, Friedrich
1958 *The Condition of the Working Class in England.* Translated and edited by W. O. Henderson and W. H. Chaloner. Stanford: Stanford University Press.
1972 *The Origin of the Family, Private Property and the State.* New York: International Publishers.

Erasmus, Charles John
1952 Changing Folk Beliefs and the Relativity of Empirical Knowledge. *Southwest Journal of Anthropology* 8:411-428.

Evans-Pritchard, E. E.
*1967 The Morphology and Function of Magic: A Comparative Study of Trobriand and Zande Ritual and Spells. In John Middleton, ed., *Magic, Witchcraft and Curing,* pp. 1-22. Garden City, N.Y.: Natural History Press.
1974 *Man and Woman among the Azande.* New York: Free Press.

*Fairley, N. Hamilton
1949 Malaria: The Life Cycle. *British Medical Journal,* October 15, pp. 825-830.

Falade, Solange
    1971   Women of Dakar and the Surrounding Urban Areas. In Denise Paulme, ed., *Women of Tropical Africa,* pp. 217-229. Berkeley: University of California Press.

*Fenwick, A.
    1969   Baboons as Reservoir Hosts of *Schistosoma Mansoni. Transactions of the Royal Society of Tropical Medicine and Hygiene* 63:557-563.

Fiennes, Richard
    1965   *Man, Nature and Disease.* Ithaca, N.Y.: New American Library of the World.

Fiennes, R. N., and Riopelle, A. J.
    1969   Communicable Diseases: Hazards for Man and Models for Research. In W. I. B. Beveridge, ed., *Using Primates in Medical Research,* pt. 2: *Recent Comparative Research,* pp. 93-103. Primates in Medicine, vol. 3. Basel, Switzerland: S. Karger.

*Flegel, Kenneth M.
    1974   Changing Concepts of the Nosology of Gonorrhea and Syphilis. *Bulletin of the History of Medicine* 48:571-588.

Food and Agriculture Organization
    1967   *Freedom from Hunger Campaign.* Basic Study no. 6. FAO Bulletin.

Ford, Clellan Stearns
    1964   *A Comparative Study of Human Reproduction.* Yale University Publications in Anthropology no. 32. New Haven: Yale University Press.

Forer, Raymond
    1962   Cross-Cultural Contact and Venereal Disease. In World Forum on Syphilis and Other Treponematoses, *Proceedings, . . . ,* pp. 393-398. Public Health Service Publication no. 997. Atlanta: U.S. Department of Health, Education, and Welfare, Public Health Service.

Foulks, Edward F.
    1972   The Arctic Hysterias of the North Alaskan Eskimo. In David H. Maybury-Lewis, ed., *Anthropological Studies,* no. 10. Washington, D.C.: American Anthropological Association.

Fowler, Melvin L.
    1975   A Pre-Columbian Urban Center on the Mississippi. *Scientific American* 233(2): 92-101.

Fox, J. Robin
    1964   Witchcraft and Clanship in Cochiti Therapy. In Ari Kiev, ed., *Magic, Faith and Healing: Studies in Primitive Psychiatry Today,* pp. 174-200. New York: Free Press of Glencoe; London: Collier-Macmillan.

Fracastoro, Girolamo
    1934   *The Sinister Shepherd: A Translation of Girolamo Fracastoro's Syphilidis sive, De morbo gallico libri tres* by William Van Wyck. Los Angeles: Primavera Press. (Originally published in 1530.)

Frank, Jerome D.
    1973   *Persuasion and Healing: A Comparative Study of Psychotherapy.* Rev. ed. Baltimore: Johns Hopkins University Press.

Frankenberg, Ronald, and Leeson, Joyce
    1976   Disease, Illness, and Sickness: Social Aspects of the Choice of Healer in a Lusaka Suburb. In J. B. Loudon, ed., *Social Anthropology and Medicine,* pp. 223-258. New York: Academic Press.

*Freed, Stanley A., and Freed, Ruth S.
   1967   Spirit Possession as Illness in a North Indian Village. In John Middleton, ed., *Magic, Witchcraft and Curing*, pp. 295-320. Garden City, N.Y.: Natural History Press.

Fribourg-Blanc, A., and Mollaret, H. H.
   1968   Natural Treponematosis of the African Primate. In W. I. B. Beveridge, ed., *Using Primates in Medical Research*, pt. 2: Recent Comparative Research, pp. 113-121. Primates in Medicine, vol. 3. Basel, Switzerland: S. Karger.

Friedl, Ernestine
   1974   *Women and Men: An Anthropologist's View*. New York: Holt, Rinehart and Winston.

Frisch, Rose E., and McArthur, Janet W.
   1974   Menstrual Cycles: Fatness as a Determinant of Minimum Weight and Height Necessary for Their Maintenance or Onset. *Science* 185:949-951.
   ——— , and Revelle, R.
   1970   Height and Weight at Menarche and a Hypothesis of Body Weights and Adolescent Events. *Science* 169:397-399.

Fuchs, Stephen
   1964   Magic Healing Techniques among the Balahis in Central India. In Ari Kiev., ed., *Magic, Faith and Healing: Studies in Primitive Psychiatry Today*, pp. 121-138. New York: Free Press of Glencoe; London: Collier-Macmillan.

Gann, Thomas W. F.
   1918   *The Maya Indians of Southern Yucatan and Northerly British Honduras*. Bureau of American Ethnology Bulletin, no. 64. Washington, D.C.: Smithsonian Institution.

Garine, I. de
   1974   Tabu, Food, and Society. *World Health*, February-March, pp. 44-49.

*Garner, M. F., Hornabrook, R. W., and Backhouse, J. L.
   1972   Prevalence of Yaws on Kar Kar Island, New Guinea. *British Journal of Venereal Diseases* 48:350-355.

Garrison, Fielding H.
   1929   *An Introduction to the History of Medicine*. 4th ed. Philadelphia: W. B. Saunders Co.

Gasparini, Giuseppe
   1962   Program for the Eradication of Endemic Syphilis. In World Forum on Syphilis and Other Treponematoses, *Proceedings* . . . , pp. 157-166. Public Health Service Publication no. 997. Atlanta: U.S. Department of Health, Education, and Welfare, Public Health Service.

Geddes, W. R.
   1969   *Nine Dyak Nights*. New York: Oxford University Press.

Gelfand, Michael
   1964   Psychiatric Disorders as Recognized by the Shona. In Ari Kiev, ed., *Magic, Faith and Healing: Studies in Primitive Psychiatry Today*, pp. 156-173. New York: Free Press of Glencoe; London: Collier-Macmillan.

Gessain, Monique
   1971   Coniagui Women (Guinea). In Denise Paulme, ed., *Women of Tropical Africa*, pp. 17-46. Berkeley: University of California Press.

Gigioli, George G.
 1968 *Malaria in the American Indian.* Washington, D.C.: Pan American Health Organization, Advisory Commission on Medical Research.

Gillies, Eva
 1976 Causal Criteria in African Classifications of Disease. In J. B. Loudon, ed., *Social Anthropology and Medicine*, pp. 358-395. New York: Academic Press.

*Gillies, M. T., and Wilkes, T. J.
 1965 A Study of Age Composition of Populations of *Anopheles Gambiae* Giles and *Anopheles Funestus* Giles in Northeast Tanzania. *Bulletin of Entomological Research* 56:237.

Goff, Charles W.
 1953 New Evidence of Pre-Columbian Bone Syphilis in Guatemala. In R. B. Woodbury, ed., *The Rivers of Zacculeu, Guatemala*, I, 312-319. Richmond, Va.: William Byrd Press.
 1967 Syphilis. In Don Brothwell and A. T. Sandison, eds., *Diseases in Antiquity*, pp. 279-294. Springfield, Ill.: Charles C. Thomas.

Goldsmith, Edward I.
 1969 The Current Role of Non-Human Primates in Surgical Research. In W. I. B. Beveridge., ed., *Using Primates in Medical Research*, pt. 2: *Recent Comparative Research*, pp. 41-51. Primates in Medicine, vol. 3. Basel, Switzerland: S. Karger.

Goldstein, M. S.
 1957 Skeletal Pathology of Early Indians in Texas. *American Journal of Physical Anthropology* 15:299-307.
 *1969 Human Paleopathology and Some Diseases in Living Primitive Societies: A Review of the Recent Literature. *American Journal of Physical Anthropology* 31:285-295.

Goodale, Jane C.
 1971 *Tiwi Wives: A Study of the Women of Melville Island, Northern Australia.* Seattle: University of Washington Press.

Gray, Louis H.
 1958 Circumcision. *Hastings' Encyclopaedia of Religion and Ethics*, III, 659-680.

Gregg, J. B., Steele, J. P., and Holzhueter, A.
 1965 Roentgenographic Evaluation of Temporal Bones from South Dakota Indian Burials. *American Journal of Physical Anthropology* 23:51-62.

Gresham, G. A., and Howard, A. N.
 1969 Cardiovascular Diseases. In W. I. B. Beveridge, ed., *Using Primates in Medical Research*, pt. 2: *Recent Comparative Research*, pp. 1-8. Primates in Medicine, vol. 3. Basel, Switzerland: S. Karger.

Grin, E. I.
 1961 Endemic Treponematoses in the Sudan. *Bulletin of the World Health Organization* 24:229-238.

Guerra, Francisco
 1964 Maya Medicine. *Medical History* 8:31-43.

Guthe, Thorstein
 1964 Measure of the Treponematoses Problem in the World. In World Forum on Syphi-

lis and Other Treponematoses, *Proceedings* . . . , pp. 11-20. Public Health Service Publication no. 997. Atlanta: U.S. Department of Health, Education, and Welfare, Public Health Service.

Guthrie, Douglas
1958 *A History of Medicine.* London: Thomas Nelson and Sons.

Hackett, C. J.
1963 On the Origin of the Human Treponematoses (Pinta, Yaws, Endemic Syphilis and Venereal Syphilis). *Bulletin of the World Health Organization* 29:7-41.

Hackett, L. W.
1937 *Malaria in Europe: An Ecological Study.* London: Oxford University Press.

Haga, H.
1959 Studies on Natural Selection in ABO Blood Groups with Special Reference to the Influence of Environmental Changes upon the Selective Pressure Due to Maternal-Fetal Incompatibility. *Japanese Journal of Human Genetics* 4:1-20.

Haggard, Howard W.
1929 *Devils, Drugs and Doctors: The Story of the Science of Healing from Medicine-Man to Doctor.* New York: Harper and Bros.

Hammond, Dorothy, and Jablow, Alta
1976 *Women in the Cultures of the World.* Menlo Park, Calif.: Cummings Publishing Co.

Handelman, Don
1977 The Development of a Washo Shama. In David Landy, ed., *Culture, Disease, and Healing: Studies in Medical Anthropology*, pp. 427-438. New York: Macmillan Publishing Co.

Harris, R. I.
1949 Osteological Evidence of Disease amongst the Huron Indians. *University of Toronto Medical Journal* 37(2):71-75.

Harrison, Barbara
1971 *Conservation of Nonhuman Primates in 1970.* New York: S. Karger.

Harrison, Richard J., and Montagna, William
1973 *Man.* New York: Appleton-Century-Crofts.

*Hart, Gavin
1973 Social Aspects of Venereal Disease: I. Sociological Determinants of Venereal Disease. *British Journal of Venereal Diseases* 49:542-547.

*Hendrickse, R. G.; Hasan, A. H.; Olumide, L. O.; and Akinkunmi, A.
1971 Malaria in Early Childhood. *Annals of Tropical Medicine and Parsitology* 65:1-20.

Hiraizumi, Yuichiro
1964 Prezygotic Selection as a Factor in the Maintenance of Variability. *Eugenics Quarterly* 11:241-242.

Hochstein, Gianna
1968 Pica: A Study in Medical and Anthropological Explanation. In Thomas Weaver, ed., *Essays on Medical Anthropology*, pp. 88-96. Southern Anthropological Society Proceedings, no. 1. Athens: University of Georgia Press.

Hodann, M.
1937 *History of Modern Morals.* London: William H. Heinemann Co.

Hoeppli, Reinhard
  1959 *Parasites and Parasitic Infections in Early Medicine and Science.* Singapore: University of Malaya Press.

Hoffer, Carol P.
  1975 Bundu: Political Implications of Female Solidarity. In Dana Raphael, ed., *Being Female: Reproduction, Power and Change*, pp. 155-163. Paris: Mouton Press.

Hogbin, Ian
  1970 *The Island of Menstruating Men.* Scranton, Pa.: Chandler Publishing Co.

*Hollingsworth, Dorothy, and Russell, Margaret, eds.
  1974 *Nutritional Problems in a Changing World.* New York: John Wiley and Sons, Halsted Press.

*Hooton, E. A.
  1930 *The Indians of Pecos Pueblo: A Study of Their Skeletal Remains.* New Haven: Yale University Press.

Howard, Leland O., Dyar, Harrison G., and Knab, Fredrick
  1912- *The Mosquitoes of North and Central America and the West Indies.* 4 vols. Wash-
  1917 ington, D.C.: Carnegie Institute of Washington.

Hrdlička, Ales
  1914a Pathology of Ancient Peruvians. *Smithsonian Institution Miscellaneous Collection* 61:57.
  *1914b *The Most Ancient Skeletal Remains of Man.* Report of the Smithsonian Institution for 1913. Washington, D.C.

Hsiung, G.-D., Black, F. L., and Henderson, J. R.
  1964 Susceptibility of Primates to Viruses in Relation to Taxonomic Classification. In J. Buettner-Janusch, ed., *Evolutionary and Genetic Biology of Primates*, II, 1-23. New York: Academic Press.

Hudson, Ellis Herndon
  1962 Villalobos and Columbus. *American Journal of Medicine* 32:578-587.
  1963 Treponematosis and Anthropology. *Annals of Internal Medicine* 58:1037-1048.
  1965 Treponematosis and Man's Social Evolution. *American Anthropologist* 67: 885-901.
  1972 Diagnosing a Case of Veneral Disease in Fifteenth Century Scotland. *British Journal of Venereal Diseases* 48:146-153.

Huffman, Ray
  1931 *Nuer Customs and Folklore.* London: Oxford University Press.

*Hume, John C.
  1964 Problems in Diagnosing Syphilis and Other Treponematoses throughout the World. In World Forum on Syphilis and Other Treponematoses, *Proceedings . . .*, pp. 214-220. Public Health Service Publication no. 997. Atlanta: U.S. Department of Health, Education, and Welfare, Public Health Service.

Janssens, Paul A.
  1970 *Paleopathology: Diseases and Injuries of Prehistoric Man.* London: John Baker.

Jaramillo-Arango, Jaime
  1950 *The Conquest of Malaria.* London: William Heinemann Medical Books.

Jarcho, Saul, ed.
  1966 *Human Paleopathology: Proceedings of a Symposium on Human Paleopathology.* New Haven: Yale University Press.

Jaspan, M. A.
  1976   Health and Illth in Highland South Sumatra. In J. B. Loudon, ed., *Social Anthro-*
         pology and Medicine, pp. 259-284. New York: Academic Press.

Jelliffe, Derrick B., and Jelliffe, E. F. Patrice
  1975   Human Milk, Nutrition and the World Resource Crises. *Science* 188:557-561.

Johnson, Donald R.
  1969   Malaria Eradication: What Has It Achieved? *Mosquito News* 29:523-531.

Jones, W. H. S.
  1909   *Malaria and Greek History.* Manchester: University Press.

Jordan, Brigitte, and Fuller, Nancy
  1974   Mothers and Midwives: Contemporary Maya Indian Childbirth Practices in Yuca-
         tan, Mexico. Paper read at 73rd Annual Meeting of the American Anthropological
         Association, Mexico City.

*Jozef, P. H.
  1964   The Changing Social Role of the Yemenite Mori. In Ari Kiev, ed., *Magic, Faith*
         and Healing: Studies in Primitive Psychiatry Today, pp. 364-383. New York: Free
         Press of Glencoe; London: Collier-Macmillan.

Judson, Franklyn N.
  1976   Update in Sexually Transmitted Diseases. *Journal of the American Medical*
         Women's Association 31(1):11-19.

Kaplan, Bernice A., ed.
  1976   *Anthropological Studies of Human Fertility.* Detroit: Wayne State University
         Press.

Kaplan, Bert, and Johnson, Dale
  1964   The Social Meaning of Navaho Psychopathology and Psychotherapy. In Ari Kiev,
         ed., *Magic, Faith and Healing: Studies in Primitive Psychiatry Today*, pp.
         203-229. New York: Free Press of Glencoe; London: Collier-Macmillan.

Katona-Apte, Judit
  1975   The Relevance of Nourishment to the Reproductive Cycle of the Female in India.
         In Dana Raphael, ed., *Being Female: Reproduction, Power and Change*, pp.
         43-48. Paris: Mouton Press.

Katz, Richard
  1976   The Painful Ecstasy of Healing. *Psychology Today* 10(7):81-86.

Katz, Solomon H., and Foulks, Edward F.
  1970   Mineral Metabolism and Behavior: Abnormalities of Calcium Homeostasis. *Ameri-*
         can Journal of Physical Anthropology 32:299-304.

*Keeske, Randi D.
  1976   Premenstrual Emotionality: Is Biology Destiny?*Women and Health*, May-June,
         pp. 11-14.

Kerley, Ellis R., and Bass, William M.
  1967   Paleopathology: A Meeting Ground for Many Disciplines. *Science* 157:638-644.

Kessler, Evelyn S.
  1976   *Women: An Anthropological View.* New York: Holt, Rinehart and Winston.

Kiev, Ari, ed.
  1964   *Magic, Faith and Healing: Studies in Primitive Psychiatry Today.* New York: Free
         Press of Glencoe; London: Collier-Macmillan.

*Kimber, Clarissa
 1974   Curing Mediums and Medicinal Plants in the Valley of Texas. Paper read at 73rd
        Annual Meeting of the American Anthropological Association, Mexico City.

Kitchen, S. F.
 1949a Symptomatology: General Considerations. In Mark F. Boyd, ed., *Malariology*, II,
        966-994. Philadelphia: W. B. Saunders Co.
 1949b Falciparum Malaria. In Mark F. Boyd, ed., *Malariology*, II, 995-1016.
        Philadelphia: W. B. Saunders Co.

Kluckhohn, Clyde, and Leighton, Dorothea
 1962   *The Navajo.* Garden City, N.Y.: Doubleday, Anchor Books.

Kolata, Gina Bari
 1974   !Kung Hunter-Gatherers: Feminism, Diet and Birth Control.   Science 185:
        932-934.

Krogman, W.
 1940   The Pathologies of Prehistoric and Protohistoric Man. *Ciba Symposium*
        2:432-443.

Laderman, Carol
 1975   Malaria and Progress: Some Historical and Ecological Considerations. *Social
        Science and Medicine* 9:587-594.

*La Fay, Howard
 1975   The Maya, Children of Time. *National Geographic* 148:728-767.

Lambo, T. Adeoye
 1964   Patterns of Psychiatric Care in Developing African Countries. In Ari Kiev, ed.,
        Magic, Faith and Healing: Studies in Primitive Psychiatry Today pp. 443-453.
        New York: Free Press of Glencoe; London: Collier-Macmillan.

Landes, Ruth
 1971   *The Ojibwa Woman.* New York: W. W. Norton and Co.

Landy, David
 1974   Role Adaptation: Traditional Curers under the Impact of Western Medicine.
        American Ethnologist 1:103-127.
 ——————— , ed.
 1977   *Culture, Disease, and Healing: Studies in Medical Anthropology.* New York:
        Macmillan Publishing Co.

Langagne, Alfredo E.
 1964   Program for the Eradication of Pinta (Spotted Sickness) in Mexico. In World
        Forum on Syphilis and Other Treponematoses, *Proceedings . . .* , pp. 171-177.
        Public Health Service Publication no. 997. Atlanta: U.S. Department of Health,
        Education, and Welfare, Public Health Service.

Langdon-Davies, John, ed.
 1965   *The Slave Trade and Its Abolition—A Collection of Contemporary Documents.*
        New York: Viking Press.

Lapin, Boris A.
 1969   Experiments in Monkeys with Human Leukaemia. In W. I. B. Veveridge, ed., *Using
        Primates in Medical Research*, pt. 2: *Recent Comparative Research*. Primates in
        Medicine, vol. 3. Basel, Switzerland: S. Karger.

Last, Murray
 1976   The Presentation of Sickness in a Community of Non-Muslim Hausa. In J. B.

Loudon, ed., *Social Anthropology and Medicine*, pp. 104-149. New York: Academic Press.

*Latham, Michael C.
  1975   Nutrition and Infection in National Development. *Science* 188:565.

Laurentin, Anne
  1971   Nzakara Women. In Denise Paulme, ed., *Women of Tropical Africa*, pp. 121-178. Berkeley: University of California Press.

Lawick-Goodall, Jan van
  1971   *In the Shadow of Man.* Boston: Houghton Mifflin Co.; New York: Dell Publishing Co.

Lee, Richard B.
  1968   What Hunters Do for a Living; or, How to Make Out on Scarce Resources. In R. B. Lee and I. DeVore, eds., *Man the Hunter*, pp. 30-48. Chicago: Aldine Publishing Co.

Leff, S.
  1953   *Social Medicine.* London: Routledge and Kegan Paul.

Leighton, Alexander H.; Lambo, T. Adeoye; Hughes, Charles C.; Leighton, Dorothea C.; Murphy, Jane M.; and Macklin, David B.
  1963   *Psychiatric Disorders among the Yoruba.* Ithaca: Cornell University Press.

Lessa, William A.
  1966   *Ulithi: A Micronesian Design for Living.* New York: Holt, Rinehart and Winston.

Lévi-Strauss, Claude
  1967   The Sorcerer and His Magic. In John Middleton, ed., *Magic, Witchcraft and Curing*, pp. 23-41. Garden City, N.Y.: Natural History Press.

Lewis, Gilbert
  1976   A View of Sickness in New Guinea. In J. B. Loudon, ed., *Social Anthropology and Medicine*, pp. 49-103. New York: Academic Press.

*Lieban, Richard W.
  1962   The Dangerous IngKantos: Illness and Social Control in a Philippine Community. *American Anthropologist* 64:306-312.

Lindsey, S., and Chaikoff, I. L.
  1966   Naturally Occurring Arteriosclerosis in Nonhuman Primates. *Journal of Atherosclerosis Research* 6:36-61.

Ling Shun-shêng, and Ruey Yih-fu.
  1947   *Hsiang-hsi Miao-tsu Tiao-ch'a Paoko* [A Report on the Investigation of the Miao of Western Hunan]. Shanghai: Shanghai Institute of History and Philology, Academia Sinica.

Livingstone, Frank B.
  1971   Malaria and Human Polymorphisms. *Annual Review of Genetics* 5:33-64.

Lomholt, Gunnar
  1972   Syphilis, Yaws, and Pinta. In A. Rook, D. C. Wilkinson, and F. J. G. eds., *Textbook of Dermatology*, I, 634-679. Oxford: Blackwell Scientific Publications.

*Looney, Ralph
  1972   The Navajo. *National Geographic* 142:740-781.

Loudon, J. B., ed.
  1976   *Social Anthropology and Medicine.* New York: Academic Press.

Lowenberg, Miriam E.; Todhunter, E. Neige; Wilson, Eva D.; Savage, Jane R.; and Lubawski, James L.
    1974   *Food and Man.* 2nd ed. New York: John Wiley and Sons.
Lozoff, B., Ramath, K. R., and Feldman, R. A.
    1975   Infection and Disease in South Indian Families—Beliefs and Childhood Disorders. *Human Organization* 34:354-358.
*Maclean, Una
    1972   Some Aspects of Sickness Behavior among the Yoruba. In J. B. Loudon, ed., *Social Anthropology and Medicine*, pp. 285-317. New York: Academic Press.
McClelland, G. A. H.
    1973   Some Man-Made Mosquito Problems in Africa and Prospects for Their Rational Solution. *Proceedings, 5th Tall Timber Conference on Ecological Animal Control by Habitat Management.* pp. 27-41. Tallahassee, Florida.
*McClintock, Martha K.
    1971   Menstrual Synchrony and Suppression. *Nature* 222:224-245.
MacDonald, George
    1957   *The Epidemiology and Control of Malaria.* London: Oxford University Press.
McGregor, I. A.
    1964   Studies in the Acquisition of Immunity to *Plasmodium Falciparum* Infections in Africa. *Transactions of the Royal Society of Tropical Medicine and Hygiene* 58:80-92.
Madsen, William
    1964   Value Conflicts and Folk Psychotherapy in South Texas. In Ari Kiev, ed., *Magic, Faith and Healing: Studies in Primitive Psychiatry Today*, pp. 420-440. New York: Free Press of Glencoe; London: Collier-Macmillan.
Majno, Guido
    1975   *The Healing Hand: Man and Wound in the Ancient World.* Cambridge, Mass.: Harvard University Press.
Malcolm, Sheila
    1954   *Diet and Nutrition in American Samoa.* New Caledonia: South Pacific Commission.
Malinow, M. R.
    *1965   Atherosclerosis in Subhuman Primates. *Folia Primatologica* 3:277-300.
    _____, and Maruffo, C. A.
    1966   Naturally Occurring Atherosclerosis in Howler Monkeys (*Alouatta Caraya*). *Journal of Atherosclerosis Research* 6:368-380.
*Mandel, William
    1971   Soviet Women and Their Self-Image. *Science and Society* 35:286-310.
Mannix, Daniel P., with Cowley, Malcolm
    1962   *Black Cargoes: A History of the Atlantic Slave Trade, 1518-1865.* New York: Viking Press.
Martin, M. Kay, and Voorhies, Barbara
    1975   *Female of the Species.* New York: Columbia University Press.
Martinez del Rio, Pablo
    1953   A Preliminary Report on the Mortuary Cave of Candellaria, Coahuila, Mexico. *Bulletin of the Texas Archaeological Society* 24:208-252.

Marwick, M. G.
   1967   The Sociology of Sorcery in a Central African Tribe. In John Middleton, ed.,
          Magic, Witchcraft and Curing, pp. 101-126. Garden City, N.Y.: Natural History
          Press.

Mason, J. Alden
   1971   *The Ancient Civilizations of Peru.* Baltimore: Penguin Books.

Mather, Increase
   1864   *Early History of New England.* Edited by S. G. Drake. Boston: S. G. Drake.

Matsunaga, E., and Hiaizumi, Y.
   1962   Prezygotic Selection in ABO Blood Groups. *Science* 135:432-434.

Mayer, Jean
  *1968   *Overweight: Causes, Cost, and Control.* Englewood Cliffs, N.J.: Prentice-Hall.

   1973   The Relationship of Nutrition to Brain Development and Behavior. A position
          paper of the Food and Nutrition Board. Washington, D.C.: National Academy of
          Sciences, National Research Council.

Mayr, Ernst
   1978   Evolution. *Scientific American* 239(3):47-55.

Mead, Margaret
   1928   *Coming of Age in Samoa.* New York: W. Morrow and Co.

Meagher, E.
   1977   Navajo Medicine Men Stir Benefit Dispute within Miners' Union. *Los Angeles
          Times*, June 19, p. 3.

*Meggers, B. J.
   1954   Environmental Limitation on the Development of Culture. *American Anthro-
          pologist* 56:801-824.

Mensforth, Robert, P.; Lovejoy, C. Owen; Lallo, John W.; and Armelagos, George J.
   1978   The Role of Constitutional Factors, Diet, and Infectious Disease in the Etiology
          of Porotic Hyperostosis and Periosteal Reactions in Prehistoric Children. *Medical
          Anthropology* 2(1):1-59.

Middleton, John, ed.
   1967   *Magic, Witchcraft and Curing.* Garden City, N.Y.: Natural History Press.

Miles, James S.
   1966   Diseases Encountered at Mesa Verde, Colorado. In Saul Jarcho, ed., *Human Paleo-
          pathology: Proceedings of a Symposium on Human Paleopathology*, pp. 91-97.
          New Haven: Yale University Press.

Miller, Dorothy A.
   1977   Evolution of Primate Chromosomes. *Science* 198:1116-1124.

Miller, Joseph
   1929   Some Diseases of Ancient Man. *Annals of Medical History*, n.s. 1:394-402.

Mischel, Frances
   1959   Faith Healing and Medical Practice in the Southern Caribbean. *Southwest Journal
          of Anthropology* 25:407-417.

Modell, Walter
   1968   Malaria and Victory in Vietnam. *Science* 162:1346-1352.

358

Møller-Christensen, Vilhelm
 1967 Evidence of Leprosy in Earlier Peoples. In D. Brothwell and A. T. Sandison, eds., *Diseases in Antiquity*, pp. 295-306. Springfield, Ill.: Charles C. Thomas.

Moodie, Roy L.
 1923 *Paleopathology: An Introduction to the Study of Ancient Evidences of Disease.* Urbana: University of Illinois Press.
 1926 Pleistocene Examples of Traumatic Osteomyelitis. *Annals of Medical History* 8:413-418.

Moody, Paul Amos
 1970 *Introduction to Evolution.* 3rd ed. New York: Harper and Row.

Moore, M. Brittain, Jr.
 1963 The Epidemiology of Syphilis. *Journal of the American Medical Association* 186:831-834.

Morse, Dan
 1969a *Ancient Disease in the Midwest.* Springfield, Ill.: State of Illinois.
 1969b The Origin of Treponematosis. *Peoria Academy of Science, Proceedings* 2:27-34.

Moseley, John E.
 1965 The Paleopathologic Riddle of "Symmetrical Osteoporosis." *American Journal of Roentgenology, Radium Therapy and Nuclear Medicine* 95:135-142.
 1966 Radiographic Studies in Hematologic Bone Disease: Implications for Paleopathology. In Saul Jarcho, ed., *Human Paleopathology: Proceedings of a Symposium on Human Paleopathology*, pp. 121-130. New Haven: Yale University Press.

Mosley, James W., chief
 1965 *Chimpanzee-Associated Hepatitis.* Hepatitis Surveillance Report no. 23. Atlanta: U.S. Department of Health, Education, and Welfare, Public Health Service, Communicable Disease Center.

*Moss, N. Henry, and Mayer, Jean
 1977 *Food and Nutrition in Health and Disease.* New York: New York Academy of Sciences.

*Moulder, James W.
 1962 *The Biochemistry of Intracellular Parasitism.* Chicago: University of Chicago Press.

Murphree, Alice H.
 1968 A Functional Analysis of Southern Folk Beliefs Concerning Birth. In Thomas Weaver, ed., *Essays on Medical Anthropology*, pp. 64-77. Southern Anthropological Society Proceedings, no. 1. Athens: University of Georgia Press.

Murphy, Jane M.
 1964 Psychotherapeutic Aspects of Shamanism on St. Lawrence Island, Alaska. In Ari Kiev, ed., *Magic, Faith and Healing: Studies in Primitive Psychiatry Today*, pp. 53-83. New York: Free Press of Glencoe; London: Collier-Macmillan.

Nadel, S. F.
 1946 A Study of Shamanism in the Nuba Mountains. *Journal of the Royal Anthropological Institute* 56 (pt. 1): 25-37.

Nag, Moni
 1968 *Factors Affecting Human Fertility in Nonindustrial Societies: A Cross-Cultural*

Study. Yale University Publications in Anthropology no. 66. Reprinted ed., New Haven: Human Relations Area Files Press.

Najjar, Mahmoud Y. El-
1977   Maize, Malaria and the Anemias in the Pre-Columbian New World. *Yearbook of Physical Anthropology* 20:329-337.

Nash, Manning
1967   Witchcraft as Social Process in a Tzeltal Community. In John Middleton, ed., *Magic, Witchcraft and Curing*, pp. 127-133. Garden City, N.Y.: Natural History Press.

National Research Council, Committee on Food Habits
1945   *Manual for the Study of Food Habits*. National Research Council Bulletin #111. Washington: National Academy of Sciences.

Neel, James V.
1971   Genetic Aspects of the Ecology of Disease in the American Indian. In F. M. Salzano, ed., *The Ongoing Evolution of Latin American Populations*, pp. 561-590. Springfield, Ill.: Charles C. Thomas.

————; Andrade, A. H. P.; Brown, G. E.; Eveland, W. E.; Goobar, J.; Sodeman, W. A., Jr.; Stollerman, G. H.; Weinstein, E. F.; and Wheeler, A. H.
1968   Further Studies of the Xavante Indians: IX. Immunologic Status with Respect to Various Diseases and Organisms. *American Journal of Tropical Medicine and Hygiene* 17:486-498.

————, and Chagnon, Napoleon
1968   The Demography of Two Tribes of Primitive, Relatively Unacculturated American Indians. *Proceedings of the National Academy of Science* 59:680-689.

————, and Salzano, Francisco M.
1967   Further Studies on the Xavante Indians: X. Some Hypotheses-Generalizations Resulting from These Studies. *American Journal of Human Genetics* 19:554-574.

————; Salzano, F. M.; Junqueira, P. C.; Keiter, F.; and Maybury-Lewis, D.
1964   Studies on the Xavante Indians of the Brazilian Mato Grosso. *American Journal of Human Genetics* 16:52-140.

*Nerlove, Sara B.
1974   Women's Workload and Infant Feeding Practices: A Relationship with Demographic Implications. *Ethnology* 13:207-214.

*Neubarth, Raymond G.
1954   *Dental Conditions in School Children of American Samoa*. New Caledonia: South Pacific Commission.

*Newman, Marshall T.
1975   Nutritional Adaptation in Man. In Albert Damon, ed., *Physiological Anthropology*, pp. 210-252. London: Oxford University Press.

Newton, Niles
1975   Birth Rituals in Cross-Cultural Perspective: Some Practical Applications. In Dana Raphael, ed., *Being Female: Reproduction, Power and Change*, pp. 37-41. Paris: Mouton Press.

Ngubane, Harriet
  1976   Some Aspects of Treatment among the Zulu. In J. B. Loudon, *Social Anthropology and Medicine*, pp. 318-357. New York: Academic Press.

Nicholls, L.
  1921   *Malaria and the Lost Cities of Ceylon.* Indian Medical Gazette 56:121-130.

Noguer, W., Wernsdorfer, W., and Kouznetsov, R.
  1976   The Malaria Situation in 1975. *WHO Chronicle* 30:486-493.

Nurge, Ethel
  1958   Etiology of Illness in Guinhangdan. *American Anthropologist* 60:1158-1172.
  1975   Spontaneous and Induced Abortion in Human and Non-Human Primates. In Dana Raphael, ed., *Being Female: Reproduction, Power and Change*, pp. 25-35. Paris: Mouton Press.

O'Conor, G. T.
  1969   Cancer—A General Review. In W. I. B. Beveridge, ed., *Using Primates in Medical Research*, pt. 2: *Recent Comparative Research*, pp. 9-22. Primates in Medicine, vol. 3. Basel, Switzerland: S. Karger.

Orgel, M. Norman
  1964   Education about Venereal Disease in Schools. In World Forum on Syphilis and Other Treponematoses, *Proceedings* . . . , pp. 481-483. Public Health Service Publication no. 997. Atlanta: U.S. Department of Health, Education, and Welfare, Public Health Service.

Ortiz de Montellano, Bernard
  1975   Empirical Aztec Medicine. *Science* 188:215-220.

Pales, L.
  1929   Maladie de Paget préhistorique avec note additionelle du Professeur R. Verneau. *L'Anthropologie* 39:263-270.
  1930   *Paléopathologie et pathologie comparative.* Paris: Masson.

Pan American Health Organization, Advisory Committee on
          Medical Research
  1968   *Biomedical Challenges Presented by the American Indian.* WHO Scientific Publication no. 165. Washington, D.C.

Pariser, Harry
  1964   A Plea—Put Syphilis Back in Differential Diagnosis. In World Forum on Syphilis and Other Treponematoses, *Proceedings* . . . , pp. 227-228. Public Health Service Publication no. 997. Atlanta: U.S. Department of Health, Education, and Welfare, Public Health Service.

Park, George K.
  1967   Divination and Its Social Contexts. In John Middleton, ed., *Magic, Witchcraft and Curing*, pp. 233-254. Garden City, N.Y.: Natural History Press.

*Parramore, Thomas C.
  1970   Non-venereal Treponematosis in Colonial North America. *Bulletin of the History of Medicine* 44:571-581.

Parran, Thomas
  1937   *Shadow on the Land: Syphilis.* New York: Reynal and Hitchcock.

*Passmore, R., Nicol, B. M., and Rao, M. Narayana, with
          Beaton, G. H., and Denmayer, E. M.

1974   *Handbook on Human Nutritional Requirements.* Geneva: World Health Organization.

Pauling, Linus
 1970   *Vitamin C and the Common Cold.* San Francisco: W. H. Freeman. (Paperback ed., New York: Bantam, 1971.)

Paulme, Denise, ed.
 1971   *Women of Tropical Africa.* Translated by H. M. Wright. Berkeley: University of California Press.

Peters, W.
 1975   Guest Editorial. *Journal of Tropical Medicine and Hygiene* 78(8):167-170.

Petersen, F. D.
 1959   *Ancient Mexico.* New York: G. P. Putnam's Sons.

*Pinto, Lucille B.
 1973   The Folk Practice of Gynecology and Obstetrics in the Middle Ages. *Bulletin of the History of Medicine* 47:513-522.

Poirier, Frank E.
 1975   Socialization of Non-Human Primate Females: A Brief Overview. In Dana Raphael, ed. *Being Female: Reproduction, Power and Change*, pp. 13-18. Paris: Mouton Press.
 1977   *In Search of Ourselves: An Introduction to Physical Anthropology.* 2nd ed. Minneapolis: Burgess Publishing Co.

Pratt, Harry D., Barnes, Ralph C., and Littig, Kent S.
 1963   *Mosquitoes of Public Health Importance and Their Control.* Public Health Service Publication no. 772. Atlanta: U.S. Department of Health, Education, and Welfare, Public Health Service, Communicable Disease Center.

*Press, Irwin
 1971   The Urban Curandero. *American Anthropologist* 73:741-756.

*Prince, Raymond
 1964   Indigenous Yoruba Psychiatry. In Ari Kiev; ed., *Magic, Faith and Healing: Studies in Primitive Psychiatry Today*, pp. 84-120. New York: Free Press of Glencoe; London: Collier-Macmillan.

Prothero, P. Mansell
 1965   *Migrants and Malaria.* London: Longmans Green and Co.

Pusey, William Allen
 1933   *The History and Epidemiology of Syphilis.* Springfield, Ill.: Charles C. Thomas.

Puttkamer, W. Jesco von
 1975   Requiem for a Tribe: Brazil's Kreen Akrores. *National Geographic* 147:254-283.

Quimby, George I.
 1974   Habitat, Culture and Archaeology. In Y. A. Cohen, ed., *Man in Adaptation: The Biosocial Background*, pp. 429-434. Chicago: Aldine Publishing Co.

Ramalingaswami, V.
 1975   Nutrition, Cell Biology and Human Development: The Jacques Parisot Foundation Lecture, 1975. *WHO Chronicle* 29:306-312.

Raphael, Dana, ed.
 1975   *Being Female: Reproduction, Power and Change.* Paris: Mouton Press.

Rappaport, Roy
   1967   *Pigs for the Ancestors.* New Haven: Yale University Press.

Reed, D., Struve, S., and Maynard, J. E.
   1967   Otitis Media and Hearing Deficiency among Eskimo Children: A Cohort Study. *American Journal of Public Health* 57:1657-1662.

Reed, T. Edward
   1966   The Evidence for Natural Selection Due to Blood Groups. In *Proceedings, World Population Conference, Belgrade,* II, 298-502. New York: United Nations.

Reemstma, K., McCracken, B. H., and Schlegel, J. U.
   1964   Reversal of Early Graft Rejection after Renal Heterotransplantation in Man. *Journal of the American Medical Association* 187:691-696.

Reining, Priscilla, and Tinker, Irene, eds.
   1975   *Population: Dynamics, Ethics and Policy.* Washington, D.C.: American Association for the Advancement of Science.

Ritzenthaler, Robert E.
   1970   *Prehistoric Indians of Wisconsin.* Milwaukee: Milwaukee Public Museum.

Roche, A. F., and Falkner, F., eds.
   1973   *Nutrition and Malnutrition.* Advances in Experimental Medicine and Biology, vol. 49. New York: Plenum Press.

Rogler, Lloyd H., and Hollingshead, August B.
   1961   The Puerto Rican Spiritualist as a Psychiatrist. *American Journal of Sociology* 67:17-21.

Ross, Milton
   1976   Current Status of Syphilis and Other Venereal Diseases. *Journal of the Florida Medical Association* 63(1):74-77.

Ross, Ronald
   1904   *Researches on Malaria.* Stockholm: Kungl. Boktryckeriet, P. A. Norstedt.

Ruffer, M. A.
   1921   *Studies in the Paleopathology of Egypt.* Chicago: University of Chicago Press.

Russell, Paul F.
   1952   *Malaria: Basic Principles, Briefly Stated.* Oxford: Blackwell Science Publications.
   1955   *Man's Mastery of Malaria.* London: Oxford University Press.
   1956   Malaria: World-wide Distribution, Prevalence and Control. *American Journal of Tropical Medicine and Hygiene* 5:937-965.

Sachs, Ralph R.
   1964   Effect of Urbanization on the Spread of Syphilis. In World Forum on Syphilis and Other Treponematoses, *Proceedings . . . ,* pp. 153-156. Public Health Service Publication no. 997. Atlanta: U.S. Department of Health, Education, and Welfare, Public Health Service.

St. Clair, R. W.; MacNintch, J. E.; Middleton, C. C.; Clarkson T. B.; and Lofland, H. B.
   1961   Changes in Serum Cholesterol Levels of Squirrel Monkeys during Importation and Acclimatization. *Laboratory Investigation* 16:828-838.

Salzano, F. M., Neel, J. V., and Maybury-Lewis, D.
   1967   Further Studies on the Xavante Indians: I. Demographic Data on Two Additional Villages; Genetic Structure of the Tribe. *American Journal of Human Genetics* 19:463-489.

Sambon, L. W.
  1901   The History of Malaria: A Medico-Literary Causerie. *The Practitioner* 66:348-359.
Sanders, William T.
  1973   The Cultural Ecology of the Lowland Maya: A Reevaluation. In T. Patrick Culbert, *The Classic Maya Collapse*, pp. 325-365. Albuquerque: University of New Mexico Press.
Sarkad, Umasankar
  1975   Malaria Rides Again. *Journal of the Indian Medical Association*, 65(6):185-186.
Saul, Frank P.
  1972   *The Human Skeletal Remains of Altar de Sacrificios: An Osteobiographic Analysis.* Papers of the Peabody Museum of Archeology and Ethnology, vol. 3, no. 2. Cambridge, Mass.: Peabody Museum.
Schaefer, A. E.
  1966   Observations from Exploring Needs in National Nutrition Programs. *American Journal of Public Health* 56:1088-1096.
Schamberg, Ira Leo
  1964   Syphilis Resurgent. In World Forum on Syphilis and Other Treponematoses, *Proceedings ...*, pp. 221-226. Public Health Service Publication no. 997. Atlanta: U.S. Department of Health, Education, and Welfare, Public Health Service.
Schmidt, K. E.
  1964   Folk Psychiatry in Sarawak: A Tenatative System on Psychiatry of the Iban. In Ari Kiev, ed., *Magic, Faith and Healing: Studies in Primitive Psychiatry Today*, pp. 135-155. New York: Free Press of Glencoe; London: Collier-Macmillan.
Schultz, Adolph H.
  1972   *The Life of Primates.* New York: Universe Books.
Scrimshaw, Nevin, and Young, Vernon R.
  1976   The Requirements of Human Nutrition. *Scientific American* 235(3):50-64.
Sebrell, William H., Jr., Haggerty, James H., and the Editors
         of Life
  1967   *Food and Nutrition.* New York: Time Inc.
Seifrit, Emma
  1961   Changes in Beliefs and Food Practices in Pregnancy. *Journal of the American Dietetic Association* 39:455-466.
Shannon, R. C.
  1942   Brief History of *Anopheles Gambiae* in Brazil (1). *Caribbean Medical Journal* 4:123-128.
Sherfey, Mary Jane
  1966   *The Nature and Evolution of Female Sexuality.* New York: Random House.
Shipley, A. E.
  1908   *Pearls and Parasites.* London: John Murry.
Sigerist, Henry E.
  1943   *Civilization and Disease.* Ithaca: Cornell University Press. (Paperback ed., Chicago: University of Chicago Press, 1962.)
  1951   *A History of Medicine*, vol. 1: *Primitive and Archaic Medicine.* New York: Oxford University Press.

Silverman, Julian
1967   Shamans and Acute Schizophrenia. *American Anthropologist* 69(1):21-31.
Silverman, P. H.
1977   Malaria Vaccines. *Science* 196:1156.
Skultans, Vieda
1976   Empathy and Healing: Aspects of Spiritualist Ritual. In J. B. Loudon, ed., *Social Anthropology and Medicine*, pp. 198-222. New York: Academic Press.
Smith, G. Elliot
1930   Introduction to Cyril P. Bryan, *The Papyrus Ebers*. London: Bles.
Smith, Harriet
1974   *Prehistoric Peoples of Illinois*. Chicago: Field Museum of Natural History.
Snow, Charles E.
1948   *Indian Knoll Skeletons*. Reports in Anthropology, vol. 4, no. 3, pt. 2. Lexington: University of Kentucky.
*Solecki, R. S.
1975   Shanidar IV, a Neanderthal Flower Burial in Northern Iraq. *Science* 190:880-881.
Southam, Anna L., and Gonzaga, Florante P.
1965   Systemic Changes during the Menstrual Cycle. *American Journal of Obstetrics and Gynecology* 91(1):142-165.
Spencer, Dorothy M.
1941   *Disease, Religion and Society in the Fiji Islands*. New York: J. J. Augustin. (Reprint ed., Seattle: University of Washington Press, 1966.)
Stewart, T. D.
1940   Some Historical Implications of Physical Anthropology in North America. Essays in Historical Anthropology of North America. *Smithsonian Miscellaneous Collection* 100:15-50.
*1950   Pathological Changes in South American Indian Skeletal Remains. In J. H. Steward, ed., *Handbook of South American Indians*, VI, 49-52. Bureau of American Ethnology Bulletin 143.
1960   A Physical Anthropologist's View of the Peopling of the New World. *Southwestern Journal of Anthropology* 16:259-273.
*1969   The Effects of Pathology on Skeletal Populations. *American Journal of Physical Anthropology* 30:443-450.
————, and Spoehr, Alexander
*1967   Evidence on the Paleopathology of Yaws. In D. Brothwell and A. T. Sandison, eds., *Diseases in Antiquity*, pp. 307-319. Springfield, Ill.: Charles C. Thomas.
Stout, C., and Lemmon, W. B.
1969   Predominant Coronary and Cerebral Atherosclerosis in Captive Nonhuman primates. *Experimental and Molecular Pathology* 10:312-322.
Strathern, Marilyn
1972   *Women in Between; Female Roles in a Male World: Mt. Hagen, New Guinea*. London: Seminar Press.
*Stuart, George E.
1972   Who Were the "Mound Builders"? *National Geographic* 142:782-801.
*Sussman, Max
1967   Diseases in the Bible and Talmud. In D. Brothwell and A. T. Sandison, eds., *Diseases in Antiquity*, pp. 209-221. Springfield, Ill.: Charles C. Thomas.

Taylor, C. B., Ho, H. J., and Liu, L. B.
  1973   Recent·Advances in Arteriosclerosis and Cholesterol Metabolism in Primates. In
          W. P. McNulty, ed., *Nonhuman Primates and Human Diseases*, pp. 127-149. New
          York: S. Karger.

Temkin, O.
  1945   *The Falling Sickness.* Baltimore: Johns Hopkins Press.

Thomas, William L., ed.
  1956   *Man's Role in Changing the Face of the Earth.* Chicago: University of Chicago
          Press.

Tietze, Christopher, and Lewit, Sarah
  1977   Legal Abortion. *Scientific American* 236(1):21-27.

Titterington, P. F.
  1935   Certain Bluff Mounds of Western Jersy County, Illinois. *American Antiquity*
          1:6-46.

*Tizard, Jack
  1974   Can the Brain Catch Up? *World Health*, February-March, pp. 10-15.

Tobias, P. V.
  1962   Sapiens and Peking Man: A Re-examination of the Kanam Mandible. *Actes du IVe
          Congrès Panafricain de Préhistoire et de l'Etude de Quaternaire.* Tervuren,
          Belgium, Annales du Musée Royal de l'Afrique Centrale, Série in-8°, Sciences
          Humaines, no. 40, p. 345.

Traeger, J.
  1969   Transplantation of Kidneys from Chimpanzees to Man. In W. I. B. Beveridge, ed.,
          Using Primates in Medical Research, pt. 2: *Recent Comparative Research*, pp.
          52-54. Primates in Medicine, vol. 3. Basel, Switzerland: S. Karger.

Turner, Victor
  1964   A Ndembu Doctor in Practice. In Ari Kiev, ed., *Magic, Faith and Healing: Studies
          in Primitive Psychiatry Today*, pp. 230-263. New York: Free Press of Glencoe;
          London: Collier-Macmillan.

Vallois, H.
  1937   La Durée de la vie chez l'homme fossile. *L'Anthropologie* 47:499-532.

Vastesaeger, M., and Delcourt, R.
  1966   Some aspects of Spontaneous and Experimental Cardiovascular Disease in Old
          World Monkeys and Pongidae. In R. N. T.-W. Fiennes, ed., *Some Recent Develop-
          ments in Comparative Medicine*, pp. 179-194. New York: Academic Press.

Walker, Alan, and Leakey, R. E. F.
  1978   Hominids of East Turkana. *Scientific American* 239(2):16, 54-66.

Wallace, Anthony F. D.
  1967   Dreams and the Wishes of the Soul: A Type of Psychoanalytic Theory among the
          Seventeenth Century Iroquois. In John Middleton, ed., *Magic, Witchcraft and
          Curing*, pp. 171-190. Garden City, N.Y.: Natural History Press.
  1972   Mental Illness, Biology and Culture in Psychological Anthropology. In Francis
          L. K. Hsu, ed., *Psychological Anthropology,* pp. 363-402. Cambridge, Mass.:
          Schenkman Publishing Co.

Warshaw, Leon J.
  1949   *Malaria: The Biography of a Killer.* New York: Rinehart and Co.

Waugh, M. A.
 1972   Studies on the Recent Epidemiology of Early Syphilis in West London. *British Journal of Venereal Diseases* 48:534-541.

Weiner, Joseph S.
 1971   *The Natural History of Man.* New York: Universe Books.

Weinstein, E. David, Neel, J. V., and Salzano, F. M.
 1967   Further Studies on the Xavante Indians: VI. The Physical Status of the Xavantes of Simões Lopes. *American Journal of Human Genetics* 19:532-542.

Wells, Calvin
 1964   *Bones, Bodies and Disease: Evidence of Disease and Abnormality in Early Man.* New York: Frederick A. Praeger.

Whisson, Michael G.
 1964   Some Aspects of Functional Disorders among the Kenya Luo. In Ari Kiev, ed., *Magic, Faith and Healing: Studies in Primitive Psychiatry Today*, pp. 282-304. New York: Free Press of Glencoe; London: Collier-Macmillan.

Wilkinson, Richard
 1975   Techniques of Ancient Skull Surgery. *Natural History*, October, pp. 94-101.

Willcox, R. R.
 1960   Evolutionary Cycle of the Treponematoses. *British Journal of Venereal Diseases* 36:78-91.
 *1972   A World-wide View of Venereal Disease. *British Journal of Venereal Diseases* 48:163-176.
 1974   Changing Patterns of Treponemal Disease. *British Journal of Venereal Diseases* 50:169-178.

Willey, Gordon, and Shimkin, D. B.
 1971   The Collapse of Classic Maya Civilization in the Southern Lowlands: A Symposium Summary Statement. In C. Lamberg-Karlovsky and J. A. Sabloff, eds., *The Rise and Fall of Civilizations,* pp. 104-118. Menlo Park, Calif.: Cummings Publishing Co.

Williams, Herbert U.
 1932   The Origin and Antiquity of Syphilis: The Evidence from Diseased Bones. *Archives of Pathology* 13:779-814, 931-983.

————, with Rice, John P., and Lacayo, Joseph Renato
 1927   The American Origin of Syphilis. *Archives of Dermatology and Syphilology* 16:683-696.

Wintrobe, Maxwell M.
 1962   *Clinical Hematology.* 5th ed. Philadelphia: Lea and Febiger.

Withington, Edward T.
 1894   *Medical History from the Earliest Times: A Popular History of the Healing Art.* London: Scientific Press.

Wood, Corinne Shear
 1970   A Multiphasic Health Screening of Three Southern Californian Indian Reservations. *Social Science and Medicine* 4:579-587.
 1974   Preferential Feedings of *Anopheles Gambiae* Mosquitoes on Human Subjects of Blood Group O: A Relationship between the ABO Polymorphism and Malaria Vectors. *Human Biology* 46:385-404.

1975   New Evidence for a Late Introduction of Malaria into the New World. *Current Anthropology* 16(1):93-104.

————, Harrison, Caroline Dore, and Weiner, J. S.

1972   Selective Feeding of *Anopheles Gambiae* According to ABO Blood Group Status. *Nature* 239:165.

World Forum on Syphilis and Other Treponematoses

1964   *Proceedings of the World Forum on Syphilis and Other Treponematoses (Washington, D.C., September 4-8, 1962).* Public Health Service Publication no. 997. Atlanta: U.S. Department of Health, Education, and Welfare, Public Health Service.

World Health Organization

1963   Problems of Malaria Eradication. *WHO Chronicle* 17:368-375.

1971   Malaria eradication in 1970. *WHO Chronicle* 25:498-504.

Wright, A. Dickson

1971   Venereal Disease and the Great. *British Journal of Venereal Diseases* 47:295-306.

*Wright, D. J. M., and Grimble, A. S.

1974   Why Is the Infectious Stage of Syphilis Prolonged? *British Journal of Venereal Diseases* 50:45-49.

Zinsser, Hans

1934   *Rats, Lice and History.* Boston: Little, Brown and Co. (Paperback ed., New York: Bantam, 1965.)

INDEX

Digitalis, 307
Dimetrodon, 6
Dinka, 232
Dinosaurs, 5, 6, 7, 8, 9, 13
Diphtheria, 333
Distemper, 164
Diviners, xvii, 341; functions of, 309, 311, 323; techniques of, 323-325
Dobuans, 109
Douala, 66
Dusun, 139
Dysentery, 200

Ear disease, 166-167
Ecuador, 309
Edaphosauri, 5, 6
Edward VI (England), 219
Eggs: folklore and prohibitions, 66, 76; nutritional value, 80, 82, 84, 92
Egypt: arthritis in, 27, childbirth in, 144; female circumcision in, 111; gum disease in, 14; iron deficiency anemia in, 183; syphilis in, 235
Elephants, 14
Empedocles, 264
England (Britain), 67, 89-90; arthritis in, 26; and cauterization, 38; and malaria, 267-269; and slavery, 197-198; syphilis in, 235
Eocene epoch, 47
Epidemic: and population size, 24; in non-human primates, 43-44; in New World, 176, 189, 192, 207; of syphilis, 210-213
Epilepsy, 24
Episiotomy, 146
Erotomania, 111
Erythrocytes, 251, 255-256, 287
Eskimo, 94-95, 139, 311, 331; women, 108; ear disease, 166-167; and shaman, 304, 311, 313
Esper, E.J.C., 10
"Evil eye," 328-330
Eyes, 80-81, 180

Family planning, xiii, 104, 128, 133, 155

Fiji, 75, 121, 134, 136, 139, 150
Filariasis, 42
Fish, 92, 283; nutritional value, 79, 80, 82, 84; prohibitions on consumption, 64, 65, 66, 76, 153
Fleming, Alexander, 216
"Fletcherism," 99
Food. *See individual listings*
Food-sharing, xii, 98
France, 235
Francis I (France), 219
Frascatoro, Girolamo, 213, 215

G-6-P-D deficiency, 248, 271
Gamma globulin, 258-259
Gastro-intestinal disease. *See* Intestinal parasites; Diarrhea
Ge-speakers, 202-208
Geophagy, 131
Germany, 49, 67, 213
Ghana, 75, 259, 284
Gibbons, 43
Gnau-speakers, 306
Gonorrhea, 333
Gorillas, 42, 43, 48
Greece, 34, 125, 159; kwashiorkor in, 75; malaria in, 264, 269, 283; and menstruation, 114; syphilis in, 220
Guaiac, 216
Guam, 135
Guatemala, 177, 181, 207; malnutrition in, 69; smallpox in, 191; syphilis in, 237
Guinea, 111, 122
Gum disease, 175; in antiquity, 14; in *Australopithecus*, 14; causes, 26; in *Merchyhippus*, 14; North American Indians and, 183, 185; in non-human primates, 42
Gunantana, 136
Gururumba, 112, 113
Guyana, 319

Haruspication, 323-324
Havasupai, 129, 328
Hawaiians, 139
Healers: categories of, 310, 321;

contributions to modern medicine, 307-308, 334; as entertainment, 301-305; holistic healing techniques, 306, 329, 355; innovative methods, 332, 333; as judges, 295-297; recognition by governments, 332; scope of function, xvii, 294-305, 330-332; selection of ailments to treat, 309-310. *See also* Diviners; Herbalist; Shaman; Spiritualist
Hebrew, 147
Hehe, 309, 310, 314
Hemoglobin: abnormal, 281; C, 249, 271; D, 249; E, 207, 249, 271; K, 249; O, 249; levels in blood, 287
Hemp, 316
Henry VIII (England), 219
Hepatitis, 48, 309
Herbalist, xvii, 325-327
Herpes, 49
Hindu: food prohibitions, 64; and menstruation, 115; and rickets, 92
Hippocrates, 80, 327
Histoplasmin, 207
Holland, 277
Home base, xi
Hominy, 86
Homo erectus, 15; appearance, 19-20; life span, 25; pathologies, 20; violence of, 20
Homo habilis, 19
Homo sapiens, xiii, xiv, 16, 24, 28; culture, 40; evolution, 41; life span, 17
Homosexuality, 243-244
Hookworm, 183, 200
Hopi, 116, 130
Hormones, 106, 110
Horses, 12, 14
Hottentots, 96, 137, 144, 146
Hrdlicka, Ales, 166, 173, 181
Hupa, 114
Huron, 170
Hutterites, 154
Hypercalcemia, 94
Hypervitaminosis D, 39, 94

372